K. STEVEN WHITING, Ph.D.

HEALTHY LIVING

MADE EASY

The Only Things You Need To Know About
Diet, Exercise and Supplements

all the Best

D1451174

Morgan James Publishing · NEW YORK

HEALTHY LIVING
MADE EASY

ISBN: 1-60037-129-9 (Paperback)
ISBN: 1-60037-128-0 (Hardrback)

Published by:

MORGAN · JAMES
THE ENTREPRENEURIAL PUBLISHER ™
www.morganjamespublishing.com

Morgan James Publishing, LLC
1225 Franklin Ave Ste 32
Garden City, NY 11530-1693
Toll Free 800-485-4943
www.MorganJamesPublishing.com

Interior Design by:

Rachel Campbell
rcampbell77@cox.net

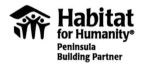

Habitat
for Humanity®
Peninsula
Building Partner

WHAT OTHERS SAY

"If you've been looking for authoritative information on nutrition and secrets of a longer, healthier life, you've found the right book. Dr. Whiting, in "Healthy Living Made Easy", presents accurate and practical information that you won't find anywhere else. It is the most authoritative source of information on nutrition and healthy lifestyle available, and should be required reading for anyone in the healthcare field."

Spencer P. Thornton, M.D., FACS
Clinical Professor of Ophthalmology
University of Tennessee Health Science Center

"This comprehensive and engaging book is destined to become one of the wellness reference bibles on many health-conscious consumers' book shelves."

Dr. Burton Goldberg
Author – The Definitive Guide to Alternative Medicine

"Dr. Whiting has finally taken the complex area of nutrition and put it into a simple, straightforward text that anyone can understand. His no-nonsense approach is practical and logical. It should motivate everyone to take charge of his or her life and health care. His integration of diet, exercise and supplementation just makes sense, so this book should be a best seller."

Jeffrey Anshel, OD
Author – Smart Medicine For Your Eyes

TABLE OF CONTENTS

INTRODUCTION

I have been in the health industry, in many arenas, for over 30 years. During that time, there have been more books written about better health, eating right, the benefits of exercise, and the need for dietary supplements, than almost any other subject. At any given time, you can find dozens of books on one or more of these subjects. In fact, virtually everything that has ever been written about one's physical health, can likely be distilled down into a combination of the big three, diet, exercise and supplements.

Yes, there are such factors as stress management, relaxation techniques, meditation, etc. All of these are extremely important in a high stress society, but for the most part, these are personal pursuits that can vary greatly from person to person.

On a purely physical level, diet, exercise and the use of supplements are things the majority of us at least try to do with some regularity.

The problem with most of the books written in this field is that they are often too complicated and demand, either, too much time, money or far too many changes in ones lifestyle.

The result of this complexity is that people tend to bounce from one 'program' to another, looking for ways to improve their health and extend their lives, but because of factors such as cost, time, and complexity, frequently give up or change what they are doing. The end result, of course, is that they fail to reap the benefits they seek because they don't stick with anything long enough.

It is not uncommon to hear people saying, " I'm doing low Carb", or "I'm doing low fat". Others say, " I'm eating organic", or "I'm following macrobiotics". When it comes to exercise, we also look for something better, "I'm pumping weights", or "Aerobics are better". "I workout 5 hours a week, but it's hard to fit it in", or " I know I should get more exercise, but there never seems to be time". When it comes to supplements our choices are even greater. "I take a good multiple every day", or "I'm so confused as to which supplements to take". Still others confess that, "I am taking so many things that it seems all I do is swallow pills"!

In the areas of diet and supplements and to a lesser extent with exercise, we have a situation of 'too much information', rather than a lack of knowledge. This combined with the fact that our society has more people over the age of 50 than at any other time in history, we have a population that is seeking a better quality and quantity of life, but has little direction as to how to accomplish this goal.

In the past decade, our Research Centers, both in the United States and in Europe, have worked with many thousands of individuals, helping them to design lifestyle programs aimed at increasing the quality and quantity of their lives ahead. Over and over again, the objections raised and the reasons for abandoning the programs are consistently the same. Participants point out that lack of direction, complexity of the programs, cost, and excessive restrictions are the biggest problems in implementing most health-building programs.

If we distill all the information in the many books written on health, we come back to the healthy diet, regular exercise and dietary supplements to embellish the diet. Why then, should these relatively simple three present so much confusion and take up so much time?

When we speak of diet, in this sense, we are of course speaking of a healthier diet rather than a diet for weight management. We will reserve that humongous topic for another book! Even if we limit our discussion of diet to what is healthier, there are still many points of view. While each of these undoubtedly holds value, they certainly are not for everyone. Many of these eating programs propose recommendations that are impractical or unappealing to most. The end result is that, over time, people simply abandon these restrictive diets and return to their previous way of eating, which is often very unhealthy. According to the United States Congress, in their research for the passage of the Dietary Supplement Health and Education Act (DSHEA) several years ago, the Standard American Diet (SAD) was found to be one of the most detrimental ways of eating on the planet!

Very few people are unaware of the unhealthy state of our food, yet remain unclear as to how to address this problem. Most of us want to eat better, most of us think about eating better a fair amount of the time, but only the very few will be willing to follow most of the extreme dietary recommendations of the more popular healthy eating programs, and the point is that you don't have to. Extensive research shows that if we would change but a few of our eating habits, the rewards in the form of better health and longevity would be immense. It will be my goal to illustrate how you can implement these changes into your diet and still enjoy most of your favorite foods, in moderation.

Exercise has often been coined as the longest four-letter word in the English language! As with eating better, most of us know that we need to get more exercise but we don't. Why? The biggest reasons why seem to be related to time. We join a gym or health club and then don't make time to use it. We somehow, fall under the impression that in order for exercise to be of benefit, we must slave at it for hours every week. This is simply untrue. Again, science shows us that as little as 30 minutes three or four times per week, can produce profound changes in the internal health and physiology of the human body. In order to reap those benefits however, the program must have the elements of fun, fast, and effective built right in. In my years in the health field, I have been a power lifter, bodybuilder, and fitness coach. I have owned fitness centers and have worked with some of the largest fitness chains in the world. This experience has taught me that exercise need not take up ten percent of your life! We will provide you with guidelines for either choosing a facility to exercise or, if you prefer, how to build an effective exercise program at home.

The third leg of our triad of better health is the dietary supplement. According to U.S. statistics, just over half of the population takes some form of dietary supplement on a regular basis. Yet, in the area of supplements, 'to much information' is the rule rather than the exception. A visit to your local health food store will quickly illustrate this point. Their shelves are filled, often with hundreds of bottles of vitamins, minerals, protein powders, amino acids, antioxidants, phytonutrients, etc., etc. For most of us, this can be a daunting and intimidating experience. Which products are best? Which products are right for me? Do I need more vitamin C? Which is the best calcium supplement to help prevent bone loss? Are there natural supplements that could help my arthritis, diabetes, or prostate problems? The questions can go on and on.

Again, according to the United States Congress, in their research for the passage of DSHEA, it was illustrated that at least fifty percent of all chronic, degenerative diseases could be prevented if we simply got a little exercise and took a broad-spectrum dietary supplement regularly. It seems simple, but it isn't. Why? There are hundreds of products and almost as many points of view on which supplements are best and why. In spite of all of this abundance, there remains, basic truths, which can be used in choosing a supplement program that would be right for you.

We know that the body requires key nutrient groups, which must be provided on a regular basis to the living system of the body. We know that factors such as absorption, ratio and potency are also important. Further, we know that certain select nutrients, in larger doses, can have a preventive and healing effect on many chronic, degenerative disease conditions. In fact, there have been more clinical studies published in peer-reviewed medical journals on the role of natural nutrients on disease pathology than there are for drugs! Still, in spite of this copious amount of information, we still have special interest groups, such as the larger drug companies, the American Dietetic Association and the American Medical Association, who deny the effectiveness or even the validity of supplements at all. Is it any wonder that so many are confused by so much information.

In the thirty years that I have been in this industry, I have seen many profound changes. I have seen dietary supplements go from almost underground status to that of a thriving industry, improving the lives of many millions. Through our Research Centers, we have developed lifestyle evaluation programs that address not only diet and exercise, but provide us with key information about a client and his/her state of internal biochemistry. It is this biochemistry of the body that supplements impact directly. Through our evaluation process, we are now able to design custom supplement programs to meet the needs of people, regardless of their present state of health or lack thereof.

Surprisingly, this is not as difficult as it may seem. All living bodies need the basic nutrient intake, this we have called Full Spectrum Nutrition, the art of supplying all the known nutrients, in the right potencies and ratios to each other for maximum absorption and subsequent benefit. After this baseline of Full Spectrum has been met, we can look to science and the many tens of thousands of clinical studies, which tell us which nutrients, in higher potencies, will likely benefit people with specific health challenges. This is concept we call Targeted Nutrition —using key nutrients, which have been shown to help prevent, manage or even reverse many chronic health conditions. Through Targeted Nutrition, we can isolate just the nutrients shown by science to exert a positive effect on a particular condition, increase their potency to therapeutic levels, and not have to mega dose all other nutrients at the same time.

Through this isolated, targeted approach, we can greatly simplify ones supplement program. It is not unusual for people to be taking 10 or 15 or more supplement products at a time. They are taking vitamin C, B complex, antioxidants, phytonutrients and their favorite herbs. While all these likely have benefits, the cost and convenience of these programs may discourage people from continuing them for the long haul. There is an easier way! Through the concept of Full Spectrum and Targeted Nutrition, supplement programs can be designed, even for those with multiple health concerns, which are simple and relatively cost effective. I will show you how to choose a Full Spectrum nutrition supplement. Once this has been implemented in your life, I can show you how to customize your supplement program to meet any individual needs you may have.

Part two of this book addresses those individuals who have already developed specific chronic degenerative diseases. We will take a look at many of the major health conditions currently threatening the quality and quantity of life for many millions of people. We will show you how you can prevent, manage and yes, even reverse many of these conditions by re-adjusting your body chemistry back to that of a healthy individual through a concept we have come to call Targeted Nutrition.

The final chapter of this book is a virtual encyclopedia of over 250 of the most common health conditions and concerns for which we have listed the key, targeted nutrients, which clinical studies have shown to be of positive benefit in the prevention, management, or even reversal of the problem. This compendium is the result of reviewing thousands of peer reviewed clinical studies appearing in dozens of medical journals from around the world.

My goal in writing this book was to provide not only factual based information, but a program that was actually doable by virtually anyone. Of what value is information if it isn't applicable to our lifestyle? Making the simple changes in diet, exercise, and supplements necessary to improve the quality and potential quantity of life ahead does not have to be difficult, in fact it is not difficult. A healthier lifestyle need not consume endless time and money in its pursuit. There are very few changes or modifications necessary to achieve better health for you and your family. Let me show you how easy it really is.

PART ONE

THE TRILOGY OF GOOD HEALTH

There is an old saying that "Good Things Come In Threes." In the world of Nature, everything always comes in 'threes'. In fact many scientists call this concept 'Nature's Mathematics.'

In nature, one and one never equals two, but always three. Hot and cold air, for example, creates our weather. Force on an object equals movement. Male and female equal a third offspring. Since the human body is a product of these natural forces, it would stand to reason that the concept of 'threes' would play a role in maintaining it.

If we look at the body, we can see that its needs are very basic. Thanks to a very complex internal biochemistry, our bodies can function pretty much, on their own. When we put ourselves into one extreme state or another, the body has the ability to alter the biochemistry within and adjust to the imbalance, thereby restoring internal equilibrium. In fact, this very process takes place hundreds of thousands of times per day completely without our knowledge.

As our society has become more and more technological, the pace and stress of our lives has grown. The result of this increased stress has caused the body to work harder and harder in an attempt to maintain a healthy internal environment. For this reason, emphasis upon stress management, elimination and the overall simplifying of our lives is realizing greater and greater importance.

Stress management is an internal effort and must take place within each individual. While the management of stress is essential and we will discuss it later in this book, our focus right now is upon those things that the body needs outside of its own self, to maintain health and wellness. Upon thorough review, it may be found that there are, once again, three factors that are essential to the health and well-being of the human body.

This 'trilogy' consists of macro-nutrition, protein, fats, carbohydrates, fiber and water. Next come the micronutrients, of which there are at least 100, including vitamins, minerals, amino acids, fatty acids, antioxidants, and phytonutrients. Lastly, but certainly not in the least, the body requires action, motion, exercise.

It may be argued that the middle category of micronutrients can be obtained from consuming foods, which provide the macro-nutrients. There may have been a time when this was true, but not for many decades. Modern farming techniques, food processing, transportation and storage all rob our food of essential micronutrients, making it impossible to live a healthy life without supplementation.

Here we have our 'Trilogy of Good Health'. Through Diet, Exercise and proper Supplementation, we have the best opportunity to provide the body with everything it needs from the external world around it.

Failing to provide these simple, yet essential factors, can, over time, lead to the disease and ultimate premature death of the human body. It would seem that something so easy and a good diet, regular exercise and the taking of supplements would be a no brainer, but not so. Our society has changed and as such, each succeeding generation changes with it – and often not for the better.

Our diet, often referred to as the Standard American Diet (SAD) more often than not, contains a complete imbalance between protein, carbohydrate and fat. Further, the processed, junk food diet has now replaced healthy fats and carbohydrates with altered, man-made counterparts, which are wreaking havoc with the internal chemistry of the human body.

Modern technology has created a generation of sedentary vegetables, couch potatoes whose idea of exercise is their index finger on a remote control switch. Our youth are growing up in an era of electronic entertainment, where there is no longer a need or desire to exercise and partake in physical activities. Virtually every sport conceivable can be played, with the greatest of realism, on a computer or television screen.

The concept of nutrient supplements is still all too new to millions of people. The food industry, the most powerful lobby in government, would have us believe that we can get all the nutrients we need from the lifeless junk food that they peddle into our bodies. Yet, a simple analysis of the content of these foods, show that the exact opposite is the case.

In fact, the food industry goes to great financial lengths to conceal the deficits caused by modern food processing and storage. A timely case in point is that of trans fats. Now that food manufacturers are required to list the amount of trans fats on Nutrition Facts boxes, all of a sudden you see hundreds of foods carrying the proud label saying 'contains no trans fats!'

If the food makers had the technology to eliminate dangerous trans fats from our foods, why didn't they do so years ago? Simple answer? Economics.

This over-processing of most of our foods has, along with other factors of our modern age, caused a gross depletion of the micronutrients, the vitamins, minerals and other nutrients so essential for our internal chemistry. Without adequate intake of these micronutrients, the chemistry of the body does not have the raw materials it needs to carry out the millions of chemical processes that are required to keep us healthy and well.

Through the avoidance of these three simple things, we have removed ourselves from the natural world from which we have come. The end result, in spite of all the technology and advancements in medicine, is the greatest epidemic of chronic, non-infectious disease in the history of mankind.

This section of the book is designed to show you why these factors are important and how you can bring them back into your routine once again, with minimal impact on the rest of your life.

Diet need not be a boring drudgery. Exercise need not take up hours and hours of your already busy schedule. Supplementation need not be complicated and expensive. By approaching these facets of good health in the right manner, you will be amazed at the difference these small changes can make. Let's get started.

Diet

CHAPTER 1: THE VERY MENTION OF THE WORD 'DIET' CAN instill fear and anger in people. In fact, for many, the term diet is a 'four letter word' of great disgust!

This is because we often associate the term 'diet' with something totally different called weight loss. Diet, when used in the context of 'I'm going on a diet', is a restriction of some short, designed to reduce the amount and/or variety of food consumed for the purposes of weight loss.

When I speak of the term diet here, I am referring to what a person consumes on a daily basis. Is the diet 'balanced', providing the right ratios of protein, fats, carbohydrates and fiber? Is the diet made up of smart choices or poor choices? How are the foods we eat prepared? Do we cook at home or eat out most of the time? How is the food prepared in our favorite restaurants?

These questions define the term diet as we use it here. In this chapter we will discuss how you can learn to make simple choices at the supermarket and in restaurants, to help you eat much healthier.

What's Wrong With Our Daily Diet?

I was speaking with an owner of a fitness center recently and we were talking about the Standard American Diet (SAD)! And how it adversely affects human health. I was telling her about the late Adele Davis, one of nutrition's early pioneers, and her favorite saying of "you are what you eat", meaning that if you eat good quality foods you will be healthier and if you eat processed foods you will be less than well.

Her response to this was 'well, if that's true, then I'm cheap, fast and easy!!' After over 30 years in the health field, very little sets me back, but as funny as that was at the moment, after thinking about it a while, it concerned me that someone in the health and fitness business would still be eating that way herself!

This led me to think about why so many of us, even those who should and do know better, eat such a poor diet so much of the time. My conclusion was that there is just no guidance as to how to eat.

There seems to be two thoughts, the major line of thinking is 'eat whatever, unless you have to lose weight'. The other is 'give up everything that is familiar and tastes good and sit in the corner and chant and eat tofu.'

Each thought is an extreme way of approaching food and neither is healthy or necessary. It is in these extremes, however, wherein lies our problem.

Since the majority of people don't know what constitutes a healthy diet and their image of such is the 'tofu' concept, they simply 'try' and eat well, most of the time failing. Eating healthy is not nearly as difficult as you may think. In this chapter we will show you how you can take just a few simple steps to change your food choices and by so doing, statistically, increase your health and longevity tremendously, and yes, it will be easier than you think.

I am not the type of nutritionist who thinks you should avoid all your favorite foods, even if some of them are not very healthy. By moderating their intake, and by making some positive changes in other areas, you should be able to eat just about any food, at least occasionally.

The two great downfalls of what has come to be called the Industrialized Diet, are the over processing of foods and the over consumption of foods made from them.

The adulteration of our food begins in the fields on which it is grown. Improper fertilization has resulted in soils almost totally devoid of trace minerals (more on that later). Foods are picked green, allowing time for storage and transit to markets. Once purchased, food is further adulterated by over cooking, drying, freezing, canning and yes even juicing.

Each step is robbing our food of key components such as enzymes, phytonutrients, vitamins & minerals. It is for this reason that I so strongly feel that we cannot be optimally healthy with our present diet, unless we resign ourselves to take a broad spectrum dietary supplement that provides us with all the baseline nutrients no longer contained, in adequate amounts, in our foods. We will discuss this concept in chapter 3 and show you how easy this is.

Food Basics

Every food we consume is made up on one or more of the four basic groups: proteins, fats, carbohydrates and fibers. Convenience foods or more commonly (and accurately) called 'junk foods', can be made up of combinations of foods and additives not found in nature.

These man-made foods or food artifacts as I call them, are something created in a laboratory, made up of unnatural combinations of our food groups mixed together with chemicals and additives that are unknown to the healthy human body.

Incomplete proteins, adulterated, altered fats, and concentrated, refined sugars lead to the production of junk food. More about those foods later; first let's take a look at real food and see why each group is important to us in its natural state. A basic understanding of the four main food groups will help you to make wiser choices as we proceed.

Protein, Fats, Carbohydrates and Fiber

PROTEIN – We should discuss protein first as it is the most essential food for the human body. In fact the term protein is of Greek origin and means 'of first importance.' The body uses protein, in the form of amino acids, to build and maintain every cell. It is estimated that several billion cells die in your body daily. These must be replaced with new cell material, made up almost exclusively from protein. Protein is also used to carry out the myriad of metabolic reactions that take place every minute within your body.

There are two types of protein naturally found in foods:

COMPLETE PROTEINS. All proteins must be digested and broken down into individual amino acids. There are two groups of amino acids, essential and non-essential. By this, we don't mean to imply that some amino acids are not needed, but rather the body can manufacture most amino acids, which is why we call those non-essential, as long as it has the 8-10 basic amino acids, which it cannot make. Those we call the essential amino acids because they must be obtained from whole protein foods. The essential amino acids include leucine, isoleucine, valine, methionine, threonine, lysine, histidine, phenylalanine, tryptophan, and arginine.

The only food in which these essential amino acids may be found in adequate amounts, is in animal source protein foods. Meat, chicken, fish, etc., contain 100 percent of each of the essential amino acids.

INCOMPLETE PROTEINS. Foods containing protein, but lacking in one or more of the essential amino acids are called incomplete proteins.

These foods provide amino acids and protein but one or more of the essential amino acids is either missing or present in too small amounts to make the protein bio-available to the body. These proteins are most often vegetable proteins. This does not mean that vegetable proteins are of no use. It does mean however, that they must be combined with other proteins at the same time, to provide the missing amino acids.

There is a principle in the biochemistry of proteins called "The All Or None Law Of Protein Utilization." This means that any given protein food will be limited in the amount of protein that it can provide to the human body by the level of the lowest amino acid. Since complete proteins provide 100 percent, we have the potential of getting 100 percent protein utilization from those foods. Incomplete proteins, on the other hand, are limited to the level of the lowest essential amino acid present. Incomplete proteins provide the essential amino acids at varying levels from 100 percent.

In a practical sense, if a vegetable protein has only 60 percent of one of the essential amino acids, say methionine, that means that only 60 percent of the protein in that food will be useable by the body. The rest will be unavailable and pass out with the waste matter. This is why if you intend to rely on primarily vegetable proteins in your diet, it is essential that you learn to combine these proteins, at the same meal, to ensure that all essential amino acids are present at the same time.

Since protein deficiency is responsible for many complications to both health and longevity, including premature aging, making sure we ingest adequate amounts of high quality protein should be our first dietary goal.

Everyone needs adequate protein, regardless of age. Some specific age groups need more protein than others. Protein requirements are outlined below:

Age Period	Daily Intake
One to three years	40 grams
Four to six years	50 grams
Seven to nine years	60 grams
Ten to twelve years	70 grams
Thirteen to twenty years	75-100 grams depending on activity level
Male Adult	80-100 grams
Female Adult	70-90 grams

Female Pregnant   80-100 grams

Female Lactating   100-120 grams

The level of activity can also affect protein needs. If you are exercising regularly, especially with resistance, it is essential to ensure adequate protein intake. A deficiency of protein while resistance training can result in flabby tissues, especially if weight loss is also involved. One of the best ways to prevent that flabby look after significant weight loss is continue to exercise AND ensure adequate protein intake.

Signs of Protein Deficiency

Specific conditions and situations directly linked to protein deficient diets include:

Dizziness

Nausea

Lowering of hemoglobin levels (affects immune system)

Increase fluid retention (edema)

Growth retardation in children

Reduced absorption of fat-soluble nutrients (vitamins A, D, E, and K)

Loss of liver enzyme activity

Retarded spermatogenesis in males

Cataracts

Acid and alkaline imbalance in the digestive system

Loss of antibody production (immune function)

Poor skin tone

Premature aging

There has been considerable controversy with regard to the possible benefits verses the possible harm of the high protein diet. It has long been the norm to limit sick people to diets low in protein and bland in taste. There is no time in our lives when we need the life-supporting body building benefits from good, high quality protein than when the body is under siege with a health challenge.

The amino acids we derive from quality protein in our diet will be used to rebuild muscle and organ tissue. Additionally, other amino acids will be used in the formation of hormones and other chemicals that the body needs for health and repair.

In spite of all the diet programs to regularly come in and out of vogue, the lower carbohydrate, higher protein diet remains one of the most effective weight loss concepts for millions of people. The reason for this is that while it is very easy for the body to store carbohydrates as fat, it is very difficult to do so with proteins.

If you are thinking about dieting for weight loss purposes, you should consider taking our Weight Management Test to determine how your body handles different food groups. If you are primarily carbohydrate intolerant, a higher protein diet will likely work much better for you than one that counts only calories. If you are unsure as to whether you lean towards being calorie sensitive or carbohydrate intolerant, you can take our free evaluation questionnaire, which may be found on The Institute's website: www.healthyinformation.com

Fats

Fats provide the most concentrated source of energy of all the food groups. They are also among the most misunderstood of foods. Fats are absolutely essential for the well being of the body. Fats are responsible for building the sheaths around nerves; they are also active participants in a variety of bodily reactions. Fats are an excellent source of energy, but must be consumed with prudence. Each gram of fat provides 9 calories of energy, compared with 4 calories for both proteins and carbohydrates.

Fats serve as carriers of fat-soluble nutrients while keeping calcium readily available to bones and teeth. Fats are needed for proper protein digestion and absorption, which is why fats are frequently found together with proteins in natural foods.

There are two types of fats:

SATURATED FATS. These are usually found in animal products and tropical oils such as coconut and palm oils. Saturated fats may be recognized by the fact that they are generally, solid at room temperature and because of their molecular structure, are very stable.

Saturated fats are very misunderstood. We have been told that they are at the cause of heart disease and other bodily ailments. This is not true. In fact, saturated fats provide far more protection for the heart and blood vessels than most other fats.

Clinical studies, over the past decades, continue to prove that saturated fats, in moderation, are far healthier for our heart and vascular system than vegetable oils, which can very easily become rancid and form damaging, dangerous free radicals.

I know this smacks in the face of most everything you have heard about fats but remember that our grandparents and great grandparents consumed saturated fats almost exclusively, since there were no processed, packaged vegetable oils in their time, and they had a fraction of the cholesterol problems and heart disease that we have today.

Mary G. Enig, PhD., a Clinical Nutritionist specializing in research on the nutritional aspects of fats and oils, has made some remarkable discoveries that bear mentioning. In her landmark research report on cancer and dietary fat, she revealed that during the sixty-year period of the studies, there was a positive correlation between vegetable fat consumption and increased cancer, while there was a negative correlation between increased cancer and animal fat!

Further, Dr. Enig reminds us that while there is so much emphasis placed upon the benefits of HDL cholesterol, trans fatty acids, generated from oxidized vegetable oils, lower this 'good' cholesterol dramatically, while raising the 'bad' LDL cholesterol.

Research conducted over the past three decades continues to show that our indiscriminate use of vegetable oils, in concentrated forms, has greatly compromised our state of health. Works such as the pioneer book, Supernutrition for Healthy Hearts, by Richard Passwater, PhD, presented, clearly, why vegetable oils present such a health risk to humans. Another major work, Fats and Oils, The Complete Guide to Fats and Oils in Health and Nutrition, by Udo Erasmus, also lays out the benefits and risks of various types of fats.

While this information about vegetable oils verses olive oil and butter may seem shocking and 'new' to you, science has known this for several decades. The food industry doesn't want you to know this because they have invested billions in the vegetable oil business and can sell these oils at many times the profit margin of other fats and oils. If you don't believe me, just look at how fast the food industry dumped trans fats when they were required to list them on food labels!

UNSATURATED FATS. These fats are usually found in vegetables and grains. They have a very open molecular structure, which makes them generally, liquid at room temperature. The structure of these fats makes them highly susceptible to damage from oxidation. This occurs when the concentrated oils are exposed to the air. Oxidation and subsequent rancidity, is dramatically accelerated when the fats are heated to high temperatures as in cooking and frying. Once these oils become oxidized, they form compounds called free radicals. The specific free radicals formed from oxidized vegetable oils are responsible for the damage that occurs to the arteries of our body, leading to atherosclerosis, the basis of most heart disease.

Interestingly enough, if you graph the consumption of concentrated vegetable oils and the incidence of heart disease, they both increase at almost the same rate!

Other sub-groups of unsaturated fats are trans fats and hydrogenated fats. These may be found when liquid vegetable oils are chemically changed to form margarines and shortening. Evidence is now conclusive that oxidized vegetable oils and most especially hydrogenated oils and trans fats, are some of the most dangerous substances in our diet.

If you wish to use a liquid vegetable oil, there is one that is safe. Olive oil, used in Mediterranean countries for Centuries, is what we call a mono-unsaturated oil. This means that its molecular structure is such that it is not readily susceptible to oxygenation and hence few damaging free radicals are formed. It is safe for use in cold food preparation as well as for heating as in cooking and even frying. Those that think they don't like the taste of olive oil should try the extra virgin variety, which has almost no taste to it at all. An additional benefit in using olive oil is that it has the ability to raise HDL cholesterol (the good one).

Carbohydrates

The carbohydrates make up the largest group of foodstuffs consumed by most people. Carbohydrates are the quickest energy fuel of the body. The more active we are, the greater our need for carbohydrates. The problem with the Standard American (SAD) diet is that it provides highly concentrated, overly refined carbohydrates that deliver far more units of energy than the body can possibly utilize in such a short period of time. This results in the need to convert these sugars into stored energy or body fat.

All carbohydrates, regardless of whether they are sugars, starches, whole grains, vegetables, etc., will eventually be digested and reduced to the one simple sugar that the body uses for energy namely glucose.

As carbohydrates are converted to glucose, this sugar enters the bloodstream to be used as a source of immediate energy. If those energy requirements are not needed, blood sugar must rapidly be removed.

Insulin, from the pancreas, is secreted into the bloodstream with the primary purpose of converting glucose, or blood sugar into stored sugar called glycogen. This is done, by adding one molecule of water to glucose. Once this chemical change has taken place, glycogen can then be stored in the body, primarily in the muscle tissues and the liver, for later use.

Since the diets of most people contain enormous amounts of refined, concentrated carbohydrates that convert to glucose rapidly, and since we are generally, very inactive most of the time, the amount of stored glucose in the form of glycogen, can increase rapidly. Once the storehouses for glycogen are full, and more and more sugar forming foods are consumed, the body must find another storage site for the excess sugars.

Through further action of insulin on glucose, the excess is converted to another substance called triglyceride. Triglycerides are then stored in our fat cells for future use.

The problem with this concept is that there never comes a time for 'future use.' We always seem to have an abundant and excess supply of sugar-forming foods in our diet, so rather than converting body fat back into useable energy, we keep adding to our storehouse of reserves, the end result, of course, is the epidemic problem of obesity, and all the related health challenges that face our society today.

It is for this reason that choosing healthier carbohydrates is essential. The more complex a carbohydrate, the slower it digests and converts to blood glucose. This, in turn, reduces the amount of insulin produced and subsequently the amount of glucose being converted to triglycerides and stored as body fat.

There are two basic groups of Carbohydrates:

COMPLEX CARBOHYDRATES. These foods include some fruits, whole grains and some vegetables. Complex carbohydrates are always found in their natural state. Over cooking or processing breaks down the complexity of the food, making it more and more easily digestible.

When it comes to carbohydrate consumption, the longer a carbohydrate takes to digest, the better it is for us. Carbohydrate foods such as whole grains, can take up to 3 or more hours to fully digest. This gives the body the chance to utilize the glucose formed from their breakdown, more readily.

SIMPLE OR REFINED CARBOHYDRATES. Simple carbohydrates would include many fruits and some vegetables. While they are easier to digest and break down, they often are well tolerated by most people due to the fact that they don't provide an excessive amount of glucose. Refined carbohydrates on the other hand, are altered so that they are not only very easy to digest, but usually provide very high concentrated amounts of glucose entering the bloodstream rapidly.

Refined sugars and white flour products, the staple of the SAD diet, convert to blood sugar almost immediately, causing repeated spikes in both blood sugar and insulin. You can illustrate this to yourself very easily. Take a piece of white bread, made from highly refined white flour and place it in your mouth. Chew on it, but don't swallow right away. In just a few seconds that bread will start to taste sweeter and sweeter, as the enzyme in your saliva already starts to break the simple starch down into sugar. An excessive consumption of refined carbohydrates as in the SAD diet is the single greatest cause of the overweight and obesity epidemic we see around us everywhere.

Overall, the carbohydrate group of foods is of the least importance to the body's health and well-being. In short, we need a lot less carbohydrate foods on a daily basis than is provided by the SAD diet. This excess, as we will see later, is not only making us fat, but is at the root of many epidemic, chronic degenerative diseases.

Fiber

As food is digested and the waste matter from that process makes its way out of the body, organs like the colon and bowel are responsible for gathering this waste and preparing it for elimination. In fact, most of the body's waste material and potential toxins are passed through the colon and bowel tract. The time that it takes for waste matter to enter and pass through the colon is called the tract or transit time. The normal transit time for feces is about twenty-four hours.

Modern diets, consisting of over-processed foods and lifeless foods with no enzyme activity also often contain little or no fibrous material. All the natural fiber of foods such as grains has been removed in the refining stages. Because of this lack of bulking fiber, it is not uncommon for many people to have a transit time of forty-eight to ninety-six hours!

This additional time of fecal retention sets up the perfect conditions for toxic materials to form and the body begins to drown in its own waste. Constipation, an all too common condition, is the ultimate in tract retention and almost all people who suffer from this condition are also very toxic as a result. While there can be underlying medical causes for these problems, the vast majority of those suffering from these elimination problems is due simply to a lack of adequate fiber in the diet.

Cellulose and hemicellulose are common fibrous materials found in a variety of foods in their natural states. These materials are referred to as insoluble carbohydrates because the body has no enzymes to break down these structures. Seeds, nuts, grains, and many vegetables are protected from their environment by a tough layer of fibrous cellulose.

Most of this material is coarse, even rough, and provides a natural cleansing or scraping of the human intestinal wall as it passes along the tract.

The SAD diet, by its refined nature, provides very little natural fiber. This lack of bulking material can lead to a variety of problems including constipation, diarrhea, hemorrhoids, varicose veins and phlebitis.

Digestion Of Foods

Now that you have a basic understanding the primary food groups, a discussion of the digestive process is in order. How does your body take these various foods and break them down into useable components for fuel and bodybuilding? It is important to have an understanding of how your digestion works. With this, you will be able to see how you can adjust your diet to improve your digestion and eliminate digestive problems, while still being able to enjoy most of your favorite foods.

The first concept to understand is that of food combining. You may have heard about this, and even seen complicated charts governing everything you eat. This, for the most part is totally unnecessary. In fact the concept of food combining can be reduced to one simple, easy rule:

Do not combine concentrated proteins, together with concentrated carbohydrates at the same mea.

Sounds easy enough right? It is. All this means is that if you are going to have a big steak, or a chicken dish or seafood, do not consume concentrated proteins such as potatoes, refined rice, refined grain product or sugars with it, at the same time. Why?

Foods do not digest in the same place and under the same conditions within the digestive tract. Protein foods digest in the stomach, in an acidic environment. Acids, produced by the stomach, break down proteins into individual amino acids so that they may be used by the body for tissue rebuilding. Carbohydrates, on the other hand, digest in the small intestines in a rather highly alkaline chemistry. Since acid and alkaline are opposites, foods that digest in these different environments should be kept separate.

In fact, the combining of concentrated proteins and refined carbohydrates together is the single greatest cause of digestive disturbances such as heartburn, gas, bloating, etc.

Here is what happens. Let's say you have a big steak, a salad, which is a good combination, but then you top it all off with a large piece of chocolate cake, with a scoop of ice cream. All of this enters your stomach at the same time. The stomach senses the presence of protein and begins to secrete gastric acids to digest it. In this acidic environment, the cake and ice cream cannot digest since it needs and alkaline condition, so it sits in your stomach, fermenting at 98 degrees Fahrenheit for up to 4 hours while the steak is digesting. During this period of time, the concentrated carbohydrates can slow the production of stomach acids, creating feelings of fullness, bloating and upper intestinal gas.

In order to relieve this uncomfortable situation, we often run for either over the counter or prescription anti-acids. These are effective because they completely neutralize all the stomach acid present. Once this happens, your body thinks that the digestion of proteins is finished and it opens the valve in your stomach and dumps the entire contents into the small intestine.

Here, in an alkaline environment, the cake and ice cream finally begins its digestive process, but the partially digested steak, which was interrupted by the anti-acid you took, now cannot complete the digestion process because the small intestine is too alkaline.

The end result of taking these anti-acids is that you successfully exchange upper intestinal gas for lower intestinal gas, which is socially less acceptable!

By separating concentrated proteins and concentrated, refined carbohydrates, you can avoid these many digestive problems. How can this be practically done? Easy! If you are going to have a large amount of protein, combine it with vegetables, salads, and very complex carbohydrates such as whole grains. This should constitute one meal. If you want to have concentrated sugars or starchy foods, eat them alone at another meal. This one simple rule can make a great difference in our overall health.

Enzyme Action

While the food combining rule is certainly easy enough, there are situations wherein this is not always practical or circumstances where we simply want to eat a 'full course' meal. Enter the enzyme supplements.

Digestive enzymes, which are either found, naturally, in fresh, living foods or are manufactured in the body, are responsible for breaking down the foods we eat into useable elements. All foods, in their natural state, have enzymes, designed to break them down. The over-ripening of fruits and veggies to the point of complete breakdown is the action of enzymes in those foods at work.

The problem we have, presented by the SAD diet, is that we rarely consume foods in their raw, natural state. Foods are processed, canned, frozen, cooked or otherwise heated. Each of these changes the chemistry of the food and destroys most if not all of the enzymes.

You can illustrate this easily for yourself. Take a fresh tomato and place it in your kitchen window or on your counter. Next to it place a small dish and in it put some canned stewed tomatoes. Leave them both. In a short time, the fresh tomato will become softer and softer, eventually completely liquefying. This is the action of enzymes. The canned, cooked tomatoes however, will not liquefy, they will simply mold. Molds take over to breakdown the food when there is no longer any enzyme activity remaining. This happens because the heating of the tomatoes in the canning process has destroyed all the living enzymes previously contained in them.

We refer to these processed foods as 'dead foods' because enzymatic action is life – the life chemistry of that food. Once it is gone, the food becomes lifeless or 'dead.'

Over-consumption of these dead, lifeless foods for years or decades places a tremendous burden on the human digestive system. When you eat these foods, the body must produce the missing enzymes in order to break down the food. If not, these foods would putrefy, and 'mold', making us extremely ill.

The production of enzymes in the body begins in the stomach and is stimulated by the presence of the stomach acids. After years of having to produce high amounts of enzymes, the digestive system begins to slow, producing less stomach acids and hence less enzymes. The end result of course, is poor digestion of proteins, due to a reduction of stomach acids and subsequent poor digestion of carbohydrates due to missing enzymes. This, by the way, is the single greatest cause for heartburn, acid reflux and all the other names we have for these conditions.

If you suffer from digestive problems, in addition to separating your proteins and refined carbohydrates whenever possible, consider taking a multi-purpose digestive enzyme product that provides the precursor agents for building enzymes that digest proteins, carbohydrates and fats. A good enzyme formula will also contain betaine hydrochloride, the natural stomach acid.

The Greatest Dietary Evils

At the beginning of this chapter, I assured you that eating well would not be difficult. I told you that you don't have to give up your favorite foods and eat nothing but salad and tofu. This is true. In fact, there are very few things in the diet that, in moderation, are truly contributing to potential disease and a shortened lifespan. We are about to discuss these now.

You will see that in almost every case, there is a healthier substitute for what should be reduced or eliminated. By controlling your consumption of these few things, you can, statistically, reduce your risk of developing chronic degenerative diseases such as heart disease, cancer, diabetes and arthritis, by more than 50 percent!

The Big Four

VEGETABLE OILS – Do not, repeat, do NOT use any vegetable oils willingly, unless it is olive oil. You will get rancid, oxidized vegetable oil, filled with trans fats and hydrogenated fats every time you eat fried foods in most restaurants. For this reason, you should try and consume the majority of your fried foods at home, where you can cook them in either olive oil or good old-fashioned lard. In restaurants, choose grilled, baked or broiled selections to avoid these terrible oils.

SUGARS – Sugar makes things taste great and we all like sweets, but it is important to limit your intake of refined sugars. Whenever possible, choose fresh fruit as a desert and save that banana split or chocolate brownie for a special occasion. It is not necessary to deny yourself any food that you really enjoy, but by moderating the intake, you will improve your health and likely enjoy that food much more. Choose your poison. If you really like ice cream, than choose that and leave another sugary food, like donuts, alone. We can't have it all and remain healthy, but we can have some of almost anything.

REFINED STARCHES – White flour and the dozens of products made from them, also need to be moderated. Choose instead, breads, rolls, etc., made from whole grain flour with all the fiber left. These foods will break down much more slowly and eliminate the constant spiking of blood sugar and insulin. Many restaurants offer whole grain alternatives to white baked goods, just ask.

OVER-PROCESSING – The last of the big four is the easiest of all. Instead of giving in to the urge to cook, or juice living fruits and vegetables, try eating them raw, or at the very least stir fried (in olive oil!) so that they are still partially raw. This will preserve the enzymes as well as the vitamins and minerals naturally present in these foods.

Choose fresh foods instead of frozen or canned whenever possible. It is not difficult to prepare fresh foods since they should not be over-cooked anyway. The perceived convenience of canned and frozen foods is an illusion, they don't really save any time at all and they are almost completely dead due to the destruction of their natural enzymes.

Quality Foods

Remember a time when fresh fruits and vegetables tasted like what they were? For many that answer is 'probably not.' Unless you grew up on a farm or lived in a rural enough area to grow some of your own produce, most of us have no real idea of what fresh fruits and vegetables can really taste like. Why is this?

Much of the taste and in fact, nutritional value of foods are developed during the last days of ripening. Since virtually all commercially grown food is harvested 'green' in order to allow for storage and transportation time, these nutrients and much of the flavor of foods is altered when it is separated from the plant and from the soil.

We will talk about nutrients a little later on. Right now I want to concentrate on helping you make some simple choices that will greatly enhance both the taste and value of the foods you consume.

It's true that unless we live in an area where we can grow our own food, we are pretty much reliant on mass harvested product. Still, we can make wiser choices here. Almost all cities have markets that offer 'organic' produce, those grown without excessive chemical additives such as pesticides and herbicides. In some cases these may be better sources.

Even if you cannot find this level of produce in your area, you can still pick and choose from what is available. Try and purchase produce as ripe as you can. It's better to go to the market a bit more often.

Surviving the Supermarket

It has been said that if you only shopped the outside walls of the supermarket, you would be much better off. In general this is true because most markets set up their fresh foods, produce, dairy and meat sections against the outside walls of the building. The aisles are most often reserved for things that are not edible or should not be consumed. These items include the obvious such as pet foods, paper goods, cleansers and the like. Where we often get into trouble is down those aisles that pretend to offer food such as the canned goods aisle or the frozen food section. While these foods are often convenient, they carry very little food value except for highly concentrated, empty calories.

RULE NUMBER ONE WHEN GOING TO THE MARKET: MAKE A LIST BEFORE YOU GO! This way you will have a guide as to what you really need and may be less temped to pick up things along the way.

RULE NUMBER TWO: NEVER GO TO THE SUPERMARKET HUNGRY. You will buy much more than you or your budget need and you will be tempted to buy many more convenience foods because you're hungry right now.

RULE NUMBER THREE: THINK ABOUT WHAT YOU PUT INTO YOUR SHOPPING CART BEFORE YOU DO SO. Learn to take just a quick glance at the nutrition facts boxes on foods. They can tell you a lot.

Once you have learned these few new, simple changes, going to the supermarket will be just as fast and just as easy as ever before. You can go back to autopilot. Just remember a few simple choices:

If you choose foods from these groups choose:

Butter instead of margarine

Lard instead of shortening

Olive oil instead of any other vegetable oil

Whole grain bakery goods instead of those from bleached white flour

Fresh fruits and veggies instead of frozen or worse yet, canned.

Reserve high sugar foods for treats and not staples

See, the list is short and easy. The scientific evidence strongly supports the fact that with these few simple changes, you can reduce the risk of developing a chronic degenerative disease by at least 40 percent!

If you want to understand one of the major causes of the chronic disease epidemic facing our society, you merely have to visit a major supermarket and as you shop, take a look into the shopping carts of your fellow shoppers. Most of what is inside will break our simple rules for a better diet.

Remember, you don't have to give up any of your favorite foods, just make the simple changes above and enjoy everything you like. If what you really like contains high amounts of sugar or refined carbohydrates, simply use moderation and make these foods a welcome treat or reward rather than the mainstay of your diet. That, my friends, is the easy approach to a healthy diet!

Exercise, Made Easy!

CHAPTER 2: THE HUMAN BODY WAS MEANT TO MOVE. ONE look at its construction, and this becomes obvious. Our bodies have the most complex system of joints, which allows us range and direction of motion like no other living thing. Muscle and connective tissue are attached so as to give us the widest possible range of motion.

Because of this design, we know that our present lifestyle, in front of computers, televisions, and behind desks and on soft couches is not what our bodies were built for. Since the body was designed for motion and movement, it therefore, relies on that motion to assist it in maintaining the health and well-being of itself. We have come to call that movement or motion exercise.

The benefits of exercise to the human body are numerous. Exercise directly improves digestion and hence absorption of calories and nutrients from foods, while improving eventual elimination of wastes. A lack of exercise produces a sluggish digestive system, which usually results in a lack of energy.

Exercise increases endurance, which translates to increased energy. It promotes a higher muscle to fat ratio, increasing strength. Exercise helps to balance blood fats, specifically triglycerides, the most dangerous of all blood fats. Exercise reduces and helps us to manage stress and anxiety, which are at the core of almost all diseases and disorders in the body. In addition to the many physical benefits of exercise, it also affects our brain chemistry by elevating levels of 'feel good' hormones such as endorphins, reducing moodiness and depression.

Of all the factors that can positively affect your health, exercise certainly sits at the top of the list. In fact, studies have shown that regular exercise is a greater factor in health and longevity than are your cholesterol levels, blood pressure or even obesity. Naturally, a regular fitness program will positively affect many of these other factors as well.

Exercise is good for you and it is also satisfying and rewarding. Already I am sure that there are millions of people who are disagreeing with that statement! Why? Well, exercise and the physical conditioning of the body are interesting phenomenon. When we don't get enough physical activity, we are tired, often with aches and pains, stiffness sets in and our energy levels continually decline. The more these things occur, the less we feel like exercising! You can see that it is a downward spiral, the less active we are, the less motivated to be active we become. This leads to a greater and greater sedentary lifestyle, which, in turn, leads to more fatigue and inactivity.

Like all cycles of the body, whether it's constantly eating improperly, as we discussed previously, or whether it's a lack of physical activity, which leads to lethargy, each can be reversed, but it is often the starting that is most difficult. The reason for this is that we are often starting from a position of bad habits and physical exhaustion. This is not a position that will often inspire exercising!

How do we begin? Let's start with a brief discussion of the excuses we have for not exercising. Firstly, it's difficult. Yes, it can be, especially in the beginning. To solve this problem, you must find an activity that you enjoy or that you can learn to enjoy. You must not overdo it in the beginning. Doing so will only make you more tired as well as stiff and sore. Starting out slowly is the key to overcoming this objection.

Another favorite objection to being active is that ' we just don't have enough time.' Well if you feel you need to spend ten or twelve hours a week on your exercise program, you are dead wrong. In fact doing so will produce the very opposite results you are likely looking for.

Only highly trained, professional athletes can train at that level of intensity and derive benefit and even they must take time off regularly. You may be surprised at how well your body will respond to relatively little exercise. Excellent fitness can be obtained in as little as two hours a week. If you are interested in an above average level of physical fitness, you can accomplish this in about four hours per week.

The key to overcoming this objection, and keeping your fitness program at four hours or less, per week, is to exercise smart and not long. We will show you how you can build such programs, depending on what you wish to achieve, and yes, it will be easy!

Before we show you how to build an exercise program that will be easy and effective, a review of the types of exercise and their purposes will help you to understand the descriptions that follow. There are two basic types of exercise, aerobic or endurance and anaerobic or strength building. Very few exercise programs can address both completely, but we can find a happy medium and design a program that will address both to some extent.

Aerobic exercise improves the body's ability to utilize fuel more effectively, while increasing oxygen to the cells of the body. Aerobic exercise detoxifies the body, rapidly helping to eliminate cellular toxins. Activities that go on for sustained periods of 20 minutes or more are considered aerobic for the most part. Endurance exercises such as swimming, bicycling, jogging, power walking and rowing are examples of exercises that will benefit the cardiovascular system.

Anaerobic or strength exercises help to increase muscle strength and size by resistance. When we lift a weight or other resistance, it tears down the fibers of the muscle. When the muscle rebuilds, it does so a little stronger and a little bigger than before to meet the resistance level or work load. Weight training, pulleys and cables, even sit ups, using your own bodyweight for resistance, will build strength.

There is another category of exercise often referred to in the texts called range-of-motion exercise. These activities would be exercises that allow for movement to the fullest extent of the joint or muscle capability. Stretching, yoga, tai chi and similar activities place emphasis upon expanding the range-of-motion. I feel that if your exercise program is designed properly, it will incorporate these qualities and the need to pursue these activities would be for enjoyment.

Common Misconceptions About Exercise

There has been so much written about exercise and, like with eating healthy and taking supplements, we often become overloaded with too much information. As a result of this, we sometimes form thoughts about what constitutes a healthy lifestyle and they are totally off the track. Here are some common thoughts about exercise that many people share, yet are not quite accurate.

THOUGHT: If I can make myself exercise, then I can eat anything I want and still get in shape.

REALITY: Not quite so. True, if you are exercising regularly, your diet can probably be a bit less strict, but if your goal is to lose weight and get into shape, what you eat will actually be more important and you should go back to chapter 1 and review the easy guidelines to healthier eating. Also, you should never 'make' yourself exercise. As you will see later, that can set you up for failure. You must prepare for exercise *before* you start. That way, you will not have to force yourself, but you will actually look forward to it.

THOUGHT: My primary goal is to lose weight, so I should do only aerobic exercises to burn calories.

REALITY: If you want to lose weight, especially if you are 40 pounds or more overweight and if you actually want to look good afterwards, you must do a combination of endurance and resistance exercise. Resistance exercise increases metabolism, which directly helps with weight loss.

Further, strength training shapes the body and tones the tissues, helping to prevent that flabby appearance, which can occur after significant weight loss. In fact, if the truth were to be known, resistance exercises, done correctly, can cause greater weight loss than endurance activities because of the action on the metabolism. A balance of both, are needed for fitness.

THOUGHT: As a women, if I lift weights, I will get big muscles.

REALITY: If only it were that easy! Bodybuilding or muscle building takes a great deal of effort. As a women, you simply don't have the hormones necessary to build large muscles. Tone yes, firm yes, but to build bulk, you need key hormones, which are not present in your body in sufficient quantities to develop large muscles. Fat takes up much more space or bulk than lean muscle, so by lowering fat percentages and slightly increasing muscle mass, you will shape up and actually look much trimmer.

THOUGHT: I exercise 3 days a week. If I kick it up to 5 or 6 days a week, I will achieve my goals faster.

REALITY: Over-exercising often produces more negative results than benefit. There are several reasons for this. Muscles grow and strengthen during periods of rest, not exercise. In this case, resting is more important than exercising. All types of exercise will be changing the physiology of not only your muscles, but also your heart and vascular system, lungs, oxygen capabilities and your ability to detoxify. As with all changes, the body requires time to adjust to them. If you push yourself too hard, you will likely become exhausted both physically and mentally, and this will cause you to quit, putting you back in the same place you were before.

Preparing for exercise

Believe it or not, what you do before you start your exercise program will be of greater benefit than you can imagine. It is essential to be in the right frame of mind before you begin. This will ensure your long-term success rather than yo-yo exercising. Like dieting to lose weight, people often go on yo-yo exercise programs, attacking exercise like an enemy, thinking more is better, only to burn out rather quickly and stopping altogether. Once the guilt and the gut set in, they are back on the diet and in the gym again, until they burn themselves out.

It is essential that you make exercise, like eating better, your friend and not your enemy, so before you start any exercise program, prepare your mind, your psyche for the experience. We can do this in several ways.

First of all you must decide that a healthier lifestyle is what you want. If not, keep living the way you have been and see where it will take you. When you are sick enough, fat enough, tired enough and disgusted enough to do something about your state of health, then you will be ready. Sadly, for many people, this is when they have already traveled down the road of poor health a considerable distance. Fortunately, the body is an amazing machine and it wants to be well, in spite of us. Give it a little help and it will reward you tenfold.

So, then, the first thing you must do is make the choice to live a healthier lifestyle. As we said in chapter one, you don't have to give up anything to be healthier, just moderate the consumption of some foods, frequently replacing them with others. The same is true of exercise. You don't have to figure out how you are going to find an extra 10 hours a week to devote to your fitness program. Just find 2 hours to start with, then, if you really want to take your fitness to the highest level, find another 2 hours.

Once you have made the decision that living a healthier lifestyle is more important than constant self-abuse, then you need to focus on why you want to make these changes. Do you want to feel better, look better, have more energy, reverse existing chronic diseases, be alive to see your grandchildren grow up, and meet their children. Whatever motivation is important to you, find it and make a list on paper, that you can see and read frequently.

The last step you need to take before actually starting to exercise is to mentally prepare to workout. The importance of this was driven home to me upon reflecting back on my many years in gyms. Currently I own two women's fitness centers, and as such, work a lot with women. Many years ago, when I was pursuing the sports of bodybuilding and power lifting, I was almost exclusively surrounded by men. The difference between the two groups and environments taught me a great deal about human nature and to some extent, the differences between the sexes.

For most men, their workout was a "testosterone thing." Since it was primarily a male environment, and men tend to use their hormonal aggression to exercise, I found that they often achieved results faster than women, putting in the same amount of time. It has often been noted, for example, that men can lose weight faster than women. While there are hormonal and other physical factors at work, it is more than that. Men tend to approach their exercise program, whatever it is, with greater emotional and mental intensity than women.

When most men workout, they have already psyched themselves up before they get started. When most women exercise, it is often, although not exclusively, done with little mental preparation. In my women's fitness clubs, I frequently notice that this time serves as a social outlet for many women, which in and of itself is great. We just have to remember that we are also there to accomplish other important goals such as fitness, weight loss, etc. I find myself reminding my ladies that they need to focus on their exercises, feel them mentally as well as physically.

Why is this important? If you are not present with your mind as well as your body, if you are not exercising in your head as well as with your arms and legs, you will have a much greater chance of failing and not meeting your goals. You should never workout without first having thought about it. Think about why you are doing this. Remind yourself of your goals. Think about all the good things that your workout will do for you and how it will slowly change your body into the image you want. Think about how your body was made to be in motion and how that activity will help to prevent or reverse any chronic disorders you are dealing with. I bet you didn't think that there was so much to think about!

This thought process, often referred to as 'psyching up', does more than put you in the right frame of mind. Mentally preparing for your workout sets mind and body on the same path and when you mentally understand and can visualize both the reasons why you are doing this and what you want to achieve, your chances of quitting are much less.

Maximizing Your Exercise Sessions

We are about to provide you with guidelines to help you build your own exercise program, according to your goals, but first there are a couple of 'tricks' I have learned over the years of being in this industry that will help you maximize the results you achieve.

Firstly, the best time to workout, if possible is in the morning. This doesn't mean that working out at other times of the day is not good, but if you can, a morning workout will increase the fat-burning effects, especially if you workout before eating. If weight loss is a primary factor for you, consider trying to schedule your workouts in the morning, before eating.

Next, try not to eat for one hour after your workout. Chances are, you will not be hungry right after working out anyway. Drink water, but try to avoid eating immediately after exercising. When you do eat, make sure the first meal after your workout contains a substantial amount of protein. Protein is the only food that can rebuild lean muscle and promote fat burning.

Next, remember to take supplements. We will be talking about the need for supplementation in the next chapter, however right now you need to know that when you exercise and especially if you are also going to be following a weight loss diet, your need for supplemental nutrients increases.

Both weight loss diets and exercise excrete nutrients from the body at a faster rate. Further, when you restrict either quantity or variety of foods as in weight loss, your chances of getting the baseline nutrients you need becomes considerably less. Since the body sees nutrient deficiencies as a form of starvation, a lack of supplementation can cause an increase in appetite.

Dozens of nutrients are also involved in rebuilding tissues challenged by your workouts. In order to get maximum benefits from your exercise program, you must take a Full Spectrum dietary supplement every day. The next chapter will show you how easy that is to do.

Lastly, if you have not exercised significantly in some time and you are over 35 years old, consider a visit to your health care provider to ensure that there are no underlying reasons why you either should not exercise or should restrict the extent of exercise. Once you get the OK, there is nothing stopping you but you. Prepare your list of reasons why you want to do this, reviewing daily and prepare to change your looks and your life.

Options for Exercising

There are several ways you can go about designing and implementing your workouts. Much of this depends on your personal preference. Some people feel more comfortable and motivated by going to a gym or fitness club. The camaraderie and support from other members and the staff is frequently the boost they need to keep going. Others prefer the convenience of exercising at home.

If you will plan to workout at home, you will need to invest in at least a small amount of equipment. This can be anything from an exercise cable to a couple of sets of dumbbells, to a home gym. Gary Heavin, founder and CEO of Curves International, the largest fitness franchises in the world, has a complete home workout using your body's resistance and a flexible cable, available in many sports shops. His complete routine may be found in his book *Curves: Permanent Results Without Permanent Dieting*, published by Putnam.

If you want to invest a little more in your home fitness center, there are many 'home gyms' on the market. These come in simple machines that can fit under the bed when not in use, to more elaborate systems of pulleys, cables and resistance. My personal favorite is the equipment made by Bowflex. After spending over ten years in gyms with free weights, I find the Bowflex machines to provide the most intense workouts with minimal time. Their newer machines don't even require the changing of cables and the weight is adjusted by a series of power rods, each with a different resistance.

Whatever you choose, your goal is to fit a combination of aerobic and anaerobic or endurance and resistance exercise into one 30 minute session. You don't want to go longer than this in the beginning, especially if you have not exercised for some time. Doing so will only over-work your muscles and burden you mentally. Starting out slowly will allow your mind and body to adjust to the new lifestyle. You can always add some time and extend your workouts later if you choose, but as you will see, this is rarely necessary.

In order to achieve both endurance and resistance exercise at once, it is important to pick a level of resistance that you can do at a steady ongoing pace. If the resistance is too much, it will tire you too quickly.

Here is the basic outline of any workout. You only need to decide if you are going to use something as simple as a flex cable for resistance or something a bit more elaborate such as a home gym. If you are planning to attend a fitness center or gym, the following basic workout outline should still apply, as it is an excellent starting point.

Your Workout Outline

Every workout should contain resistance exercises for the major muscle groups. These should be able to be done at a pace that also provides endurance or aerobic benefit. Consult the guidebook or instructions for your piece of equipment as to how to perform the exercise/s for each muscle group, or ask a staff member at your exercise facility to help you design a program that fits into this outline.

THE WARM UP: THERE IS A LOT OF CONTROVERSY AROUND THE BENEFIT OR EVEN THE NEED FOR WARMING UP. Generally speaking, the more out of shape you are, the greater will be the need for warming up. The warm up need be no longer than 3 or 4 minutes. Simple twisting at the waist, a couple of knee bends, toe touching and reaching above your head with your outstretched arms should be sufficient.

ENDURANCE/RESISTANCE TRAINING: FOR EACH MUSCLE GROUP LISTED, YOU SHOULD PLAN TO DO 15 TO 20 REPETITIONS PER SET AND YOUR GOAL SHOULD BE 3 SETS PER MUSCLE GROUP. You want to try and cluster your upper body exercises together in a group and your lower body exercises in another grouping. This keeps the blood, which is nourishing your muscles, in one particular area of the body at a time.

UPPER BODY:

1. Chest Press
2. Shoulder Press
3. Back Pull down or Row
4. Biceps (upper arm)
5. Triceps (back of upper arm)

LOWER BODY

1. Lower Back Raise
2. Squat or Knee Bend
3. Leg Curl
4. Leg Extension

You should choose a resistance, whether it be a bungee cable, pulleys, weights or hydraulics, that you can complete at least 15 repetitions with, without becoming too fatigued. If you can't, then you need to reduce the amount of resistance until your body becomes stronger.

In order to incorporate endurance factors into your workout you should be able to repeat the exercise after about 30 seconds rest between sets. If you find this difficult in the beginning, reduce the amount of resistance until you can comfortably complete the three sets of at least 15 repetitions in a row with about 30 seconds rest in between.

Stretching

For most people, it is a good idea to stretch after working out. Doing so will enhance the benefit of your overall workout and prevent muscle cramping and injury. (Note: if you suffer from repeated muscle cramps during and after your workouts, or at night, it may be a sign of an electrolyte imbalance between the key minerals calcium, magnesium and potassium. You may wish to increase your intake of these minerals, especially at night, before bed. See the next section on supplements for guidelines)

Stretching exercises should include:

1. Lunges
2. Calf Raises
3. Arm Extension Overhead
4. Waist Twists
5. Knee Pulls

Again, your fitness guide or instructions for whatever equipment you have chosen to use, will offer illustrations and instructions for stretching. If you are going to be attending a facility, ask them for their guidelines to stretching after your workout.

Repeated clinical studies continue to show that 30 minutes or so, of combined resistance and endurance exercise can produce excellent results if repeated 3 or 4 times per week. That's just 1 ½ to 2 hours of time per week! Easy!

Moving Forward

As you progress, you will find that you can increase the amount of resistance and still keep the endurance pace without becoming winded. This is a sign that both your cardiovascular system, as well as your muscles, are becoming strengthened and toned. By increasing the resistance, in whatever manner your equipment dictates, you will increase the size and density of your muscles. More lean muscle mass equals a faster metabolism, which equals less body fat.

It is impossible for me to lay out specific exercises for you as these will depend on the type of equipment you chose to use. What we have provided is a guideline, which you can apply to any equipment, either at home or in an exercise facility. The important thing to remember is to follow this basic outline, at least for the foreseeable future. Trying to do too much, too fast, will only result in exhaustion, excess stress in trying to fit it all in, and ultimate failure. Remember, we said we were going to make these changes in diet, exercise and supplements easy, so don't go out and make it difficult!

Staying With It For The Long Haul

The key to any health-building program, whether it be changes in your diet, taking up exercise, or adding supplements, lies in doing it regularly and doing it for the long haul. Starting an exercise program, only to stop again after a month, will produce very little result.

Whether you stick with your workouts or not, is almost exclusively controlled by your mind and not your body. Sure you may be a bit sore for the first few workouts, but people rarely quit because of this or any other physical reason. The failure occurs in the brain, deep inside our thoughts. Here are some ways in which you can keep yourself motivated and your mind on the right track.

KEEP YOUR GOALS OUT FRONT: Remember that list of we asked you to make of the reasons why you wanted to be fit? Don't stuff it in a drawer somewhere. Keep it posted where you can see it and be sure to read it at least once a day, even on the days when you are not working out. Knowing why you are doing something, especially if it is for a greater purpose than self, will do a great deal to keep you focused and on track.

CHANGE NEGATIVES INTO POSITIVES: Negativity or adversity, rains into everyone's life to one degree or another. During the tough times, you will need to feel your best to handle situations that may arise. Neglecting your workouts because of 'other problems' can be one of the worst things you can do. Then, more than even at other times, you need the benefits, such as the stress management, better sleep, clear thinking and greater resilience that you derive from your exercise program.

If you find yourself surrounded with negative people, places, or circumstances, be sure to sit down and totally separate those issues from the health-building activities you are doing. By keeping them completely separate, you will prevent one from tarnishing the other.

TRY NEVER TO LIE TO YOURSELF: We all tell lies, some of them are just little white ones and some are real whoppers. I am not trying to validate or condemn these either way. What I want to stress to you is that you should not lie to yourself. That my friends, is pathological!

Each time you miss a workout, or eat junk food more often than you agreed on, you are lying to yourself. You're telling yourself, 'I will start again next week,' or, 'after I take care of all these other problems, I will get back into my health program.' We say these things because we have mentally, lumped our health-building program into the same category as our other responsibilities and problems. Re-read the section above and remember that you MUST keep your better eating habits, exercise program and supplement program separate from everything else. By keeping these things in their own category, you will not choose between them and 'something else.'

Choose which problems you are going to deal with, prioritize which tasks you will do and in what order, choose which social obligations you will fulfill, but NEVER put your health program into any of these categories. Those are not choices, they belong to drinking water, eating and sleeping, they are not choices, they are simply done.

STOP SEEING YOURSELF AS PERFECT – SEE YOURSELF AS BETTER: WE ALL HAVE A VISION, PERHAPS AN ILLUSION, OF HOW WE WANT TO LOOK AND FEEL.

Oftentimes, this is may not be reality. Focus on how much better you feel and how much better you are looking instead of on some illusion that may or may not be attainable. Focus on the progress you have made right now, the changes you have made, right now and how much better you look and feel right now.

By staying in the present, you can stay motivated. Looking ahead to distant goals often frustrates us and can set us up for failure. Your body will change, your health will improve, so look to what you have done so far and let it be the inspiration for tomorrow.

Whichever exercise program you choose, once you have your three days a week committed to habit and routine, you can then think about expanding your exercise program further, but only if you wish. Any additions to physical activities at this point should be made up of things you really enjoy doing.

If, for example, you enjoy taking an early morning walk or a sunset walk in the evening, by all means do so. If you enjoy swimming, or biking, add it in on a time permitting basis. It's ok to do these things sporadically, but never do these activities instead of your 3-day workouts. Remember, those are in a totally separate category and are never compromised.

By adding activities on a time available basis, you can increase your overall exercise by doing things that are truly fun.

If you wish to take your workouts to a higher level and can commit to 4 hours a week down the road then you simply increase your basic three workouts a week from 30 minutes to 45 minutes, slowing down the pace to a 90 second rest between sets.

This will allow you to increase the resistance of each exercise and concentrate on building greater muscle density. Then, in order to pick up the endurance benefit sacrificed by the longer rest time between exercise sets, take the remaining time and schedule three

30 minute cardio or endurance activities such as biking, jogging, treadmill or other such sustained pace exercises.

Even with this expanded program, you will be devoting under 4 hours a week to your fitness. Keep in mind however, that you NEVER have to increase this over your three 30 minute workouts in order to achieve incredible results. Remember it's not how long you workout or how often, but rather how smart and how long you stick with it that will count in the end.

In closing this simple discussion of exercise, it, like many things in life, is a matter of attitude. If you exercise because it's good for you or you want to lose 20 pounds, you will set yourself up for failure. Why? Simply because those motivations are either negative or temporary.

Instead you should be exercising and eating better and taking supplements for a purpose greater than yourself, because you want to be able to live all your life to the fullest, including your last twenty years.

And lastly, if you should find yourself in need of further motivation to live a healthier lifestyle, simply volunteer at your local old age or convalescent home for a day. When you see what can happen to the human body when it is not cared for, it can be a very sobering sight.

Remember, don't make any of this difficult, it's really very easy!

The Role of Dietary Supplements In Health and Longevity

CHAPTER 3: CURRENT STATISTICS CONFIRM THAT AT ANY given time, about fifty percent of us take some form of dietary supplement on a regular basis. Further surveys reveal that the majority of us that do take supplements, do so without any real knowledge of what we are doing.

This is not surprising considering that the supplement industry has become increasingly complicated. I can think of no other field of science where new information is coming out at such a rapid rate than that of nutrition and in particular, its role in the prevention and management of various disease conditions.

Every week on Medline, the website for the National Library of Medicine, there are dozens of new studies examining the role of natural dietary supplements, vitamins, minerals, amino acids, antioxidants, etc., in health and longevity.

Much of this information never makes it to the public eye, but that which does, usually comes in the form of new supplements, which line the shelves of health food stores. The average consumer, wanting to do the best they can for themselves, often finds the health food store shelves overwhelming to say the least. There are hundreds of products on the shelves in dozens of categories. Each one, we feel, must have some potential benefit, but how do we choose? How do we answer the many questions that should be asked such as which products are best, which supplements do I need, how do I know where to begin, and how much is this going to cost?

Each of these questions is valid and deserves an answer. The answers to these questions may vary greatly, depending upon whom you ask. There are many different viewpoints on supplementation of the diet; all of them carry truth. Our job is to glean that which is best for us, for our bodies. In order to help with this job, a little basic knowledge of why we need to supplement, what every human body needs as a foundation of good nutrition, and how to begin to put together a personal supplement program, will undoubtedly be helpful.

Remember, supplementation, like eating better and exercising, does not have to be complicated, nor does it have to be time consuming or expensive. With a little background information, you will find that the benefits of taking the right dietary supplements can be made easy!

Why Do We Need Supplements?

This question has been the source of an ongoing argument between biochemical nutritionists and the American Dietetics Association for at least the past 40 years.

Dieticians, who have generally aligned themselves with the medical model, preach the tenant that 'we can get all the nutrients we need from a good, balanced diet.' Biochemical, or Orthomolecular nutritionists stand firm on the premise that 'industrialized diets are so depleted in nutrients, due to food processing, that no one can get even the minimum requirements of many essential nutrients.'

Which position is right? Science, over the past 60 years or more, would lead us to believe that the latter position is most accurate. Back in the 1930's and 40's, it might have been a bit easier to 'eat well' and meet basic nutrient intake requirements. Today however, this is much more difficult.

Why are we so nutrient deficient? What has happened to our food? We, who live in modern, industrialized nations, have more choices and volume of foods today than ever before. We have endless restaurants, massive supermarkets, often open 24 hours a day, each filled with seemingly unlimited choices. How then, can we be so much more nutrient deficient than previous generations? The answer is simple, quantity does not equate to quality.

In order to understand what really happened to our food and how it has lost much of its nutrient content, we need to take a little trip back in time, back to the days when the European settlers, having established themselves along the East Coast of America, began to get the itch to move westward.

As settlers migrated west, families or groups of families, would stake claim to lands, build housing and set up farming. In those days, little thought was given to care for the land and after several years of farming, the land became less and less fertile, losing key minerals required for abundant crops. The result was that the families would abandon the farms and move further westward, seeking new and fertile lands. These would then be farmed to death and the migration would continue. It wouldn't be until decades later that farmers would learn how to care for the land and replace lost nutrients, thereby keeping the farmlands 'alive.'

America began to employ farming techniques, long practiced, at that time, in Europe, namely replacing nutrients in the soil by composting and the use of animal fertilizers. This ended the need to constantly seek new farmlands and the families stayed, the population grew and cities and towns began for form across the country. America and in fact many nations, produced some of the highest quality food since commercial food farming began.

During that period, people were among the healthiest at any recorded time. With the exception of infectious diseases, which often took people's lives prematurely, our great grandparents and their parents, were some of the healthiest people of relatively modern times.

Enter Big Business and Big Profit

As nations flourished and the populations grew, the demand for greater and greater supplies of food became apparent. The United States Department of Agriculture was established, in part, to provide ongoing support to farmers to meet this growing demand for 'more food.'

As methods of refrigeration and other storage developed, farmers could ship their foods to wider and wider geographic areas before spoilage took place. This increasing market allowed farmers to plant larger acreage of crops. Before you knew it, farming and food production became a big business.

As demands for more and more food production increased, large investment groups began buying up the smaller farms, consolidating them into vast expanses of land, under one ownership. The days of the individual farmer were fading and food production had become the domain of big business.

Profit is important to everyone and is, in fact, essential to the survival of enterprise, but as mega corporations infiltrated the food production industry, their drive for greater and greater profits became obsessive. Food and soil chemists were hired to research better ways to increase production. The UDSA was petitioned to assist in finding ways to decrease cost and increase the yield per acre of farmland. This focus led to the first major blow to the quality of food we consume today.

As chemists analyzed the chemistry of plants, they discovered that by using just three basic nutrients, but in high quantities, they could increase not only the yield per acre of crops, but they could also shorten the growing season of many foods, thereby allowing farmers to often plant and harvest another time before winter weather set in. Armed with these two benefits, the farming industry became massively powerful and swallowed up further small farming operations into their conglomerate.

The three nutrients, when used in larger amounts, that produced accelerated growth and yield are nitrogen, phosphorus and potash or potassium. By manipulating these three minerals, according to each individual crop, nothing else appeared to be necessary for optimal growth and production. So well, did this new concept of NPK fertilization work, that all other, time consuming, 'old fashioned' ways of farming were quickly abandoned. No more did farmers compost, no more did they turn un-useable parts of plants back into the soil. All of this became unnecessary with the advent of NPK fertilizers.

Plants need at least 70 major and trace minerals in order to be healthy. In mineral-rich soils these are easily available. With the widespread use of the NPK – nitrogen, phosphorus and potash fertilizers, the rest of the minerals became increasingly deficient in the soils. After several years, many of these trace minerals were so deficient that the crops grown on these lands contained only a fraction of the mineral content of a few years ago. This practice of NPK farming has continued, more or less, unabated ever since. After at least 60 years of these practices, our foods are almost completely devoid of key trace minerals essential for human health and well-being.

Does Anybody Know About This?

Since this has been going on for many decades and since it so negatively affects the food chain, us included, has anyone brought this to the attention of the food industry?

You bet, but they're not listening. The food industry has become one of the largest non-governmental industries in the world and they are only interested in profits, not the health of you and I. (A recent classic example of this may be found in the new ruling for trans fats. As soon as it became a requirement to list trans fats on the food label, virtually every junk food containing high amounts of trans fats was reformulated, overnight, and new packaging was produced proclaiming the food as 'trans fat free.' This shows clearly, that the technology was there for perhaps years, to eliminate these deadly fats from our foods, but because it was cheaper to produce, nothing was done until regulation forced the hand of the food industry.)

The concept of NPK fertilization produced bigger crops, larger yield per acre, and even often allowed for an additional crop per growing cycle; why then would the food industry want to spend any more money on enriching our soils?

Back in the early 1930's a group of scientists prepared a report for the United States Congress, describing the sorry and alarming state of our food production. So important was this document that it was entered into the 74th Congress, Second Session as document number 264. Among the many points made by the scientists, was the rapidly declining mineralization of soils and food grown on those soils:

"The alarming fact is that foods – fruits and vegetables and grains – now being raised on millions of acres of land that no longer contain enough of certain needed minerals, are starving us – no matter how much of them we eat…"

"Ninety nine percent of the American people are now deficient in these minerals.…"

"Any upset of the balance, any considerable lack of one or another element, however microscopic the bodily requirement may be, and we sicken, suffer and shorten our lives.…"

"When the importance of these obscure minerals elements is fully realized the chemistry of life will have to be rewritten. No man knows his mental or bodily capacity, how well he can feel or how long he can live.…"

Today, 70 years later, the ominous warning of these words has been proven in many ways. Our life spans have not increased but marginally, in the last 50 years, in spite of tremendous advancements in medical science. The incidence of non-infectious chronic degenerative diseases, have reached epidemic proportions, affecting the lives of almost everyone alive, one way or the other.

In his landmark work, "Nutrition and Physical Degeneration", Weston A. Price, DDS, examined the dental status of primitive and modern people over a period of many years. His conclusion was that as the diet of humans progressed toward modernization, physical deterioration accelerated. He found that in the more primitive tribes, the quality and condition of the teeth of these people were excellent, even into advanced age. He further documented that as 'modern foods' were introduced in these societies, the dental status of the people began to decline in as little as ten years!

Hawaii is the most remote land mass on earth, the nearest point of land being 2500 miles away. As such, these people consumed a diet of indigenous foods, grown on rich volcanic soils. With the advent of the European and American influences in the late 1800's and again with the massive influx of 'Americanization' during World War II, many thousands of native Hawaiian people died from chronic, non-infectious conditions that were virtually unknown previously. As a result of Statehood and the complete immersion into the Standard American Diet (SAD!), Type II Diabetes is epidemic among the Hawaiians, affecting over 30 percent of the population. (The same is true for the Native Americans where Type II Diabetes is the number one health problem)

William Albrecht, PhD, in his fine work published in 1975 under the title of The Albrecht Papers, Volume One, further reminds us of the desperate state of our farmlands:

"The excessive use of chemical salts (NPK) in fertilizers is upsetting the plant nutrition."

"Modern fertilizing techniques are the art of putting salts in the ground so that the plant roots can try and dodge them."

"Insects and diseases are the symptoms of a failing crop, not the cause of it."

As a result of this last postulation, several universities have conducted experiments in raising crops on soils fertilized with mineral salts (NPK) and soils re-mineralized with organic, full spectrum minerals. The results, repeatedly, are the same. Plants grown on mineral-rich soils do not attract insects, while those growing on mineral deficient soils quickly become ravaged with insect infestation.

The bottom line is that that crops grown in healthy soils are healthy plants and healthy plants just don't taste good to insects. Insects on the other hand, are attracted to mineral-depleted plants because, in nature's scheme, they are not fit for consumption by higher life forms – animals and humans!

Instead of fixing this problem, chemical companies make millions selling pesticides and herbicides to the food industry, the residues of which remain on our food and in our soils. Ultimately, these chemicals find their way into our bodies, where an already over-worked liver must try and find a way to deal with them. Don't worry though, there is a way around this problem, and yes, it's easy!

Where Did All The Vitamins Go?

We can now see why it is essential to supplement the diet with a broad spectrum of major and trace minerals, as they are no longer present, to any degree, in our foods. What then, has become of our vitamins? According to the United States Congress, in investigation proceedings for the passage of the Dietary Supplement, Health and Education Act, back in the 1980's, "at least 50 percent of the population is getting less than 50 percent of the necessary nutrients from their foods." Many of these nutrients are from the vitamin group.

In the ideal diet, the major source of vitamins for animals and humans come from plants - fruits, vegetables and grains. Oddly enough, plants are not as dependent on the vitamins as they are the minerals, but manufacture vitamins in the latter stages of plant maturity and ripening.

For the most part, animals cannot manufacture most vitamins and humans can manufacture even less of them. Instead, we must rely on the vitamins found in fresh foods. Herein begins the problem with vitamin deficiency. Most of the foods we consume today are processed to some degree. We seem to be obsessed on doing something with our food before we eat it. We cook, steam, stew, bake, fry or juice it, but we rarely just eat it raw. This over-cooking of food is the first major blow in the destruction of the vitamins. In fact almost all vitamins and certainly all enzymes found in foods are destroyed or broken down at temperatures over 120 degrees Fahrenheit.

The next problem contributing to vitamin deficiency in foods comes from storage. As the demand for more and more foods to feed the growing populations increased, the food industry had to develop ways of storing and transporting fresh foods. No longer were foods grown in the 'neighborhood.' Populations of the highest concentration were often the furthest from any food production and as such foods had to be stored and transported, at least long enough to make it to these high demand markets.

Modern chemistry comes to the rescue once again and develops chemicals that actually put our foods in a form of suspended animation. Thus, foods are picked green, long before they are ripe, and then chemically treated to prevent further ripening. In this state, foods can be stored for months in cold storage houses awaiting supply and demand.

When these foods are ready to be shipped to retail markets, they are gassed with other chemicals to accelerate ripening, so that by the time they reach your local market, they look like they had just been fresh picked yesterday!

The result of this storage process is that since our fruits and vegetables never actually ripen on the plant, far less vitamins are produced. Then, long periods of cold storage further retard the production and retention of delicate vitamins.

Lastly, since most plants need key trace minerals to produce the vitamins in the first place and those minerals have been depleted from our farmlands, the sins of modern farming, which began long ago, are depleting greater numbers of nutrients from our modern day food supply. Again, this sounds like a big problem, which it is. Fortunately, there is an effective solution to this problem, and, yes, it's easy!

Refining And Processing – The Final Insult

Much of the industrialized diet is made up of refined over-processed foods. As we illustrated in Chapter 1, the over-processing of sugar and grains has created highly refined carbohydrates, which are found in the majority of our processed foods. In addition to contributing to the dietary problems outlined previously, the refining of these whole foods into starchy and sugary counterparts also depletes nutrients.

Consider the refining of whole wheat into white flour as an example:

Whole wheat provides many minerals and some vitamins. The following chart shows the percentage of loss of key minerals during the refining process. Further losses will occur during storage and cooking.

Calcium	60% Loss
Phosphorus	71% Loss
Magnesium	85% Loss
Potassium	77% Loss
Chromium	98% Loss
Manganese	86% Loss
Iron	76% Loss
Cobalt	89% Loss
Copper	68% Loss
Zinc	78% Loss
Selenium	16% Loss

This is just one example of how refining basic foods can further deplete essential minerals. Consider the number of foods made from these refined grains and the percentage of people who over-consume them and you will begin to get the picture of our nutrient status.

Nutrients That Protect Us In A Modern Age

There are more man-made chemical compounds in existence today than at any other time. Tens of thousands of chemicals are in our food, water, the air we breathe, and the many man-made objects in our immediate environment. Each of these sources of exposure and ingestion adds to the potential complications, which arise when the internal environment of the human body becomes excessively toxic.

Conditions like autoimmune illnesses, fibromyalgia, chronic fatigue syndrome and many others have been linked with excess toxins in the body. The liver, the organ primarily responsible for the processes of these toxins often becomes over-burdened and unable to effectively do its job. (One sign of this is the millions of people with excessively high levels of cholesterol. Cholesterol regulation is a function of the liver and can become compromised when the liver is over-burdened with toxins from the environment)

The by-products of breaking down these many toxins in the body are called free radicals. Free radicals can form as a result of many chemical actions, some of which are normal and healthy, but the free radicals formed from chemical compounds and some altered foods, as discussed in Chapter 1, can easily damage living cells and even alter the genetic structure of other cells.

The protective factors that insulate cells from free radical damage are called antioxidants. While there are many nutrients that act as antioxidants, the key players are vitamin A, beta carotene, folic acid, vitamin C, bioflavonoids, vitamin E, zinc, and selenium.

In recent years, antioxidants that protect against specific types of free radical activity have been isolated. These are of particular importance in our age of chronic, degenerative disorders. Some of the many key heavy hitting antioxidants include lycopene, quercetin, bilberry extract, grape seed extract, co-enzyme Q10, milk thistle, alpha lipoic acid, lutein and N-Acetyl Cysteine.

The problem with the antioxidants is that while they often exist in relatively high amounts in some foods, the amount of antioxidants needed to protect us from the massive amounts of free radical activity, generated by the excessive toxins in the environment, can exceed that which can be obtained from any dietary intake. Supplementing antioxidants can be complicated and sometimes costly, but don't worry, there is an easy way!

The Essential Nutrients For Optimal Health

Every day, our bodies need a wide variety of nutrients from many different categories. A deficiency of these nutrients, which are really chemicals of life, for prolonged periods, can result in the development of one or more of the many chronic diseases that are epidemic in our society today. Conditions like arthritis, diabetes, heart disease, many forms of cancer, fibromyalgia, elevated cholesterol, and complications of the menopause are all examples of conditions that can develop as a result of prolonged nutrient deficiencies.

Fifteen years ago, I compiled a list of what I believed to be the essential nutrients, required on a daily basis, for optimal health and longevity. This list has changed a little over the years, today's list now includes:

8-12 AMINO ACIDS – Essential for forming human proteins and repairing tissue structures within the body

3 FATTY ACIDS – These are necessary for the formation of numerous compounds and physical structures.

16 VITAMINS – Divided into two groups, the fat soluble and the water soluble, vitamins act as chemical catalysts for thousands of biochemical functions within the body.

70+ MINERALS – The minerals are the largest group of nutrients, made up of major minerals such as calcium and magnesium to the micro trace elements, such as zinc, chromium, selenium and many others. Minerals are involved both in structure and function of the human body and may be found as the basis for countless chemical equations in human biology.

PHYTONUTRIENTS – These are plant chemicals, compounds formed in the process of plants carrying out their life functions, which have been shown to produce chemicals necessary to our optimal health. Phytonutrients come from living plants, but are easily broken down and destroyed by processing and over-cooking.

ANTIOXIDANTS – This category of vitamins, minerals and other nutrients protect the body from the ravages of free radical damage to living cells and genetic material of the body.

If you add these groups together, you get somewhere around 100+ nutrients per day. There are several problems involved in ensuring we meet our body's daily intake of so many nutrients.

We have already established that obtaining adequate amounts of these nutrients from foods is unlikely, even if you eat well. Therefore, supplementation is the only logical answer.

When it comes to supplements, there are several issues that can often complicate matters. In order to get all of the 100+ nutrients on a daily basis, it is often necessary to take several products. You might need a multi vitamin/mineral product, extra vitamin C, a calcium/magnesium product, a trace mineral product, a fatty acid product, a phytonutrient formula and an antioxidant product.

The first problem with this is determining how much of each formula is right for you. Secondly, it often does not take too long before your kitchen cabinet is filled with supplement bottles and it can take a fair amount of time to open, count out the pills and then swallow them all.

Over time, only the die hard will pursue and most of use give up and take only 'one or two' because it is just to complicated, not to mention too expensive! It is easy to spend $150.00 or more per person, per month in the pursuit of getting the 100+ nutrients everyday. Very few people will endure the inconvenience and expense of such a program, but don't worry, there is an easy way!

Enter The Concept Of Full Spectrum Nutrition

I first addressed this issue of the complexity of nutrient supplementation and its often-high cost back in 1991. At that time, I was working with ways of combining nutrients together to make a more complete broad-spectrum supplement. There were however, several issues to consider:

POTENCY – It was important to ensure that we had adequate amounts of each nutrient to meet the baseline needs of a wide variety of people.

COMPATIBILITY – Many nutrients do not do well in the presence of others, in that some nutrients can inhibit the absorption of others, while some nutrients tend to break down others if compounded in the same formula. In order to prevent these reactions, we had to find a way to 'insulate' one nutrient from another, through coatings that would prevent chemical reactions but still allow for digestion and absorption.

RATIO – One of the newest concepts in dietary supplementation is the concept of ratios. In nature, vitamins and minerals are found in specific ratios to each other. This is for a reason. Nutrients, especially the minerals, compete for transport across cell membranes. If there are extra high amounts of one mineral, over another, the dominating mineral can, in some cases, prevent cellular absorption of the others.

ABSORPTION – Today we know that it is not just what you eat, in the form of foods or supplements that can make you healthy, but rather how much your body is able to absorb, at the cellular level, that counts. Known factors that can affect absorption include the size of the nutrient particle, (The smaller the better) the form the nutrient takes, the ratio as mentioned above, and the pH or acid/alkaline state of the nutrients. Each of these needed to be considered and factors addressing each needed to be incorporated into the optimal dietary supplement.

After nearly two years of trial and error, experiment and failure, I finally came up with a method of combining all 100+ nutrients into one formula, one bottle, taken just once per day.

All of a sudden we had eliminated two of the biggest hurdles facing people in taking supplements, namely convenience and cost. We now had all the baseline nutrients in one formula. The nutrients were properly protected from each other to prevent unwanted chemical reactions. The pH of the formula was adjusted to match that of a healthy stomach – going a long way to enhance digestion and absorption. The potency and ratio of each nutrient had been carefully worked out, and because all the nutrients were now in one formula, the cost was a fraction of that incurred when buying many products in an attempt to get all the essential nutrients.

The only way I could get all 100+ nutrients into one formula, at the time, was to put them in a liquid suspension. There is a lot of space between the molecules of water and I found that with some coaxing, all the nutrients could be included. Because our delivery system was water, this allowed for us to adjust the particle size of the nutrients by processing them through what is called a colloidal shear. This process reduces the particles to micron size, thereby enhancing absorption.

Another benefit to using water as a medium of delivery was that we could easily adjust the pH or the acidity of the product to be acidic. In fact the liquid matches the pH of a healthy stomach exactly. This too, aids in absorption of the nutrients, especially the minerals, at the cellular level.

Once this concept was established and the first formula was stable, I developed several other formulas, using this same concept, a concept that I have since coined Full Spectrum Nutrition. Since that original development, we now have a capsule version of our Full Spectrum Formula. While we feel it does not provide as good an absorption rate as a liquid delivery system, it comes as close to completeness as any encapsulated formula we have seen on the market.

Full Spectrum Nutrition is simply providing the body with all the 100+ nutrients it needs everyday in one formula that is easy to take and meets the requirements of potency, ratio, pH and particle size for better absorption.

Who Needs Full Spectrum Supplementation?

The answer to this question is simple; if you are still breathing, you can benefit from Full Spectrum Supplements. Such Full Spectrum formulas are now available from a variety of companies, many of them are quite good.

I told you this was a 'made easy' book and what could possibly be easier than one formula, taken once per day?

What about the cost? Since all the nutrients are combined into one convenient formula, the cost is but a fraction of what it would be if you had to take 8 or 10 different formulas just to meet baseline needs. For less than a dollar a day, anyone can provide their body with the 100+ nutrients in a highly absorbable formula.

If you consider the cost of many of our other indulgences this is the cheapest thing you can do and certainly the best. Consider for example, the cost of even moderate alcohol consumption. At just $2.00 for a beer, consuming 2 beers per day results in a cost of $28.00 per week or $1,460.00 per year! How about those pack-a-day smokers? At an average of $5.00 a pack, that's $35.00 a week, or $1,825.00 per year! Think you don't have any vices well how about coffee? A double latte can cost $4.00 each. Have one a day that's $28.00 per week or $1,460.00 per year.

In each case, the things we spend money on and take for granted are all far more expensive than providing your body with a little true 'health insurance' in the form of Full Spectrum Nutrition.

The formulas we currently use at our clinics and research centers around the world are also available to everyone and certainly meet all the criteria we have previously discussed. If you should have problems finding these formulas in your area, you can contact The Institute of Nutritional Science for sources. You can email them at AskTheDoc@HealthyInformation.com

Let's continue now with a brief discussion of the vitamins and minerals so that you will have a basic knowledge of what they are and what they do once you get them into your body.

The Vitamins

Of the 100+ nutrients, 16 of them are classified as vitamins. There are two groups of vitamins, the fat soluble, which include vitamins A, E, D, and K and the water soluble, which are made up of the B complex and vitamin C.

We have come a long way in our research and information about vitamins. Considering the relatively short time vitamins have been under study, and the number of obstacles along the way, much progress has been made. Several myths were put into motion by writers and medical minds, who did not have the knowledge or understanding of how vitamins work or what effects they have on the body.

The greatest and possibly most dangerous myth about vitamins and other nutrients was the Minimum Daily Requirement (MDR). While these recommendation have been revised several times since and are now, in fact, called the Daily Values (DV) on food and supplement labels, these amounts are not only far too low to be of any real benefit, but do not match the levels being proven by hundreds of clinical studies to be optimal. These values were established back in the 1940's when our knowledge of human nutrition was in the dark ages, by comparison to today. Sadly, they have never been revised to any appropriate extent.

Vitamins are absolutely essential for growth, maintenance and reproduction of the human body. We, who work with vitamins and other nutrients, under clinical conditions are convinced of the undeniable benefits to the human condition from vitamin sufficiency.

The Fat Soluble Vitamins

The fat-soluble vitamins, A, D, E, and K are found in foods of the fatty variety, since fats are needed to transport these vitamins within the body. Vitamins in this group are stable with temperature changes and therefore are less likely to be damaged or destroyed during freezing or cooking. The problem with the fat-soluble vitamins is in the absorption. If insufficient fats are ingested in the diet, absorption of these vital nutrients is greatly reduced.

Because the fat-soluble vitamins are stored in the liver, it is essential that you ingest only natural forms of these nutrients. Synthetic forms of the fat-soluble vitamins can store in the liver to excessively high quantities producing toxic results. On the other hand, it is very difficult to over-dose on these nutrients if you always take them in their natural form.

Vitamin A

This wonderful vitamin has been, possibly, the source of more controversy and scare than any other. It has been down played, underrated, and feared for its attributed side effects, but the fact is that every medical case on record, of vitamin A toxicity occurred when the individual was taking synthetic rather than natural vitamin A!

There are two forms of this vitamin, the first being pure vitamin A and the other, which is a precursor of vitamin A called beta-carotene. It is important to note that beta-carotene is not vitamin A. It must be converted to vitamin A in the body.

Some of the many functions of vitamin A include supporting the immune system, protection of the mucosa linings of the body against infection, growth and repair of body tissues, healthy teeth and gums, the production of gastric juices for digestion, and night vision and general health of the eyes.

Vitamin A has been shown to be beneficial in supporting the body in fighting such problems as canker sores, skin eruptions, acne, athlete's foot, bedsores, boils, burns, dandruff, dermatitis, shingles, glaucoma, diabetes, colitis, sinusitis and arthritis. You will find vitamin A part of our targeted protocols for these and other conditions later in the book.

Vitamin D

Vitamin D is often referred to as the 'sunshine' vitamin since it is readily produced when the unprotected skin comes in contact with sunlight. Even though this seems common, there are many people who live in parts of the world where little or no sunlight occurs for months on end. For this reason and because the functions of vitamin D are so vital to good health, supplementing vitamin D is a wise choice.

Functions of vitamin D include growth, especially in children, development of bones and teeth, maintenance of bone density in older people, formation of key enzymes, normal heart action, stabilizing the nervous system and normal blood clotting.

The importance of vitamin D supplementation occurred in the last century with the advent of a condition called rickets, which is a bone disorder. Once vitamin D was supplemented this condition was all but eradicated.

Vitamin E

Vitamin E belongs to a group of chemical compounds called tocopherols. There are seven major forms of tocopherols, and may be listed on supplement labels as alpha, beta, delta, epsilon, eta, gamma and zeta. The most potent form of these tocopherols is the alpha form, hence this is the most frequent form of this vitamin used in supplementation.

One of the greatest benefits of vitamin E in the body is that it is a potent antioxidant, which means that it opposes the oxidation of substances, which can cause free radical formation.

Of all the vitamins, the most dangerous, in synthetic form has to be vitamin E. This nutrient must be taken only in its naturally occurring forms. The way to tell if the vitamin E in your supplement is natural is to look at the supplement facts box. If the vitamin E comes from natural, safe sources, it will be listed as d-alpha tocopherol. If the vitamin E is synthetic and as such should be avoided, it will be listed as dl-alpha tocopherol. There is just one little letter difference so beware.

Vitamin E has many biological functions within the human body. Some of these include cellular respiration of muscles, a powerful antioxidant, reduces scar tissue formation, increases formation of new blood vessels, stimulates urine secretion, assists in normalizing blood viscosity and retards muscle degeneration.

Vitamin K

Vitamin K is the last of the fat-soluble vitamins and is often referred to as the coagulating vitamin. It is not found in most supplements because it is needed in relatively small amounts and it is readily found in many foods, especially green, leafy vegetables. Vitamin K is often given in supplement form, to pregnant women to prevent hemorrhaging. Because of its clotting properties, vitamin K should not be taken by those with a tendency towards blood clots or those taking prescription blood thinners.

The Water Soluble Vitamins

Unlike the fat-soluble vitamins, the water-soluble group is generally not stored in the body tissues for any length of time. For this reason, it is essential that they be ingested on a daily basis. Any excesses of the water-soluble group of nutrients are passed out of the body via the urine. The water-soluble vitamins are made up of the B complex and vitamin C.

The B Complex Vitamins

The B complex vitamins are linked together in likeness in several chemical ways, as well as in methods of action within the body. This family of powerful nutrients is made up of B1, B2, B3, B5, B12, B13, B15, Biotin, Choline, Inositol, Folic Acid and PABA (Para Amino Benzoic Acid).

In general, the B complex group is responsible for providing energy to the body through direct involvement with the conversion of carbohydrates to glucose. They are also critical in the metabolism of fats and proteins. The proper functioning of the nervous system is also affected by the B vitamins, and a deficiency of one or more of these can lead to many problems with the nervous system, including anxiety, insomnia and nervous twitching.

Vitamin B1(Thiamine)

This nutrient, along with others in the B complex family is essential to the health of the nervous system and ones mental attitude. Functions of this vitamin include the conversion of carbohydrates to glucose, growth, fertility, feeding of the nervous system, appetite control and is needed in the metabolism of alcohol.

Vitamin B2 (Riboflavin)

This vitamin is involved in many chemical reactions within the body. It combines with other nutrients to form key enzymes. Of particular importance is the part vitamin B2 plays in the process of oxidation reduction reactions, preventing excess formation of free radicals.

Other functions of B2 include the respiration of cells, the conversion of amino acids, the metabolism of carbohydrates, the maintenance of the skin, nails and hair and support for the eye tissues.

Vitamin B3 (Niacin or Niacinamide)

This stable nutrient is often referred to by one of two different names. Niacin is the pure form of the vitamin, which contains an organic acid group in its makeup. This compound causes vasodilatation, which manifests itself as hot flashes. This flushing property is beneficial for some people and in some heath conditions. For those who don't like this effect or who don't need the flushing properties, there is another form called Niacinamide, which contains an amino acid group in place of the flushing properties.

Functions of Niacin include an active role in the co-enzymes that provide an essential ingredient in tissue oxidations, the synthesis of sex hormones, regulates the activity of the nervous system, improves circulation and reduces serum cholesterol.

Vitamin B6 (Pyridoxine)

This vitamin is one of the newer additions to the B complex group by comparison to many of the others. Vitamin B6 is very susceptible to destruction by heat and as such is one of the most deficient vitamins in the human body as most of our food is cooked.

There is a strong connection involving long-term B6 deficiencies and either hypoglycemia or type II diabetes. It has also been observed that those suffering from these conditions need much higher amounts of this nutrient to maintain acceptable levels.

One of the main functions of B6 is that it is a carrier agent, helping to transport other nutrients into the cells. It is for this reason that many specialized formulas also include vitamin B6 to help ensure absorption and transport of other key factors.

Some of the other functions of B6 include, assimilation of B12, production of hydrochloric acid in the stomach, the metabolism of many amino acids, the metabolism of fats, helps to maintain the sodium/potassium balance, facilitates the conversion of stored glycogen to useable glucose and must be present for the production of antibodies and red blood cells.

Vitamin B12

From the molecular point of view vitamin B12 is one of the most complex of all the B complex nutrients. It is important to note that neither man nor animal is able to synthesize or manufacture any vitamin B12 in the body. For this reason, supplementation with B12 is essential.

Unlike the rest of the B complex family, B12 is difficult to absorb. It is essential that the stomach produce adequate hydrochloric acid to aid in the absorption of B12 taken orally.

Recent studies have shown that B12 has an overall stimulating effect upon the immune system. A deficiency in this nutrient manifests itself in a decreased T and B cell response to infection. Other functions of vitamin B12 include the functioning of bone marrow, nervous tissue & the gastrointestinal tract. It also aids in the synthesis of many nutrients, the formation of nucleic acids and assists in the formation of red blood cells.

Pantothenic Acid

First discovered by biochemist Roger J. Williams, pantothenic acid's main function seems to be the effect it has upon the body's ability to handle stress. Excess stress can deplete the body of this essential nutrient in a very short period of time. The consumption of antibiotics also greatly reduces the levels of pantothenic acid.

Other functions of this nutrient include, prevention of stress-related fatigue. It is necessary for many metabolic processes, blood pressure and heart rate control, prevention of hypoglycemia and the prevention of arthritis.

Biotin

A lesser-known member of the B complex family, biotin's functions in the body include acting as a coenzyme, manufacture of the fatty acids, the formation of glycogen or stored sugars, the synthesis of amino acids and the formation of nucleic acids at the cellular level.

Choline

Unfortunately, choline is considered by many experts to be a rather non-essential nutrient. This is sad since choline is involved in many very important catalytic and metabolic functions within the body. Choline is the active factor in lecithin, and is a member of the lipotropic family of nutrients, which includes choline, methionine and inositol. These nutrients work together to ensure healthy liver function.

Other functions of choline include, the metabolism of fats and improved liver function. It is necessary for the production of a chemical called acetylcholine, which is essential to normal nerve function. It protects the myelin sheaths of the nerves and is a part of many hormones such as epinephrine.

Inositol

Functions of inositol are similar to that of choline and in fact, this nutrient is almost always found in conjunction with choline. It plays a role in the metabolism of fats, acts as a growth factor, feeds the brain cells and aids in the growth of hair.

Folic Acid (Folacin)

The primary role of folic acid is as a carrier in the formation of heme, which is the iron-containing protein present in hemoglobin. This is necessary for the formation of red blood cells. A deficiency of folic acid can lead to some complications of pregnancy, which is why women are advised to double their intake of this nutrient during pregnancy. Other functions of this vitamin include the stimulation of natural stomach acids, increased liver function and the prevention of macrocytic anemia.

Para-Aminobenzoic Acid (PABA)

While PABA is very much a part of the B-complex vitamin group, this food factor is still, sadly, considered by some in the industry, as non-essential. PABA has been used successfully in treating certain forms of parasitic diseases such as Rocky Mountain Spotted Fever. PABA also retards the premature graying of the hair. Other functions of PABA include increasing healthy intestinal bacteria and as a coenzyme in the breakdown of proteins, assists in the formation of blood cells, and helps to prevent loss of skin pigmentation.

While there are other, more obscure vitamins such as vitamin B13 and possibly pangamic acid, this pretty much concludes our discussion of the B complex. One last reminder on the B complex family: Each B vitamin must be taken in harmony and ratio with all the others. These nutrients work together.

Vitamin C

The last of the vitamins to be discussed is probably the most well known. Also called ascorbic acid, the importance of vitamin C was first recognized in conjunction with British sailors on long ocean voyages. After a time out of port, the majority of the men would develop a condition, which came to be called scurvy. It was discovered that scurvy developed when citrus fruits were not available. Later, of course we recognized that it was the vitamin C in the fruit that prevented scurvy.

Vitamin C became the most popular nutrient largely through the work of the late Linus Pauling, PhD. Dr. Pauling illustrated that the human body could obtain increased benefits and protection from pathogens such as bacteria and virus by often dramatically increasing the daily dose of this nutrient.

Many animals manufacture high doses of vitamin C in response to and in prevention of infection. Goats, rabbits, cats and dogs for example, manufacture amounts that would be equivalent to 10,000 mg per day in a person of 150 pounds.

Vitamin C is one of the least stable of all the vitamins. It is very sensitive to light, heat and oxygen, being easily destroyed by any or all of them.

Some of the many functions of vitamin C include, the formation of collagen protein, increased healing of wounds, acts as a natural antihistamine, maintains the strength of blood vessels, fights bacterial and viral infections, promotes the formation of hemoglobin, acts as a natural diuretic and helps the adrenal glands in the secretion of key hormones.

The Minerals

When we speak of supplements, we often think first of the vitamins, but the fact is that the largest group of essential nutrients for human health and well-being is the mineral group. There are at least 70 known major and trace minerals present in the human body. Many of these are micro trace elements, meaning that they are present in very small quantities. Quantity, however, should not be synonymous with importance since many of the micro trace minerals perform functions that are vital to our health and longevity. It is these tiny trace elements that are most often deficient due to their depletion in the soil of our farmlands.

When is comes to mineral supplementation, not all mineral supplements are created equal. Minerals are very hard to absorb and require specific chemistries to achieve this. Most of the supplements on the market today are made up of what we call elemental or 'inorganic' minerals. These are derived from rocks, soils, clays and sea beds. They are, generally, very alkaline in nature, which presents the first problem. Most minerals need to be acidic before they can be, properly absorbed by the body. These inexpensive sources of minerals are often used, by manufacturers, to save money and increase profits, but the absorption rate of most of the minerals in this form is less than 20 percent. This becomes important for example in the case of calcium. Many people, especially middle aged women, are aware of their need to supplement calcium, yet they often are taking a supplement made up of ground rocks, which will yield about a 20 percent absorption rate. This means that the 1000 mg of calcium they are taking is actually providing about 200 mg of absorbed nutrient – not enough to prevent bone loss.

Caring supplement manufacturers often pre-acidify their minerals in supplement form, thereby greatly increasing the absorption potential to the body. The process of pre-acidification is called chelation, which literally means 'to bind.' The mineral is bound with an acid, usually citric acid, malic acid or an amino acid, which makes the mineral much more bio-available to the cells of the body.

Other forms of mineral supplements that are extremely highly absorbable are those, which have been derived from organic compounds. The 'organic' minerals are extracted from plant material that had been grown on mineral-rich soils. Because these minerals are still part of more complex plant compounds, their bio-availability is extremely high.

It is important to read supplement labels and to keep in mind that not all mineral supplements are the same. Be sure that the source of the minerals in your supplements are either chelated or from 'organic' plant origins.

Major Minerals

CALCIUM. Calcium reigns as the single most abundant mineral in the body. It is involved in the formation and maintenance of bones and teeth. It plays a vital role in many biochemical activities within the body. To properly function, calcium must interact with several other nutrients, which include Vitamin D, boron, magnesium, manganese, copper and zinc, which are all necessary to ensure proper absorption of calcium.

Since calcium is often very alkaline, taking chelated forms of this mineral is essential for absorption. As we age, this becomes more important because our digestion often becomes less effective due to a decline in the production of natural stomach acids.

Functions of calcium include, building and maintaining bones and teeth, and reducing insomnia. It is needed for acid/alkaline balance, it regulates heartbeat, balances the minerals potassium and sodium for muscle tone, it assists in the clotting of blood, and aids in nerve impulse transmission.

PHOSPHORUS. This mineral is another found in relatively high amounts in the body. Supplementing with phosphorus is almost never necessary since the diet provides more than adequate amounts of this mineral. In fact excess phosphorus can displace calcium, causing a calcium deficiency.

Functions of phosphorus include, stimulating muscle contractions, and the formation of bones and teeth. It serves as a blood buffer, and is a building block in the myelin sheath surrounding all nerves.

SODIUM. This essential mineral is found almost exclusively in the body's extracellular fluids, those outside of individual cells. As an electrolyte it is involved with potassium in regulating the fluid levels of the body. Edema, or water retention, is often caused by an excess of sodium, in relationship to potassium. Since sodium is essential, very low sodium diets are not often wise or necessary. By lowering sodium intake slightly and increasing potassium intake, the balance between the two elements can be achieved. The end result is the release of unwanted, extra body fluid.

Functions of sodium include the regulation of the acid/alkaline balance. It works with potassium to detoxify and nourish individual cells, and stimulates nerve action. It aids in digestion and stimulates the production of natural stomach acids.

POTASSIUM. This mineral is found almost exclusively in the intra-cellular fluid of the body or within the cells. It can be likened to the opposite of sodium. Daily requirements of potassium are high, at least 2500 mg or more. Many doctors and nutritionists neglect the importance of supplementing this mineral because it is so prevalent in our foods. Unfortunately, the foods in which we find the greatest sources of potassium are those, which are often deficient in the SAD diet, such as fresh fruits and vegetables. Potassium is easily leached from foods during cooking. Some of the signs of potassium deficiency include nervous disorders, insomnia, irregular heartbeat, edema or water retention, and acne in adults.

Functions of potassium include, promoting normal growth and stimulating nerve impulses. It regulates bodily fluids, stimulates kidneys, aids in maintaining healthy skin and supports healthy adrenal gland function.

MAGNESIUM. The last of the really major minerals as far as shear quantity, magnesium works with both calcium and phosphorus in most of its functions. Most of the body's magnesium is found in the bones. The remaining is contained in the soft tissues as well as in internal body fluids.

Functions of magnesium include involvement in many metabolic functions. It activates enzyme systems, facilitates in the contraction of muscles and regulates the acid/alkaline balance. It is necessary for the utilization of the B complex vitamins and is needed in the conversion of glucose into energy.

The Trace Minerals

Minerals in this group are required in smaller amounts, but this does not, in any way, diminish their essential role in the human body.

IRON. This is one of the most misunderstood of minerals. Recent publicity has many people afraid of taking anything with iron in it, but the fact remains that we all need iron regularly. Excess iron intake is certainly not necessary and may lead to health issues, but media sensation often makes people go in the opposite extremes. In spite of all the negative publicity, the United States Department of Agriculture has estimated that about 35 percent of all Americans are deficient in iron.

Functions of iron include the formation of hemoglobin and the uptake of oxygen by cells. It reduces stress and free radical formation from oxidation, prevents anemia and helps to prevent constipation.

ZINC. The second largest in quantity of the trace minerals, zinc is responsible for many functions in the body, especially those of the immune system and as a constituent in the formation of sex hormones. A deficiency of this mineral results in increased fatigue, poor immune function, prostatitis in men, poor appetite, stretch marks on the skin, acne in teens and a prolonged deficiency may induce diabetes.

Functions of zinc include the absorption of B vitamins. It is necessary in the production of at least 25 key enzymes, increases the healing of wounds, and supports prostate function. It is needed in the production of sex hormones and is connected to the synthesis of DNA.

IODINE. This mineral is most commonly connected to the thyroid gland, as the body requires this nutrient in the production of thyroid hormones.

Functions of iodine include increasing energy production and the production of the thyroid hormone thyroxine. It stimulates growth and body development and regulates pulse and heart rate.

MANGANESE. The most important function of this mineral is its role in the absorption of calcium to the bones. Manganese is very poorly absorbed, but fortunately, little is needed.

Functions of manganese include the utilization of glucose, the synthesis of fatty acids, supporting nerve and brain function and pancreatic function.

COPPER. This essential trace mineral is obtained primarily from vegetables, hence the content of copper in farmlands directly determines the amount of copper in our diet. Recent studies indicate that far more people are deficient in copper than previously thought.

Functions of copper include being involved in protein metabolism, an essential part of many enzymes, the formation of the myelin sheath around nerves and assisting the body in utilizing vitamin C.

CHROMIUM. Focus on this trace mineral sharpened when its link with glucose metabolism disorders was discovered. In fact, a deficiency of chromium can lead to carbohydrate intolerance, hypoglycemia and Type II diabetes.

Functions of chromium include enzyme activity, glucose metabolism, conversion of sugars to energy, synthesis of fatty acids and amino acid metabolism.

SELENIUM. This mineral, in addition to its many elemental functions, is also a very powerful antioxidant. The amount of selenium in our diet is, again, directly related to its presence in the soils on which our food is grown. Certain areas of the country have greater selenium deficiencies than others because of the great variation of this mineral, in soils, across the country.

Functions of selenium include its major role as a powerful antioxidant, it prevents some forms of cancer, prevents premature aging, protects against heart disease by preventing free radical damage to arteries and protects against the side effects of toxic minerals.

The Micro Trace Minerals

These minerals are needed in extremely minute amounts. This again, does not mean that they are not important. They are involved almost exclusively in the bio-chemical activities of the body. When these minerals are deficient or missing from our diet, the biochemistry of the body begins to spin out of balance, the end result of which is the development of chronic disease conditions. Sadly, most supplements on the market do not provide many of these essential micro trace minerals. You will however, find them in all Full Spectrum formulations.

Many of these trace minerals are thought of as poisons, or highly toxic. This is because when they are ingested in their elemental, metallic state, they can be stored in the body, in soft tissues and eventually alter the biochemistry. Elements like aluminum, for example are essential for digestion and other processes, yet excessive amounts of elemental aluminum can be very toxic.

It is for this reason that we cannot stress too strongly the need to ensure that trace minerals in your supplements come from 'organic' sources. Plant derived trace minerals are completely safe as the body can get rid of any excesses with ease, preventing buildup.

Another interesting fact about negatively charged, organic sourced trace minerals is that they have the ability to remove their heavy metal counterparts through a process similar to chelation. Thus for example, plant based aluminum can remove heavy metallic aluminum from the body safely. This added advantage is just another reason to ensure that your supplements provide these vital trace elements – minerals we used to get from our foods before the farmlands were totally depleted of trace mineral content.

A list of the trace elements, with known biological function in the human body, are as follows:

Aluminum	Gadolinium	Nickel	Tellurium
Antimony	Gallium	Niobium	Terbium
Arsenic	Germanium	Osmium	Thallium
Barium	Gold	Palladium	Thorium
Beryllium	Hafnium	Praseodymium	Thulium
Bismuth	Holmium	Rhenium	Tin
Boron	Indium	Rhodium	Titanium
Bromine	Iodine	Rubidium	Tungsten
Cerium	Iridium	Ruthenium	Vanadium
Cesium	Iron	Samarium	Ytterbium
Chromium	Lanthanum	Scandium	Yttrium
Cobalt	Lithium	Selenium	Zinc
Copper	Lutetium	Silicon	Zirconium
Dysprosium	Manganese	Silver	
Erbium	Molybdenum	Strontium	
Europium	Neodymium	Tantalum	

Special Antioxidants For A Toxic World

We live in a world very much different from even the relatively recent days of our grandparents. In the last 50 years alone, our environment has changed more than in the last 1000 years combined. The level, number and degree of severity of the poisons in our environment have increased exponentially, exposing all of us to chemical compounds never before found in the physical universe. Each of those chemical compounds has the potential of altering the state of equilibrium within our body in a variety of ways. For this reason, we all need extra protection from this onslaught of chemical aggression.

Just when the protective antioxidants, provided in foods from nature, could no longer sufficiently protect us from the tens of thousands of man-made free radical sources, science has been able to isolate and concentrate powerful free radical fighters previously hidden deep within nature's realm. These 'super antioxidants' may very well prove to be the weapon we all need to fight off most of the chronic diseases we face today, as well as premature aging and disability. By adding the right combination of many of these latest antioxidant substances, you too, can beat the ravages of aging and forestall the many factors that compromise the quality of life as we age.

LYCOPENE. Who would have guessed that pasta sauces, ketchup and other tomato products could actually reduce your risk of getting certain types of cancers? Within these foods is a substance called lycopene, a member of the carotenoid family. Like beta-carotene, lycopene is an antioxidant with one small exception; lycopene is ten times more powerful in protecting against cancer!

Much of the current research regarding lycopene and cancer revolves around prostate cancer. It has long been observed that this dreaded cancer occurs with much less frequency in the southern Mediterranean countries such as Italy and Greece. In these countries cooked tomatoes are a dietary staple.

For some reason, which we cannot totally explain when tomatoes are cooked, the process concentrates the percentage of lycopene, making it one of the few nutrients known, which is not damaged by heating.

In a physiological sense, lycopene is the most prevalent carotenoid in the human body. One of the most concentrated sites may be found in the male prostate. It is believed that through the presence of lycopene, the human body is able to defend itself from specific cancer causing free radicals.

Other types of cancer that may be prevented through the presence of lycopene in adequate amounts include breast, lung and endometrial.

One of the reasons even people who consume large amounts of tomato products might be deficient in lycopene is that, like all carotenoids, it can only be absorbed in the presence of some fat. Therefore, the super low fat diet craze has created a situation where the incredible benefits of all carotenoids may be greatly diminished due to lack of absorption.

Other benefits from lycopene include prevention of heart disease. A recent study conducted in Israel, demonstrated that lycopene greatly increases the resistance of LDL cholesterol to oxidation. This is important because LDL cholesterol is only harmful when free radical oxygen alters the fat structure, oxidizing or literally rusting the fat.

We cannot produce lycopene within our bodies, which means that we must ingest it from foods and supplements. People who are at specific high risk such as smokers, drinkers and those with a high-risk cancer profile, should be cognizant of getting adequate lycopene daily.

Once again, like all balance within the human body, lycopene seems to work much better when combined with other antioxidants. In fact, one study, which used beta-carotene alone failed in demonstrating an anti-cancer benefit. When researchers combined the beta-carotene with lycopene and tocopherols, the results were amazing.

QUERCETIN. According to Robert C Atkins, in his book, *Dr. Atkins' Vita-Nutrient Solution,* quercetin deserves the title of 'king of the flavonoids'. This is because of its ability to affect so many areas of human health.

Quercetin is a 'secret weapon' when it comes to allergies. Millions of people suffer from a variety of allergies. Those with airborne allergies have the worst time, since they cannot escape the cause of their irritation.

Together with citrus bioflavonoids, clinical studies have shown that quercetin is better than most of the leading anti-histamines in regulating the allergic response. Still other studies are showing consistently that quercetin has the ability to block the production of a specific enzyme that neutralizes cortisone, the body's most powerful natural anti-inflammatory. At the Institute, we have tested and are now using quercetin with great success in many, previously, unmanageable allergy situations.

As with all the 'heavy hitter' antioxidants, quercetin has many applications in the body. It protects us against heart disease, the number one cause of death in America and many other countries today. Some studies indicate that quercetin's action upon the cardiovascular system may be equal to, or even greater than, that of natural vitamin E. In study after study, a high intake of this nutrient has shown a direct correlation between levels of quercetin and lower risks of cardiovascular disease and stroke.

Quercetin has another amazing ability. It can accelerate the production of specific enzymes that destroy potential carcinogens before they can do their final evil deed and convert healthy cells into cancerous ones.

In foods quercetin may be found in garlic, onions, cayenne pepper and green tea. This is one reason why these foods have had the reputation of being extra healthy. The problem is that most people do not eat a sufficient amount of these foods to ingest enough protective quercetin. Supplementation is a logical solution to this problem.

BILBERRY. Unless you have dealt with eye problems in the past, you may never have heard of bilberry. It is a distant relative to the blueberry and the cranberry.

The main benefit derived from bilberry is its ability to improve circulation and blood vessel health. This seems to apply specifically, although not exclusively, to the eye tissues. The United States military used bilberry extract back in World War II to improve the night vision of soldiers, especially air pilots. This practice is still in use to this day.

Research relative to blood vessel integrity and eyesight is quite extensive. Studies conducted in Italy have shown that bilberry can improve circulation to the eyes thereby mitigating such conditions as diabetes-caused glaucoma, day blindness, nearsightedness, and cataract formation. One such study showed that bilberry, along with vitamin E, stopped cataract formation in 97 percent of the people who took it.

Another condition, which has eluded many other methods of treatment, is macular degeneration. This problem is becoming more and more prevalent due to free radical damage to the eye tissues from smoke and other pollutants in the air. Bilberry comes to the rescue once again not only because it increases blood flow and hence oxygen to the eye tissue, but it also prevents oxidative damage on site.

The specific flavonoids in bilberry, which are called anthocyanosides, not only provide eye tissue support but help to limit calcium deposits and blood clots inside of the arteries. Because of the direct benefit exercised upon the vascular system, bilberry is also very useful in such conditions as leg swelling, varicose veins and even postpartum hemorrhoids. Lastly, bilberry helps diminish inflammation, a helpful effect in such conditions as arthritis and other inflammatory disorders.

Since bilberry is helpful in improving circulation, it is very good for wound healing. Wounds heal faster and with less infection. Bilberry works together with collagen to rebuild damaged tissues.

GRAPE SEED EXTRACT. This powerful antioxidant and anti-inflammatory is a member of the specific flavonoid group called the proanthocyanidins.

While grape seed extract demonstrates specific benefits of its own, its primary contribution to an antioxidant compound would have to be its ability to work together with other antioxidants, enhancing their potential.

There has been a debate for some time over which members of this group are better than others. The truth is that all proanthocyanidins, including cranberries, pine bark, or grape seeds contribute equally. The only difference might be the concentration. Here at the Institute, we use grape seed extract, since it is about 10 to 15 percent higher in proanthocyanidin potency than pine bark.

The earliest indication that something in the grape might be of benefit to human health came from the French. Researchers often pondered as to how the French, who consume very rich, high fatty foods, could have such a low incidence of heart disease. In fact there is very little problem with elevated, imbalanced cholesterol anywhere in France. What was special about the French, or their diet, which precluded an epidemic problem in many other areas of the world? Red wine!

Now, I realize that many people will question why we are promoting an alcoholic beverage as healthy. Sorry folks, the facts stand as they are. Obviously, if you have a biochemical problem with alcohol, you must avoid even red wine. Otherwise, two glasses of red wine per day lowers the risk of heart disease by as much as 10 times more than aspirin! This has been duplicated in no less than 7 major clinical studies.

People often ask if grape juice will produce the same effect. The answer is yes but not nearly to the same degree. The small amount of alcohol in the wine greatly increases the extraction of the proanthocyanidins from the grape. Further, the alcohol helps to calm the system and relax the arteries. In just one of the many studies on the benefits of red wine published in the Journal of Epidemiology, researchers found that after studying 24,000 middle-aged men, there was a 35 percent reduction in cardiovascular disease and a 24 percent reduction in cancer, when two to three glasses of red wine were ingested on a daily basis.

What about white wine you say? There are certainly antioxidants present in white wine but not as many as found in the red varieties. Why is this important? Well, proanthocyanidins are up to fifty times more potent than vitamin E in their free radical scavenging ability.

Some of the specific benefits, which may be derived from grape seed extract, include…

- It has the ability to cross the blood-brain barrier so it can scavenge free radicals from within brain tissue.

- It is highly synergistic with other antioxidants, such as vitamins A, C, and E, enhancing their effectiveness.

- Assists in the prevention of histamine formation, an important factor for allergy sufferers.

- Grape Seed extract protects us against radiation from all sources, including the sun, from pesticides in foods and water, and heavy metal poisoning, all of which produce free radicals in the body with great fortitude.

One final word on grape seed extract and red wine, moderation is the key here. While all the studies have shown a profound benefit from two to three glasses of wine per day, in every case, more was not better. As alcohol consumption went up, the benefits decreased proportionately. If you cannot moderate your consumption, take your grape seed extract by supplementation.

COENZYME Q$_{10}$. This amazing nutrient is really not a vitamin, a mineral or even an amino acid, yet it is absolutely essential that we have an adequate supply in order to live safely in our toxic world. Our bodies can make it in certain amounts, but frequently not sufficient to counter all the abusive substances in our environment.

One of the first observed beneficial effects of ubiquinone (Co-Q$_{10}$), was its ability to produce energy. Through this enhanced energy, individual cells of the body were able to live longer. Today we know that ubiquinone has many other abilities and can protect our body from many very destructive free radicals. Further it is a natural immune enhancer.

Some of the specific areas where Co-Q$_{10}$ has proven helpful include chronic conditions such as heart disease, diabetes, high blood pressure, obesity and even cancer.

The many benefits of Co-Q$_{10}$ are only available to us if we get the right amount of the nutrient needed. It is the feeling of many nutritionists that this level can only be sustained in the body through the use of supplements.

Since Co-Q$_{10}$ is tied into energy production, it would stand to reason that it would be most helpful to the heart. No other organ expends so much energy as our heart, which only rests between its beats. There are at least sixty studies, which support the direct benefits of Co-Q$_{10}$ on such cardiovascular conditions as cardiomyopathy, arrhythmia, coronary artery disease, congestive heart failure, mitral valve prolapse and high blood pressure.

One study showed that when potential heart transplant patients were given sufficient Co-Q$_{10}$, they no longer needed the surgery!

In another study, Co-Q$_{10}$ was given to many thousands of people suffering from congestive heart failure. The results were far more successful than any of the pharmaceutical approaches currently in use. An amazing 75 percent obtained dramatic improvements in pulmonary function, heart palpitations and edema, all with virtually no side effects.

Since we know that almost all drugs only mask the effects of a disease or disorder, often replacing those symptoms with side effects from the drug itself, Co-Q$_{10}$ is an ideal substance for all cardiovascular concerns. It has no side effects and it has consistently proven to be of greater benefit than any pharmaceutical.

It is not uncommon for people with various heart diseases to have at least 25 percent less Co-Q$_{10}$ than their healthy counterparts. According to Robert C Atkins, a holistic cardiologist, when Co-Q$_{10}$ levels fall to 25 percent of normal, the heart will stop beating!

Other areas where this wonderful substance comes to our continued rescue is with diabetes. Co-Q$_{10}$ has been found to help reduce blood sugar while protecting the heart and vascular system from the ravages of the disease.

Studies have shown that Co-Q$_{10}$ can reverse most periodontal disease, the number one cause of tooth loss in people over fifty years of age.

Very recent studies over the last two years have indicated that Co-Q$_{10}$ can help slow the progression of Parkinson's disease. This is a condition wherein the sufferer looses precious dopamine in the brain. Co-Q$_{10}$ was found to greatly slow this loss down.

While this marvelous nutrient can do so much for our well being, absorbing it is not always that easy. Once again, it is a substance that must be taken with some fat. This is another instance where the low fat fanaticism that has swept the country has caused more harm than good. This is especially true with heart disease. We were told to cut all the fat out of our diets and heart disease got worse! One reason is that the super low fat diets prevented the uptake of many of the most powerful heart protecting substances, including Co-Q$_{10}$.

MILK THISTLE. Without a doubt, the most effective of all the herbal detoxifiers has to be Silybum marianum, or milk thistle. This being the case, the organ that would logically, benefit most from such a potential must be the liver. All the toxins in the body end up in the liver to be processed before excretion. It has been said that the liver is the chemical laboratory of the body, carrying on thousands of functions at any given moment. When the liver becomes over burdened with toxic build up, it cannot do its job effectively. Silymarin, the active component in the herb, has an amazing ability to protect the liver from oxidative damage as well as boosting its detoxification abilities.

So powerful is milk thistle that in one study it cut the death rate from cirrhosis by a full 50 percent. Anyone suffering from any form of hepatitis MUST consider milk thistle as part of their treatment and management program.

The liver depends upon one specific substance in order to fulfill much of its duties. That is glutathione. This substance protects the liver from harm while serving as a base for many enzymes needed to protect other cellular structures. One example is the relationship between glutathione and cataracts. As the protein structure of the lens of the eye breaks down, new cells cannot be formed without the presence of an enzyme called glutathione peroxidase. This enzyme is made from glutathione. In fact, glutathione's importance has been recognized by scientists, for over 20 years but the problem has been in raising glutathione levels in the body.

Supplements of glutathione are not well absorbed and much of what is ingested orally, is destroyed or broken down in the digestive system. Glutathione supplements are still quite popular but, sadly, are of little benefit to the body.

Milk Thistle, along with our next magic antioxidant N-Acetyl Cysteine, actually produce glutathione in the liver, raising the levels of this vital substance tremendously.

Milk Thistle must be included in any Full Spectrum antioxidant program for it is one of the few nutrients that can serve both as an antioxidant *and* a free radical scavenger. This makes it of double benefit to us.

Another substance that is manufactured in the body with the help of milk thistle is superoxide dismutase (SOD). This is another popular antioxidant/enzyme substance, because it controls the superoxide free radical. Again, the problem has always been the delivery system. We would include superoxide dismutase because we knew it was good for us, but we also knew that much of what was ingested orally was also broken down by the digestive process.

Even enteric coated products provided little help. Now we have a way to assist the body in making superoxide dismutase in virtually all the quantities necessary and milk thistle is one of the important ingredients in that chemical process.

ALPHA LIPOIC ACID. Because of the many functions of ALA and because it can be either water or fat soluble, we often refer to this powerful free radical inhibitor as 'the universal antioxidant'. Among the many direct benefits of ALA, one of the most important is its ability to protect the body against the ravages of excess insulin as found in all hyperinsulinemia conditions, which include most obesity, carbohydrate intolerance, hypoglycemia and of course, Type II diabetes.

ALA offers protection against the free radicals, mostly from altered vegetable oils, which lead to Atherosclerosis. ALA can help to reduce and regulate cholesterol levels, exercising a lowering effect on cholesterol by as much as 40 percent.

Other important functions of ALA include protecting the body against specific types of cancers and to help detoxify and neutralize the adverse effects of toxic heavy metals, often ingested from chemicals in our environment.

LUTEIN. I have recently added this specialized antioxidant to my list of 'essentials', due to the alarming rise in vision related degenerative conditions. Cataracts, and to a greater extent macular degeneration are epidemic. In fact macular degeneration is the single greatest cause of blindness today. When the macula of the eye deteriorates, sight is gradually lost. In a study published in the Journal of the American Medical Association, we first learned back in 1994 that this deterioration was caused by a lack of antioxidant protection to the macula of the eye, leaving it vulnerable to free radical attack by peroxide radicals. Lutein was shown to almost completely prevent this free radical activity from invading the cells of the macula, thereby controlling and preventing macular degeneration.

See the appendix in the back of this book for a referral to the best eye care products we have ever seen.

N-ACETYL CYSTEINE. The most miraculous substance we have saved for last. Of all the antioxidants, common and rare, this special form of the amino acid Cysteine, is the most powerful, exercising more antioxidant potential than virtually all the other known antioxidants combined! We predict that this nutrient will become one of the biggest buzz words in the field of nutrition over the months and years to come. More and more benefits are being attributed to this amazing substance through clinical studies unfolding almost daily.

If you were to visit almost any hospital emergency room across the country, you would find they stock N-Acetyl Cysteine (NAC) and use it as an antidote for many kinds of poisoning. The most common usage is against acetaminophen poisoning, which occurs regularly due to constant over-consumption. Excess acetaminophen depletes the liver of glutathione to the point of liver failure. Large doses of NAC can so rapidly restore the glutathione levels that it can detoxify an acetaminophen overdose in a matter of a few hours.

NAC has been used medically to break down lung-clogging mucus in cases of chronic bronchitis and other respiratory disorders since the 1960's.

There are several key functions of NAC already identified, with likely, many more to follow as the nutrient is continually studied. Its primary function, along with milk thistle, is to raise the glutathione levels within the liver, protecting it from the many toxins it has to detoxify and render harmless.

It is well known that glutathione levels are much lower in people with cancer, linking a depletion of that nutrient to the immune system's inability to recognize the foreign cells.

Considering NAC's tremendous antioxidant power, it would stand to reason that it would be helpful in every chronic degenerative disease since free radical damage, causing an altered biochemistry, is responsible for virtually all chronic conditions. Recent studies however, show that it is also a powerful weapon against acute infectious attacks such as colds and flu.

In a study conducted at the Institute of Hygiene and Preventive Medicine at the University of Genoa, Italy, Dr. Silvio De Flora administered NAC or a placebo to over 250 subjects.

The conclusion was that while the NAC did not appear to prevent infection from cold or flu pathogens, only 25 percent of the NAC group developed any significant symptoms while 79 percent of the placebo group had severe flu symptoms. This means that NAC can reduce the symptoms from colds and flu by a whopping two-thirds!

There are other viruses that seasonally plague us such as rhinovirus and coxsackie virus. The researchers found that NAC was also very effective in dealing with these bugs as well. It seems that NAC is not virus or bacteria specific like many other immune products on the market. Therefore, NAC can provide a broad-spectrum of protection to ease or even eliminate the annoying symptoms of viral and bacterial related infections. This is especially good news for those in high-risk situations, such as persons with immune compromised disorders and the elderly.

In fact, overall, NAC reduced or prevented virtually all the annoying side effects of Fall and Winter ailments such as headache, achiness, nasal discharge, cough and sore throat. This pattern of improvement was observed over and over again in study after study.

NAC is a real lifesaver for those with breathing problems. In fact, conventional medicine uses NAC in many of its inhalants to ward off asthma attacks. Other related conditions in which NAC can help include adult respiratory distress syndrome, and chronic obstructive pulmonary disease (COPD).

NAC is also a potent heart supplement. Better than any pharmaceutical method, it eliminates the dangers of lipoprotein(a), which is a by product of cholesterol metabolism. The presence of lipoprotein(a) has just recently been recognized as a powerful but independent risk factor for heart disease.

NAC lowers high blood pressure due to the relaxing effect it exercises upon the blood vessels, while increasing blood flow to the extremities of the body. Researchers in Australia have demonstrated that if enough NAC is administered just after a heart attack, much more of the heart muscle remains undamaged.

Those suffering from inflammatory bowel conditions such as irritable bowel syndrome, colitis, diverticulitis etc., should take heed to the benefits of NAC. As the levels of glutathione rise in the body, these conditions seem to diminish accordingly.

In discussing the dangers of the low fat diets so popular the last twenty years or so, another problem connected with them is that they produce a deficiency of sulfur. One of the consequences of a sulfur deficiency, especially for women, is hair loss. NAC just happens to be one of the best sulfur-containing substances known.

All things considered, NAC is the most vital antioxidant for the new millennium. We will continue to poison our environment, consume diets consisting of dead lifeless foods, subject ourselves to ever-increasing radiation from electronic devices, high frequency signals, and even the sun itself, through the breakdown of the ozone layer. This being the case, NAC is the only single antioxidant that addresses every major chronic disease in our society! It may further be said that N-Acetyl Cysteine is the universal antioxidant for it activates and increases the potential of all the other antioxidants.

These powerful ingredients, any one of which could change the course of human cell life, together are an unstoppable combination, providing an unparalleled dual level of protection to all living systems.

Like other, more familiar nutrients such as vitamins, minerals and amino acids, antioxidants and free radicals are best taken in combination with each other. The total value is much greater than the mere sum of the parts involved.

According to Dr Michael Murray, "extensive research shows that a combination of antioxidants provides greater protection than does taking a high dose of any single antioxidant. Mixtures of antioxidant nutrients appear to work together harmoniously to produce the phenomenon known as synergy, where the whole is greater than the sum of the parts. In other words, when it comes to the benefits of antioxidants, one plus one equals three."

We live in a time where ignoring the problems of the food, water, and the environment around us can be very dangerous indeed. By burying our head in the preverbal sand, we only expose our backside to greater and greater threats from free radical proliferation!

For all of these reasons, we feel that these powerful antioxidants should be an integral part of every Full Spectrum formula. All of the Full Spectrum formulas developed here at The Institute contain a broad spectrum of antioxidants as part of the baseline formulation.

Designing A Custom Supplement Program For You

Well, as you can see, there are quite a lot of important nutrients playing a role in our health and well-being. At first, it may seem a bit overwhelming, but as we discussed at the outset of this chapter, through our concept of Full Spectrum Supplementation, getting all of the essential nutrients in the right potency, ratio, pH and bio-availability, has never been easier.

If you are reasonably healthy and would like to ensure that you stay that way, all you really need do is to include a Full Spectrum nutritional product once or twice per day, in your routine. Nothing could be easier! By using a Full Spectrum formula that contains all these factors, you take the guesswork out of supplementing. If you should have difficulty finding a Full Spectrum formula or are unsure as to which formula may be best for you, you may contact our research center, tell us a bit about yourself and we will happily refer you to a company that offers the best Full Spectrum product for you. The best way to contact our offices is via email at AskTheDoc@HealthyInformation.com

Further contact information for The Institute of Nutritional Science may be found in the appendix at the end of this book, together with a coupon for a substantial discount on our complete Nutrient Evaluation Program, which will enable us to design a customized program of diet and supplements just for you.

Now, if you are one of those people who are at risk for or who already have one or more chronic health conditions, you can prevent, manage or even often reverse these problems with a concept we call Targeted Nutrition. Through combining specific nutrients, in higher potencies, we can customize a supplement program that not only meets the Full Spectrum, baseline needs of everyone, but, addresses any specific health challenges you may be facing.

If you or someone you care about falls into this category and suffers from such chronic conditions as arthritis, diabetes, heart disease, prostate problems, elevated cholesterol, or other age related problems, part two of this book has been written for you!

The protocols in the next section have helped millions of people to prevent, manage or even reverse these chronic conditions, thereby increasing both the quality and quantity of their lives. They can work for you too.

INTRODCUTION

The Medical
System Worldwide

CHAPTER 4: WHILE THIS BOOK IS PRIMARILY DESIGNED TO PUT forth our easy to follow plan for achieving health and longevity through the use of methods other than conventional allopathic medicine, I must recognize that there are millions of people who already suffer from one of more of the chronic diseases our program is designed to prevent. For those, it will require additional work and more aggressive programs to rebalance the biochemistry of the human body. This is the purpose of part two of this book. Before we begin however, it is important to understand the state of our medical system and why it has failed to address the needs of those suffering from the common chronic disorders.

Hypocrites (460-377 BC), known as the Father of Medicine, defined health as the balance between the various components of a person's nature, environment, and ways of life. The Hippocratic Oath requires that the physician remember, under all circumstances, that he or she should "Of first, do no harm". Hypocrites stated "It is more important to know what sort of person has a disease than to know what sort of disease a person has". Today, we are relearning the connection between the mind and the body, and that one cannot always expect to cut, burn, and poison sick people well.

The emphasis upon understanding the patient vanished somewhere in the 1960's. As conventional medicine grew larger, it became cold and impersonal. No longer was the family physician available for house calls. Through large insurance muscle, Doctors lost their flexibility and were forced to pool resources, forming medical groups consisting of many physicians. This meant that not only did the Doctor no longer make house calls; you may not even see the same Doctor when you come back to the same office.

We boast the greatest diagnostic system in the history of medicine. Increasingly sophisticated devices, designed to diagnose disease, potential disease, and even possible disease, remove the physician farther and farther from his patients. There are more than 11 billion of these sophisticated medical tests being performed every year in the United States alone.

Not only are these medial tests out of control but the treatments have become high tech, costly and inhumane as well. The cost of maintaining the deteriorating human body has become almost unattainable.

Medical costs in the United States alone account for over 11 percent of the nation's gross national product. At approximately one trillion dollars, it equates to over $3,000 for every U.S. citizen. Other so-called 'civilized nations' are not far behind us. In the United Kingdom every citizen is spending over $450.00 annually on healthcare. In Japan it's $500.00, in France, $800.00, and in Germany nearly $1000.00! How did we get into this mess?

After the successful advent of the antibiotic in the 1940's, conventional medical practitioners rose to a God-like status, at least in their own minds. Pharmaceutical companies, riding on the success of specific key drugs, grew into one of the most financially powerful conglomerates in the world.

Today, we have a situation in which the drug companies are so powerful that they actually dictate policy in medicine through their large financial contributions to such political organizations as the American Medical Association.

They fund many medical journals through their high priced advertising. It is estimated that the pharmaceutical industry spends in excess of three billion dollars every year in order to solicit their drugs to physicians.

In a past issue of Fortune Magazine, is was uncovered that while the pharmaceutical industry claims to spend 15 percent of its sales on research and development, they spent over twice that much on advertisements appearing in medical journals, alone!

Much of the rest of their staggering advertising budget is spent on the army of drug salespeople who personally visit physicians with literature, gifts, and incentives.

A Harvard University study has shown that physicians will routinely pick up erroneous information from these 'salespeople', which is in direct contradiction to the actual clinical studies involving the drugs that they are selling.

According to Milton Silverman of the University of California at San Francisco, "In medical school, we teach students to prescribe on the basis of scientific evidence....

Five years after medical school, they are not prescribing as they were taught. They are brainwashed by detail men."

These drugs are so prolifically prescribed, that it is now believed that during any given 24 hour period, as many as 50 to 80 percent of all adults in the United States swallow a medically prescribed drug.

According to the Bureau of Statistics and published in U.S. News and World Report back in January of 1995, "Up to 2 million people are hospitalized each year as a result of significant side effects from prescription medications."

The side effects must have indeed been significant if it drove the patient to the hospital. Worse, much worse, according to the same reliable source, as many as 140,000 of those people die as a result of the side effects or reactions related to consuming those various prescription drugs!

If you factor the figure of 140,000 deaths into all the other causes of death such as heart disease, cancer etc., at 140,000 deaths, it makes prescription drugs the fifth leading cause of death worldwide!

If this atrocity were to occur in virtually any other area of professionalism, the public would have long ago demanded review and revision. So how can this occur, year after year, and no one says a word?

The answer, although complicated, goes back to the fact that allopathic medicine holds or at least has held the monopoly over health care worldwide for many decades. This has allowed them, and their counterparts such as the pharmaceutical industry, to amass such financial power that to question them seems almost impossible.

Fortunately this monopoly is breaking down. During the last 20 years, conventional medicine has lost much of the public confidence it once held due to repeated failures in properly addressing both the prevention and treatment of leading causes of disease and premature death.

The medical industry's last shining hour was the development of the antibiotic prior to 1950. Since that time very little in the way of disease eradication has been developed. Today, while infectious diseases have been reduced substantially, they have been replaced by a group of diseases called chronic degenerative diseases, which are proving to respond poorly to the standard medical model. In fact, it is estimated that at least 70 percent of all medical costs are generated by the mismanagement of these chronic conditions.

Heart disease is still the number one cause of death in spite of such invasive and expensive procedures as angioplasty and the bypass operation. Cancer, the most feared disease of the Twentieth Century, not only remains at number two, but will likely overtake heart disease as the leading cause of death within the next decade.

Other diseases such as diabetes, which has emerged from relative obscurity 100 years ago, now sits at number three. Arthritis, while not directly responsible for high numbers of fatalities, robs more people of the quality of their retirement years than at any other time in human history. Chronic prostate inflammation and complications from menopause continue to add to the burdens of aging.

As we proceed further into the new century, more and more people worldwide will cross over the 50 year old mark. In fact, in another 5 years, we will have more people alive over the age of 50 than at any time in recorded history. This vast population is the very target for chronic degenerative disease and not only has medicine failed in its management of these conditions, they have failed to properly educate the public in proven ways to prevent the occurrence of these diseases in the first place.

This dilemma has been caused by a failure to modify the standard medical model of diagnosis and treatment, as well as a realization that these very chronic conditions are what continue to support the entire medical industry.

If heart disease, cancer, arthritis and diabetes were to be suddenly eradicated from our lives, the medical industry would collapse into bankruptcy overnight. There is little hope of this occurring as long as conventional medicine continues to treat chronic diseases with the old "Standard Medical Model".

The Standard Medical Model

Whenever you, or anyone else for that matter, visit a medical doctor, you will be treated according to the 'standard medical model.' This is the way doctors have all been trained to view their patients. What is this standard medical model? It is a system of patient management that developed primarily out of the success with antibiotics.

When you apply it to infectious diseases or an emergency situation, the medical model can be a lifesaver. However, when this same line of thinking is applied to chronic degenerative disease, the results are dismal at best and a total failure most of the time.

Let's take a closer look at what has gone wrong.

The standard medical model is as follows…

1. Diagnose Disease
2. Prescribe Drugs
3. Perform Surgery

When we apply this concept to an emergency procedure for example, it works well. Let's say that you have just been hit by a car, and your leg is broken in several places. You will be very glad indeed, that there is an emergency room nearby where trained doctors can diagnose the extent of your damage, perform surgery, set bones, apply casts, and prescribe medications to prevent infection, inflammation, and pain. All will likely be well and a full recovery would be expected.

Now, what happens in the case of a chronic disease?

Let's take arthritis, for example, and apply the medical model to the management of this disease. First of all the doctor will perform an examination and perhaps run some tests. After which a diagnosis of arthritis is handed down. Next the doctor will prescribe drugs such as pain-killers and anti-inflammatory agents.

Since none of these chemicals actually addresses the *cause* of arthritis, the disease will continue to progress with time. This will necessitate the use of stronger and stronger drugs. At some point in time, the physician will make the determination that the side effects of the drug therapy are worse than the apparent benefit and will suggest that they move to stage three of the medical model and perform some surgery. In the case of arthritis, it might likely be joint replacement.

It should be seen by this example that none of the treatments or procedures outlined above did anything for the actual arthritis. Even the replacement of the joint with a plastic counterpart does not signify the end, since over time, other joints will be affected and the process and the discomfort will continue.

If you apply the standard medical model to any chronic disease condition, you will end up at the same point of no results. This is why chronic disease is the leading cause of suffering and death in our society. Until medicine is willing to look at the cause of these diseases, they will continue to rob more and more people of both the quality and quantity of their lives ahead.

As more and more of us pass the age 50 mark, we become increasingly more vulnerable to chronic disease. Since these diseases are a result of the biochemical breakdown of the living human chemistry, our chances of developing one or more of these conditions increases dramatically after the age of 45 or 50 and continues to increase with every year thereafter.

The majority of the casualties of the medical system are due to side effects of drugs, chronic disease not addressed, surgical procedures improperly performed, and the excessive use of testing procedures. These casualties occur most often in the elderly.

It is not uncommon for many older people to be taking 15 or more prescription drugs at any given time. The side effects of drug therapy increase exponentially with the number of drugs taken.

Among the older population, the use of non-steroidal anti-inflammatory drugs (NSAIDs) for arthritis, common aches and pains, and other conditions can be linked to many complications. Serious digestive problems can lead the list according to a study conducted at Emory University. The over the counter pain killers were found to cause gastro esophageal reflux disease, resulting in chronic acid injury and imbalance. The clinical study found that 35% of patients over 65 years of age showed significant damage as a result of regular use of NSAIDs.

You might think that this would discourage the practice of routinely prescribing these drugs to older people. To the contrary, a report published in the Annuals of Internal Medicine showed that doctors are not only prescribing these drugs more than in the past but that they are frequently prescribing them unnecessarily. Another study, conducted in Canada, revealed that NSAIDs were being prescribed unnecessarily as often as 41 percent of the time!

Older members of the population continue to suffer the most at the hands of medicine "gone awry". According to a study conducted in Jerusalem and presented to the American Geriatrics Society in Atlanta, Georgia in May of 1997, elderly people may not benefit from the flu shot. Yet, in spite of this study, and other credible evidence substantiating its findings, older people remain the primary recipients of the flu shot.

The study's coordinator, Haim Dannenberg of the Hadassah University Hospital revealed that the subjects who had been given repeated flu shots had *lower* antibody levels than those who had not been vaccinated! This phenomena seems to increase with age, the older participants fairing less well.

In spite of the overwhelming evidence for misuse of drug therapy on older people, pharmaceutical companies continue to target the older population in the bulk of their advertising and promotion. According to Harvard University, at least 40 percent of all older people are routinely given prescriptions for drugs they have no business taking.

Is It the Doctor's Fault?

With all of these overwhelming concerns regarding the conventional medical system, is it any wonder that millions and millions of people the world over are not only looking elsewhere for health care, but are routinely following programs other than allopathic medicine.

With this mass exodus from conventional thinking we must ask ourselves, "Is it the fault of the Doctors?"

I attended university classes with men and women whose goal was to become a physician. For the most part these were all very dedicated and sincere individuals. In fact, in my over 30 years in the health and nutrition industry, I cannot remember meeting a single medical doctor who said, "I can hardly wait to get my license so that I can go out and kill people!" Everyone starts out with the most noble of intents, with the common goal of hoping to relieve some small part of human suffering. What goes wrong?

The physician is no longer in charge of his or her own practice. They are heavily influenced by drug companies, threatened by organizations such as the AMA who are supposed to be protecting them, and overworked by an unmanageable patient workload. Is it any wonder that not one physician in 100 reads their medical journals. They simply don't have time.

In the meantime, we have to begin to learn to take responsibility for our own health care. We all need to learn how to determine when it's time to see a physician. More importantly, we must also learn how to determine whether it is in our best interests to listen to his advice exclusively, or to also seek information about some of the less invasive options available elsewhere.

Part two of this book is all about those options. As we have already established, chronic, non-infectious diseases are the main cause of ill health as we age; they also are the poorest managed forms of health problems.

It is estimated that anyone born from today forward will have a better than 90 percent chance of living to age 100 and past, but at what price? Today, the average life span is in the mid seventies, yet for many millions of people, the last 20 or 30 years of that life span is without any appreciable quality attached to it.

Instead of our retirement years being filled with the joy and activities that free time can provide, we are all congregating at doctors' offices, therapy centers, pharmacies to get the latest wonder drug, experiencing the side effects of those wonder drugs, and undergoing surgical procedures.

Quantity of life must be intrinsically linked to quality or the results are of little value. I could not agree more with the future thinkers that ages of over 100 years are well within our grasp, but the quality factor must also be equally addressed.

The quality of life a person may expect in the 'golden years' may be directly traced back to how they lived their life in the past as well as the genetics they were born with. While we can do little to change our genetic characteristics, we surely can positively affect the quality of our future years.

The human body is the most complicated chemical laboratory ever created. In all our great scientific achievement, we have barely begun to delve into its complexity. Yet, that vast chemical universe within us is almost totally self-sufficient. If we give it some quality food, pure water, and about 120 or so nutrients, it can and will take care of us very nicely.

Chronic disease is the result of a human biochemistry long out of balance. Treating the effects or symptoms of these conditions will do little to enhance the quality or quantity of anyone's life. Only when we come to the understanding of what this body of ours needs and then how to provide for those needs, will we be in a position to positively affect both quality and quantity of life ahead. The guideposts to that journey lie just ahead.

Preventing & Reversing The Disease Process

In part one, we established and explained the basics of following a good health-maintaining program. Statistics and studies prove that the guidelines provided can definitely increase your chances of preventing many chronic conditions from developing, giving you a greater quality and quantity of life ahead. What about those of you who are at higher risk for or who have already developed one or more of these chronic health challenges? Amazingly, diet, exercise, and the right supplements, called Targeted Nutrients, can prevent the development of these conditions and even reverse them many cases.

This section of the book offers guidelines for specific, targeted support when certain conditions are present. In the rest of this chapter, we highlight many of the leading chronic health conditions that affect the majority of us at any given time. I have expanded the discussion of these conditions so that you may have a better understanding of the problem, the cause and the natural way to manage or even reverse these problems.

Chapter five, which follows, is a virtual encyclopedia of health issues, from acne to vitiligo. By looking up your specific concern, you can quickly find out how diet and exercise play a role in these problems, if any, and a list of the specific nutrients involved in the prevention, management and reversal of each condition. Frequently, we can recommend specific supplement formulas, which provide the right balance of key, targeted nutrients, designed to aggressively address these problems. These are called Targeted Nutrition Supplements and if you should have problems finding these, you can contact our Research Center for help. You can email us at askthedoc@healthyinformation.com or call at 1-888-454-8464.

Before we begin our discussion of the management of these conditions, it is important that you understand one basic, but essential concept: **Only The Body Can Heal**.

No matter what ailment or health concern you may have, no matter how you choose to address your problem, after all the medications, treatments, surgeries and the like, it is still up to your body to heal itself.

Only The Body Can Heal, but it can do so only when the proper nutrients, or raw materials needed for optimal health, are present and available to the chemistry of the body on a regular and consistent basis.

When we discuss chronic health conditions, as opposed to acute bacterial and viral diseases, it is important to understand that these conditions have developed as a result of years or even decades of abuse.

When we are finally in need of medical attention for a chronic disease, it is the outcome of decades of dietary abuse, lack of exercise and nutrient deficiencies.

Medications, while often at least temporarily necessary, frequently mask symptoms but leave the cause of the problem to continue its destructive course of action inside the body. While medications are often of short-term benefit, no human body in history has ever had a deficiency of the drugs.

When finally addressing the road to better health, we need to be aware of what took us away from that path and how long we have been walking in the opposite direction. If you have developed one or more chronic conditions such as arthritis, diabetes, heart disease, prostate problems, complications of menopause or age-related complications, it is important to understand that some measure of self- discipline will be necessary to gain control over these problems.

Poor habits & our subsequent choices and abuses of life have brought us to the proverbial fork in the road. Which way we travel from here on out, depends on the right knowledge and information to guide us. The next two chapters will provide you with guidelines for managing and even reversing many of the most common health concerns of aging, but you must follow these programs in order to reap benefit from them. Thus, part two of this book will assist you in focusing on the task at hand – that being the rebuilding of a life… your life.

Focus On The Leading Chronic Conditions

Heart Disease

Heart disease and stroke take more people from their life prematurely than any other cause. These killers strike a new victim every two seconds!

During the last 20 years or so, we have followed the low fat diet. In fact, almost everything labeled 'healthy' is also low fat or non-fat. Yet, despite this fanaticism, heart disease has not diminished. To make matters worse, one of the leading factors in heart disease, obesity, has risen in greater numbers than at any other time in history!

While awareness as to the importance of such factors as diet, stress management and exercise have helped people deal with this killer, these factors have never been fully understood.

Other than by-pass surgery, are there solutions to heart disease? Yes! As with most chronic disease conditions, its cause is an altered biochemistry. When the biochemistry is corrected, the disease process is interrupted and the body is in the best possible position to help itself.

The dietary recommendations of The American Heart Association have failed miserably in curbing the epidemic of heart disease. Watch your cholesterol…Reduce the intake of animal fats….Eat margarine… Eat less protein and eat more starch. Still, heart disease is the number one killer.

It might surprise you to know that cholesterol, that evil, terrible substance, or so we are told, that supposedly gets into your arteries and kills you, has NEVER caused one case of heart disease.

Even more surprising, there has never been one clinical study to show that cholesterol has ever been at fault. Yet we are still being brainwashed about this natural, essential, fatty substance.

In order to gain control of this runaway horse called Heart Disease, we must look towards its cause. You may be both surprised and disgusted to find out that the real cause of heart disease was first identified in 1974. Yet despite this discovery, over 30 years ago, nothing has changed in the conventional medical programs ostensibly designed to prevent or manage this condition.

It's time we examined the real causes of Heart Disease and how you can intervene, at almost any stage, and begin reversing the process, which got you to that point in the first place. As with all chronic disease, Heart Disease is best prevented rather than treated.

What is The Real Cause of the Epidemic?

If cholesterol is the cause of heart disease as we have been told, the last 15 years of the low fat, low cholesterol diets should have made a marked improvement in the statistics. It has not. Diet does play a significant role in the formation of atherosclerotic plaque, but not in the way we have been taught.

What then IS the real cause of this dreaded disease?

Present research shows that deposits form on artery walls. Eventually, these arteries are occluded completely as a result of a proliferation of these cells.

This research, first conducted between 1970 and 1974 by *Dr. Earl P. Benditt* and his associates at the *University of Washington School of Medicine*, clearly shows that the cells in the artery wall proliferate because of a mutation in their DNA. This altering of the structure of DNA is caused by a variety of factors such as cigarette smoke chemicals, low-level radiation, epoxides of fatty substances, chlorine, and most importantly, free radicals from certain foods.

These data were confirmed again in 1975 through studies conducted by Dr. *Robert Heptinstall* of the *Johns Hopkins School of Medicine.*

It is this mutation of cells, which causes them to explosively multiply, eventually creating a lesion that ruptures into the inner wall of the artery.

There are many natural substances, most of them nutrients, which can help to reduce this cellular damage by protecting the artery cell DNA from oxidative and radioactive damage.

It is important to understand that no one single factor can lead to heart disease or a heart attack. But when two or more of these factors are present at the same time, disaster is a distinct possibility.

For example, autopsies performed on mummies from both Egypt and China show that many of these people had plaque build-up in their arteries, however, none of them showed signs of ever having a heart attack.

The 20th century lifestyle was characterized by lack of exercise, improper diet, poor food quality, excess stress, and environmental poisons from chemicals and radiation. These factors created an atmosphere conducive to an epidemic of Coronary Thrombosis.

To put this further into perspective, we quote from an article, which appeared in *Family Circle Magazine* in 1971. *Dr. Paul Dudley White*, an early cardiologist, stated, "First of all, I want to emphasize that heart disease truly is an epidemic today, a fact that many people seem to refuse to accept...Your generation has become so used to the specter of heart attacks, you don't even conceive of life free from this danger. But remember, when I was an intern at Massachusetts General Hospital in 1911, there was no Department of Cardiology."

When Dr. White first set up his cardiology laboratory in 1920, Coronary Thrombosis was still so uncommon, that most medical students did not know of the disease.

What About Cholesterol?

Today, professionals in the medical industry, and especially the American Heart Association, cling to the concept that cholesterol causes heart disease. Their philosophy continues to dictate that, in order to reduce heart disease, less cholesterol must be consumed.

The problem with this theory is that firstly, it does not stand up to evidence uncovered over the last twenty-five years, and secondly no clinical study has ever proven that cholesterol causes heart disease!

In fact there are numerous studies, some of them very famous, which prove just the opposite, namely that Dietary Cholesterol has nothing to do with this disease process. Even the famous *Framingham Study* proved that the cholesterol concept is a myth.

It is now known that arterial deposits are not caused by cholesterol. By the time cholesterol begins sticking to your artery walls, 90 percent of the damage has already been done. It is now well established that how much cholesterol you eat or don't eat only minimally affects cholesterol levels in the blood.

Cholesterol is a natural substance; it is formed in the body and performs a variety of life-sustaining functions. Cholesterol is responsible for liver function, nerve insulation, brain function (your brain has the greatest concentration of cholesterol in the body), and many other vital tasks.

In a healthy body, the less cholesterol that comes from diet the more the body makes and vice versa. If you have elevated cholesterol, especially if accompanied by an improper ratio of High-Density Lipoprotein (HDL) to Low-Density Lipoprotein (LDL), it is due to a liver problem.

If your cholesterol is high, or the ratios out of line, you need to support your liver. Please see the section on cholesterol for a complete program to healthily control your cholesterol levels.

The concept that dietary fat intake does not raise cholesterol levels nor does it cause heart disease is further evidenced by studies of many populations, which have little or no heart disease in spite of the fact that they follow a diet very high in saturated fats and cholesterol.

Some of these groups and studies include:

The Maasai of Tanzania

The Samburu and Punjabis of Northern Kenya

Swiss of the Loetschental Valley

Benedictine Monks

The Northern Indians

Primitive Eskimos

The Atiu and Mitiaro natives of Polynesia

Jews living in Yemen

Sweden (where heart disease is less than one-third that of the United States and their fat consumption is almost three times as high!)

Almost all of the cultures and tribes previously listed are sustained by diets high in fat, high in protein and naturally low in carbohydrates.

Fat only becomes a significant factor in the presence of sugar or highly refined carbohydrates. Even then, fat does not cause heart disease, but it can cause you to become overweight when consumed with high amounts of sugar. Obesity is a genuine factor in the development of heart disease and therefore a diet high in both fat and sugar is very unhealthy.

Low Cholesterol Diets Fail to Reduce Heart Disease

In their desperate attempt to blame cholesterol for the cause of Heart Disease, the medical industry has been on a fanatic cholesterol-fighting war for decades. To this day, Heart Disease has not been lowered through any of these efforts. Why do we stick to a concept that we know is scientifically unsound?

Their popularity grew rapidly out of the 'cholesterol scare' and is, to this day, being maintained in order to keep the sales of vegetable oils high. Yet, as we will soon see, vegetable oils actually contribute more to the pathology of Coronary Thrombosis than any other single dietary factor. Despite these findings, vegetable oils are being promoted by the American Heart Association and they advise us to use them 'for our good health'.

If everything you have been told about fats is wrong, what should you eat? How about taking a lesson from our grandparents and great grandparents? What did they eat?

Remember, before the 1900's, Heart Disease was virtually unknown, yet their diet was higher in fat than ours. They ate lard, butter, and other natural fats. Vegetable oils were not available commercially and margarine had not yet been invented.

What about eggs? The long-suffering egg has been the staple of human diets around the world for thousands of years. The late *Adelle Davis,* pioneer nutritionist, often said that the egg was the most perfect food for man. Since cholesterol doesn't cause heart disease, neither does the cholesterol in eggs. Additionally, eggs contain a substance called lecithin, which naturally metabolizes the fats in eggs including the cholesterol.

If Cholesterol is O.K., What's the Problem?

Since science has proven that cholesterol doesn't cause Heart Disease, what does? Remember the studies conducted in the 1970's at leading medical centers that we mentioned earlier? Let's take a closer look at what they found out:

* Atherosclerosis occurs only in arteries - never in veins
* Atherosclerosis occurs primarily near the junction of two arterial branches and only select arteries are usually involved.
* Cholesterol is the last substance to stick to the artery wall. By the time cholesterol arrives, 90 percent of the damage leading to the disease process has already occurred.

Let's analyze these findings in order to illustrate the real cause, and subsequently, the method for reversing this problem.

The idea that cholesterol doesn't cause Heart Disease is further supported by the fact that even though the same amount of cholesterol circulates in both the veins and arteries, **atherosclerosis never occurs in the veins but only in the arteries.** The reason this happens is the answer to the cause of the condition.

When we look at a 'cross section' of a vein, we find that it contains two layers, an inner and outer layer. An inspection of an artery, however, shows us that it has three layers, the inner and outer layer as with veins, but also a middle layer of muscle tissue.

This muscle layer is responsible for ensuring that blood leaving the heart reaches the furthest extremities while maintaining proper blood pressure. Also, under stress, this muscle wall constricts, increasing the pressure of blood and oxygen flowing to all parts of the body. But it is this same muscle wall that allows atherosclerotic plaque to begin to build.

Of all the various types of tissues found in the human body, one of the most susceptible to what we call free radical DNA damage is the muscle cell.

The Deoxyribonucleic Acid (DNA) of every cell in your body carries your genetic code. When the molecular structure of DNA cells is attacked by chemical 'free radicals', they can change, mutate, and multiply out of control.

There are numerous free radicals formed in the body under various conditions, but the specific free radical action that appears to attack arterial muscle tissue comes primarily from the oxidation of polyunsaturated vegetable oils.

Once the free radical is circulating in the blood stream, it attaches itself to the inside of the artery wall and begins to literally drill a hole into the inner layer of the artery.

Once it reaches the middle muscle layer, it attaches itself and begins to alter the structure of the cell.

As this plaque building process continues, the calcium attracts additional material from the bloodstream, including cholesterol, triglycerides, and carotene, all naturally present in healthy people.

It is important to understand that even if the cholesterol levels in the blood stream are normal or low, it will still be attracted to the calcium now lining the arteries in strategic places. This is why we say that cholesterol does not cause this disease and lowering cholesterol will not prevent or stop it!

As early as 1974, the real dangers of polyunsaturated oils (corn, safflower, peanut, sesame, and others) began to be realized.

Studies at that time involved animals and the feeding of various groups of swine. Swine were used because their cardiovascular system is similar to that of humans.

The results of the studies were shocking. Researchers found that, overwhelmingly, the pigs fed a diet of margarine and other hydrogenated fats had the greatest degree of hardening of the arteries. The next greatest group was the one fed a high sugar diet. Conversely, the group fed butter as the main fat had almost no arterial damage at all and the group fed a diet high in eggs had virtually clear arteries altogether!

The tests further showed that it was not just polyunsaturated oils and hydrogenated fats, like margarine, that were to blame, but egg substitutes as well. These products became very popular for a time during the height of the "cholesterol scare". Fortunately, their popularity is declining. Studies done on various animals fed egg substitutes showed severe upset in their blood lipid profiles and these animals all died very prematurely.

Further evidence against the use of polyunsaturated oils comes from studies done on aging and wrinkling of the facial skin. The group of test subjects who consumed high amounts of polyunsaturated oils showed marked clinical signs of premature aging, while looking physically older as well.

Yet another study involved patients who adhered to the American Heart Association's published diet, which suggests a 15 percent intake of polyunsaturated oils. The results showed that they developed a significant increase in uric acid in the blood. Elevated uric acid levels are a risk factor in heart disease and indicate the destruction of cellular nucleoprotein.

The Sugar Connection

While attention has been fixated upon the cholesterol myth regarding heart disease pathology, we have totally overlooked an increasing dietary factor, which contributes to more heart disease than cholesterol ever will.

The over consumption of sugar and sugar-forming foods in the diet may be linked to virtually every chronic degenerative disease process. Outside of the obvious connection between sugar consumption and such diseases and conditions as hypoglycemia, diabetes and obesity, sugar has been linked to arthritis, osteoporosis, and most definitely, to Heart Disease.

Triglycerides, the largest fat molecules in the blood stream, are formed exclusively from excessive carbohydrates. While these fats are normally stored in the fat cells of our bodies, they can circulate in the blood stream and reach dangerously high levels.

Work, done by *John Yudkin* and others have clearly linked the consumption of sugar with an increase in Ischemic Heart Disease as far back as 1957, yet our focus remains on cholesterol. According to the findings of Yudkin, excess sugar consumption is just as great a risk factor in the progress of coronary heart disease as is the practice of cigarette smoking.

There are eight major risk factors, which directly lead to atherosclerosis:

HEREDITY - If heart disease runs in your family you have a much greater chance of developing this condition yourself.

CALORIE IMBALANCE - Consuming the wrong type of fats and oils as well as the over consumption of sugar and sugar forming foods.

HIGH BLOOD PRESSURE - This condition damages the arteries and inner workings of the heart muscle, making them more susceptible to free radical damage and increased site cholesterol formation.

SMOKING - Cigarette smoking and the chemicals put into most cigarettes make the tars a prime source of free radical formation. Nicotine is not the problem in spite of what we have been told.

ANTIOXIDANT DEFICIENCY - These nutrients protect the cells of the body from free radical damage as well as preventing the formation of the oxidative free radical in the first place.

VITAMIN E DEFICIENCY - In the absence of adequate vitamin E, plaque formation within the arteries leads to Coronary Thrombosis.

LACK OF EXERCISE - A sedentary lifestyle further deteriorates an already damaged cardiovascular system.

STRESS - I have often said that stress is the cardinal or major cause of all disease and disorder within the body. We find it as a factor in almost every condition, and here it is again!

Stress can wreak havoc with the cardiovascular system through over stimulation of the adrenal glands. This leads to excess adrenaline in the bloodstream, which constricts arteries and accelerates free radical proliferation.

By incorporating simple routines into our lives, many of these risk factors may be eliminated or greatly reduced. Of greatest benefit is taking supplements containing the Full Spectrum of nutrients.

What About Cholesterol-Lowering Drugs?

Drugs that have been designed to lower blood levels of specific lipids such as cholesterol and triglycerides do not have any effect on preventing heart disease, nor have they ever demonstrated a benefit in preventing a recurrent heart attack.

This is confirmed by the United States Department of Health, Education and Welfare through a report from the National Heart, Lung, and Blood Institute's Coronary Drug Project.

Further, drugs most commonly used to block the absorption of cholesterol from foods can be very dangerous since they would prevent the absorption of fat-soluble vitamins, essential fatty acids and other fat-like nutrients. Also present is a serious risk of damage to the liver.

It is important to remember that the body needs fats for proper metabolism and life function. The fanatic elimination of fats from the diet, combined with drugs that further prevent fat absorption, will lead to a variety of health conditions as time progresses.

Heart Disease Prevention & Management Program

Probably one of the most important nutrients in the *prevention* of Heart Disease, from its many causes, is vitamin E.

For over 50 years, Drs. Wilfrid and Evan Shute have been achieving great results in the prevention of cardiac disease and the treatment of cardiac patients. Their program revolves around the use of vitamin E. After over 50,000 or more patients, they believe that vitamin E is essential in any cardiac program.

Vitamin E provides multi-functional benefits. Tocopherols, the active compounds found in vitamin E, provide several important benefits to the cardiovascular system.

TOCOPHEROL, an anti-clotting agent, prevents blood clots throughout the entire cardiovascular tree. It helps dissolve existing blood clots and increases the blood's supply of oxygen.

Tocopherol improves the efficiency of the heart, thereby reducing the demand for available oxygen. It also prevents scarring of the heart muscle after a heart attack and it accelerates the healing process. In addition, Tocopherol is a vasodilator and strengthens capillary permeability.

Vitamin E has also been shown to be beneficial in the treatment of angina. In a clinical study reported in the *New England Journal of Medicine*, patients given 400 IU of Tocopherol, four times per day, were able to reduce their need for nitroglycerin significantly.

Other Anti-Oxidant Nutrients

Since the prevention of free radical formation by oxidation is essential to our goal, the anti-oxidant nutrients must be a part of our program.

In addition to Vitamin E, other nutrients can also offer this much-needed protection.

VITAMIN C, an antioxidant, provides protection against free radical substances by keeping them in solution, thereby allowing the kidneys to better eliminate poisons. Vitamin C stimulates the production of the enzyme lipoprotein lipase (LPL), which acts as a cleansing agent against the artery wall. Lastly, vitamin C is essential in our over-all program, as it is a co-factor with several other ingredients in the protocol.

THE B-COMPLEX NUTRIENTS, Vitamins B1, B2, Niacin, Pantothenic Acid, B6, and PABA, are collectively synergistic and provide antioxidant benefits in their own right. They all work hard to prevent the formation of free radicals within the body.

The mineral Selenium is one of the most powerful antioxidants known. It is estimated that it provides from 200 to 500 times more antioxidant benefits than even vitamin E. both vitamin E and Selenium prevents free radical damage to tissues.

The Amazing Amino Acids

Recent research into the science of applying isolated amino acids to specific disease conditions continues to prove both beneficial and rewarding. Heart Disease and the processes by which it develops are no different.

One of the most well known amino acids relating to the cardiovascular system is L-Carnitine. This amino acid helps the body to utilize fats at virtually every level. L-Carnitine has been used, clinically, in both the prevention and treatment of Heart Disease and in other cardiac related conditions. L-Carnitine is essential in the management of congestive heart failure because it strengthens the stroke or beat of the heart and it naturally lowers or regulates blood fats as well. One note of caution: Carnitine can be purchased in two forms L and dl. DO NOT USE THE dl FORM!

Because the dl form of Carnitine is less than one/tenth the cost, most companies elect to use this form. The bottom line is that only the L form has any effect upon your heart.

Another amino acid, much less known than L-Carnitine, is called Cysteine Hydrochloride. This wonderful amino acid protects against damages caused by radiation of all types by actually terminating the free radicals through ionizing the radiation. Further, Cysteine Hydrochloride is a powerful chelating agent, attaching itself to a variety of minerals and carrying them out of the body via the urine.

Other Essential Co-Factor Nutrients

In addition to the amino acids and antioxidants, there are several other nutrients and nutrient co-factors which have been shown to be of benefit in both the prevention and treatment of heart disease.

Vitamin A must be both considered and included in any program for heart disease and cardiovascular health. This vitamin protects the mucosal linings, your body's first line of defense against invading microbes. It also increases the size of the Thymus Gland, the center of your immune system, allowing for greater antibody production. Lastly, vitamin A works with Selenium, and together they are much more powerful than either one alone.

Choline and Inositol are two B-Complex factors and together with another amino acid, methionine, they form a group of nutrients call Lipotropics. Lipotropics are responsible for metabolizing fats in the liver. If you have elevated cholesterol to an excess, it is a liver problem not necessarily a dietary imbalance. The Lipotropic group will improve liver function and lower blood lipid levels naturally without the side effects of many of the cholesterol lowering drugs. Further, Methionine is needed by the body for its powerful detoxification properties.

Another very effective free radical inhibitor, although not an antioxidant, is the mineral Zinc. Vitamin A cannot function in the body without Zinc so they must be present simultaneously in order to be effective.

The late *J.I. Rodale*, a pioneer in the modern nutrition revolution and a heart patient himself, often said that the greatest heart tonic in the world was Hawthorne Berry. He was so impressed with the ability of Hawthorne Berry to improve cardiovascular health that he wrote an entire book on the herb.

Gingko Biloba and Dimethyl Glycine are two compounds, which have the ability to increase the oxygen content of body tissues. The oxygenating benefits of a good exercise program are worthless if the cells of the body cannot absorb the oxygen from the blood stream. Gingko Biloba and Dimethyl Glycine dramatically increase the cell's ability to assimilate oxygen.

Co-Enzyme Q10 is another nutrient that we believe is vital to cardiovascular health. CoQ10 actually reduces angina and improves cardiac function. Heart patients taking CoQ10 consistently have better exercise tolerance than those who do not.

EDTA, a synthetic amino acid has the ability to enter the bloodstream and bind with the calcium aligning the artery walls. This process, called chelation, is very effective in removing deposits of calcium. Once the calcium is gone, the cholesterol and other fats cannot adhere to the insides of the arteries. Until recent years, it was impossible to administer EDTA orally as it broke down in digestion, making it almost ineffective in chelating calcium. In fact EDTA was first developed for intravenous chelation and is still used in this method, very effectively today. We now can protect the EDTA by enteric coating, allowing its use in oral chelates with great effectiveness.

If you were to go out and try to purchase all of the nutrients we have discussed it would be challenging, time consuming, and costly. In addition, ratios are extremely important in any program wherein we hope to create a 'chelating' environment. Too much or too little of certain nutrients can dramatically reduce the effectiveness of this program.

For this reason we have assembled a Master Protocol which reflects what we believe to be the ideal diet and nutrient combination in the management and promotion of cardiovascular health.

Dietary Protocol for Cardiovascular Support

If you have been diagnosed with atherosclerosis or heart disease, the following steps should be taken to modify your dietary habits as soon as possible.

1. Eliminate ALL polyunsaturated vegetable oils from your diet. This includes restaurant foods cooked in these refined oils.

2. Eliminate the use of all 'plastic' fats such as margarine, hydrogenated oils and other synthetic products, which are rapidly becoming popular.

3. Limit the calories from fat to no more than 25 or 30 percent unless you are very active.

4. Use olive oil for both cold and hot food applications/preparations.

5. Eat fruits and vegetables as close to their raw, natural state as possible.

6. Ensure that you get at least 80 grams of high quality protein every day.

7. Avoid the over-consumption of processed protein foods such as cold meats, cheeses and other foods containing nitrates.

8. Reduce the amount of refined carbohydrates and sugars in the diet.

Lastly, while not dietary in nature, begin a regular exercise program according to your fitness level and physical condition. If you have not exercised for some time, consult a professional for advice regarding what type of exercise would be appropriate for your situation. (please refer to chapter 2 on exercise guidelines)

Nutrient Protocol for Cardiovascular Support

Vitamin E	200 IU
Vitamin C (Calcium Ascorbate)	1,200 mg
Niacin	50 mg
Vitamin B6	25 mg
Vitamin B12	600 mcg
Folic Acid	800 mcg
Calcium	300 mg
Magnesium	300 mg
Choline	450 mg
Cysteine HCL	450 mg
Taurine	200 mg
Gingko Biloba	30 mg
L-Carnitine	100 mg
Dimethyl Glycine	50 mg
Co-Enzyme Q-10	20 mg
EDTA	400 mg

The exact combination, outlined in the preceding formulation, has been tested and used with excellent results since 1989. While it represents what we have found to be an optimal preventive dosage, those suffering from more acute cardiovascular conditions can achieve accelerated benefits if they increase the dosage by 50% during the first 90 days of use. Contact The Institute for more information on obtaining this formula. (See Appendix for resource information)

As with all chronic degenerative diseases, heart disease can be prevented. Once it has developed, the condition still may be greatly improved. But we must take action. Conventional medicine has been approaching these conditions in a reactive manner. They fail to see the cause of the problem, and therefore do not understand the implications involved in the prevention, management, or reversal of this deadly disease.

Every degenerative disease, without exception, is the result of an imbalance of the body's internal biochemistry. Often years, or even decades, pass before symptoms exhibit themselves and we become aware of the problem.

Through providing the raw materials needed by the body for health, and through eliminating the artificial and excessive factors provided by a modern junk food diet, we can reverse the tide towards degenerative disease. We can then focus on a course of action, which will enable us to maintain or regain optimal health.

We will now turn our attention to another chronic disease, which has become epidemic word wide, Diabetes. If you suffer from Diabetes and are also concerned about your heart health, there is a definite link between the two. Those with Diabetes have a much greater chance of developing many forms of cardiovascular disease. For optimal wellness, it is necessary to address both problems, if they exist.

Diabetes & Hypoglycemia

If someone were to ask you what the most epidemic disease of the so-called 'civilized' world was, what would be your answer? Cancer?

Cancer is certainly the most feared of modern-day diseases. You might choose Heart Disease. This condition still kills more people around the world than any other single cause. Yet, neither of these conditions is the most epidemic.

Adult Onset Diabetes or Type II Non-Insulin Dependent Diabetes, to be more currently accurate, has been the epidemic of the twentieth century, and continues unabated, into the new millenium. It is rising in numbers faster than all other chronic degenerative diseases *combined*.

Diabetes is so common that almost everyone knows someone who has the disease. According to the National Institutes of Health, there are about 12 million diagnosed diabetics in America and it is estimated that there are at least that many more undiagnosed cases.

According to 2004 statistics from the Centers for Disease Control and Prevention's Diabetes Division, 980,000 new cases are diagnosed every year. That amounts to one new case being diagnosed every 20 seconds!

To make matters worse, each year tens of thousands of diabetic Americans lose their eyesight, compromise their circulation, suffer irreversible heart damage, and/ or require the amputation of a lower limb. Each year, many of these people die prematurely due to Diabetes.

Of all these cases of Diabetes, ninety percent of them are the non-insulin dependent, Type II variety. Only ten percent are the genetically induced Type I Juvenile-Onset version.

The saddest part about these statistics is the fact that non-insulin dependent, Type II diabetes, is completely controllable and very often reversible without the need for dangerous drugs, or worse yet, the misuse of insulin. Type II Diabetes is, almost exclusively, caused by dietary abuse. It steals a long and healthy life from millions and millions of people.

Each generation produces multitudes of diabetics at younger and younger ages. We used to call this disease "adult onset", but now it is referred to as non-insulin dependent type II diabetes because it continues to manifest in younger and younger people. In fact, one of the most epidemic age groups for this disease is now between the ages of 15 and 25!

Even more common in occurrence is Hypoglycemia, or low blood sugar. It is frequently the precursor to Adult-Onset Type II Diabetes. If left unchecked, Hypoglycemia can devastate the lives of its victims. They are left with a better than a nine-to-one chance of progressing to Diabetes later in life. This condition, like Diabetes, is completely dietary induced and can be controlled. Remember that you can have the genetic tendency toward these conditions as they are well known to be hereditary, but that does not mean you must accept your fate. There is much you can do to prevent or reverse these problems. Let's find out how.

Hypoglycemia: The Undiagnosed Disorder

For many decades, Hypoglycemia was both shunned and denied by the mainstream medical profession. Millions of people went to their physicians with a long list of debilitating symptoms, only to be told that their symptoms were psychological in nature.

These patients were also advised to seek psychiatric help if their symptoms persisted. This 'mis-diagnosis' only led these people to further and further desperation. Many of them even resorted to such drastic measures as suicide. This, in turn, further fueled the argument that these people were suffering from a mental disorder.

Today, we know that Hypoglycemia or low blood sugar is both real and very common. As is the case with many chronic illnesses, Hypoglycemia was virtually unknown in the early 1900's at the turn of the last century.

This means that these conditions have escalated to epidemic proportions in less than 5 generations! Recent findings portray how severe the problem is.

At the dawn of the 20th century, the average person consumed 10 to 15 pounds of sugar per year. Today, we all consume at least our own body weight, or more, in sugars every single year!

The refining of whole wheat into white flour has produced a substance that is, chemically, one small step away from sugar. This means that eating foods made from white flour contributes to the overall consumption of sugars.

While there can be several causes for Clinical Hypoglycemia, such as excess alcohol consumption, stress, or the use of certain prescription drugs, ninety percent is the result of dietary abuse.

The symptoms of hypoglycemia are many and can come and go with great regularity. This often makes the disorder difficult to diagnose. The only scientific way to determine Clinical Hypoglycemia is through the six- hour glucose tolerance test (anything less than six-hours is non-conclusive).

The number and frequency of certain symptoms is also a valid determining factor for the presence of Hypoglycemia. Let's look at these many symptoms, keeping in mind that you may experience more than one of these symptoms at the same time.

Anxiety

Breathing (shallow and rapid)

Chill (cold and clammy)

Emotional Outbursts

Fatigue or Tiredness

Headache

Hot Flashes

Insomnia

Irritability

Mental Confusion

Nausea

Nervousness

Nightmares

Obesity (overweight by more than 25 pounds)

Physical Coordination (reduced)

Pulse Rate (elevated)

Restlessness

Sleep Disturbances (insomnia, night sweats, sudden awakening)

Tinnitus (ringing in the ears)

Tingling Sensation (in the fingers, toes, or tongue)

Vision problems (blurred or double)

Weakness

If you experience eight or more of these symptoms on a regular basis, and other possible causes have been ruled out, you can consider yourself as having instable blood sugars and possibly hypoglycemia.

There are two types of Hypoglycemia. The most common form occurs along with excess bodyweight. The second, more obscure form, produces normal or even an underweight condition. The cause of both is the same, namely excess insulin in the bloodstream, but the manner in which we manage the conditions differs slightly (see the management protocols for both Type I and Type II Hypoglycemia later in this chapter).

Medically, the cause of Hypoglycemia, Adult-Onset Diabetes and most obesity, is called Hyperinsulinemia, or excess insulin.

In the Hypoglycemic patient, the Pancreas produces excess insulin. This drives the blood sugar level down below an optimal level. This dip in blood sugar levels, over prolonged periods of time, produces the many side effects and symptoms previously listed.

Typically, when we feel weak and flushed from loss of blood sugar, our first reaction is to eat some more sugar. When we do this, the blood glucose once again rises rapidly, stimulating another insulin response, which in turn lowers blood sugar below normal again. This produces the yo-yo effect of "highs and lows" so common with Hypoglycemic individuals.

There are three phases of what we call 'Carbohydrate Intolerance'. Each level is progressively worse than the one before it and the side effects also become more severe. Let's take a closer look.

1. **Carbohydrate Intolerance:**

    This condition produces a craving for starches and sugary foods. Frequently, the subsequent consumption of starches contributes to obesity through excess insulin converting most carbohydrates to triglycerides and storing them as body fat. These individuals have a better than 10 to one chance of progressing to phase two, Hypoglycemia.

2. **Hypoglycemia:**

   As "Carbohydrate Intolerant" individuals continue to consume excess sugars and starches, periods of low blood sugar levels become more and more frequent. The symptoms previously listed begin to appear. The Hypoglycemic individual has an eight to one chance of progressing to phase three, diabetes.

3. **Diabetes:**

   This dreaded chronic degenerative disease is the final outcome for those traveling along this pathway.

The powerful hormone behind this process is called Insulin and an understanding of both what it is and what triggers its excess production is essential.

What is Insulin?

In order to more clearly understand Carbohydrate Intolerance, Hypoglycemia, and Diabetes, it is essential to understand their cause. Each condition, is caused by an excess of the hormone "Insulin", which is produced by the Pancreas.

Insulin is the glucose-regulating hormone. In healthy individuals, it is produced on an as-needed basis according to the levels of glucose present in the blood.

Many people are of the erroneous thought that insulin burns up excess glucose. It does not! Insulin serves to transport excess glucose to the body's various storage sites.

The first and normal site for glucose storage is in the liver and muscles. Insulin converts the blood glucose into a substance called Glycogen, which is 'stored sugar'. This is then transported to the liver and muscles. This is unfortunate for those following the 'sugar-filled' Standard American Diet (SAD), because the body's ability to store Glycogen is very limited.

Once all of the body's storage sites for Glycogen are full, Insulin further converts blood glucose into another substance called Triglycerides and these are then carried by insulin to the fat cells of the body. This is why most Hypoglycemics, and virtually all Type II Diabetics, are overweight.

In order to control Hypoglycemia, Type II Diabetes, and most obesity, we must control the amount of insulin present in the bloodstream.

Currently, there are no drugs that are able to reduce or limit the production of insulin. It can only be accomplished by avoiding the foods which cause an 'insulin response', which is the production of excess insulin by the body.

All sugar and sugar forming foods (carbohydrates) eventually break down into glucose. The key is the speed with which this breakdown occurs. The faster the conversion, the more insulin is secreted into the bloodstream, setting the stage for the insulin disorders of obesity, Hypoglycemia and Diabetes.

Our body needs a certain amount of glucose, but far less than the average junk food diet provides. Through this constant excess, insulin is not only over-produced but the receptor sites for that insulin become de-sensitized, requiring more and more insulin to do the job. (See the next section on Diabetes)

Unfortunately, this cycle of insulin response and production can develop into a terrible downward spiral. As more and more insulin is produced from excess sugars in the diet, more and more of it is converted to triglycerides and stored in the fat cells.

As the fat cells increase, the body becomes increasingly overweight. As the body weight rises, insulin becomes less and less effective, requiring the body to produce higher and higher amounts, which in turn cause a greater and greater weight gain, which starts the cycle all over again.

The Importance of Weight Control

After the first few weeks of infancy have passed, we have all the fat cells we will ever have. You cannot make anymore. The fat cell, however, has the ability to continue to increase in size depending upon how much stored sugar, or triglyceride, it must hold.

As the fat cells become larger and larger, their responsiveness to insulin decreases, causing the need for ever higher amounts of insulin in order to remove excess sugars from the bloodstream. Since it is the excess insulin that causes Obesity, Hypoglycemia, and Diabetes, controlling and normalizing body weight is essential in the regulation of the insulin/glucose cycle.

For those persons who are overweight and also have either hypoglycemia or diabetes, a reduction in bodyweight frequently reduces symptoms. In some individuals, a reduction in body weight eliminates the symptoms completely without any other protocol.

These individuals respond extremely well to a controlled carbohydrate diet, which counts and limits the amount of sugar-forming foods eaten each day. With a reduction in available carbohydrates, insulin production is greatly reduced. With the normalizing of insulin levels, excess bodyweight is slowly removed. Through reducing the bodyweight and the insulin production, Hypoglycemia and Diabetes are easily controlled with the help of a few assisting co-factors (see protocols latter in this chapter).

There are many effective exercise programs, which will simultaneously help accelerate fat loss and help the body to use insulin more effectively.

When we exercise, several physiological benefits occur. Muscles need energy to perform. When we exercise, we increase the need for fuel for the muscles. That fuel is glucose; therefore, exercise increases the uptake of glucose by the muscle cells. This in turn naturally reduces blood glucose levels. This means that the body needs less insulin to regulate blood sugar, reducing the peaks and valleys so common in all these blood sugar disorders.

The most effective form of exercise for this purpose, is a combination of cardio-aerobic and resistance exercise. Remember, the larger your muscle mass, the less insulin resistant you become.

Diabetes, The Final Insult of Excess Insulin

Clinically, Diabetes is *hyper*glycemia, or excess blood sugar. In the non-insulin dependent, Type II Diabetic, excess blood sugar is almost always caused by a defect in the insulin receptor sites, not by lack of insulin.

Years and years of continual dietary abuse created a situation in which there was excess sugar in the body. Insulin was then forced to convert that sugar into triglycerides and store those molecules within the fat cell.

In order to accomplish this, insulin must attach itself to "insulin receptor sites" on specific cells of the body. Through years or decades of continual dietary abuse involving excess sugar consumption, these receptor sites become de-sensitized. More and more insulin is then required to remove the excess sugar.

This is why most all Type II Diabetics have normal or even higher than normal levels of insulin in their bloodstream. Treating these individuals with drugs that increase insulin production, or treating them with insulin itself (by injection), only serves to make the disease ultimately worse.

Type II Diabetics need to reduce the amounts of sugar and sugar-forming foods in their diets. This will take the demand off of the insulin receptor sites, which constantly have to convert and store this excess sugar. This will reduce the volume of insulin in the blood stream, thereby reducing the symptoms of diabetes and the other related insulin disorders.

It is important to remember that Type II Diabetes develops slowly over the years. This is one of the reasons why this disease is so insidious. Often, by the time the disease has been diagnosed, the patient has already suffered considerable damage to nerves, blood vessels, the heart, the eyes and even the brain.

I have often called Type II diabetes the non-contagious Leprosy of the 20th century. Diabetes eats away at multiple organ and tissue systems. Slowly and steadily, inch by inch, destroying the quality of life for the sufferer.

Factors that Worsen Diabetes

In addition to the obvious dietary factor of excess sugars, which we have been discussing, there are other situations, both environmentally and chemically, which can make diabetes worse.

I have often said that stress is the cardinal cause of all illness and certainly it plays a direct role in the process of Diabetes. During periods of stress, it is not uncommon for a Diabetic to observe sudden rises in blood sugar. This phenomenon can occur even if the stress was brief but severe. Life changing events, such as the loss of a job, spouse or relative, can produce such stress as to cause the onset of Diabetes in someone who has not yet even been diagnosed with the illness.

For this reason, any program that wishes to address the complete needs of the Diabetic should include nutritional support for the nervous system as well as support for glucose metabolism.

What Do You Do Now?

Let's assume you have an insulin-induced disorder such as Obesity, Hypoglycemia, or Type II Diabetes. Where do you go from here?

With a few small modifications, the management of all these conditions is basically the same. We will do so with a combination of dietary restrictions and specific dietary supplementation.

The following section will explain the full protocol of diet and supplementation necessary for the control or reversal of your Hypoglycemia or Diabetes. The protocol will work only if you follow it exactly. Any variation from this basic program will produce less than optimal results.

Protocol for Managing and Reversing Hypoglycemia & Diabetes

Dietary Factors:

As with most chronic degenerative diseases, diet plays a significant role in the development and subsequent reversal or management of Hypoglycemia and Diabetes.

If we are ever to master these conditions, it will be essential to regulate the amount of sugar and sugar-forming foods in the diet. This is best accomplished by not counting calories but rather by counting carbohydrates.

Since all carbohydrates eventually turn into blood glucose, the amount and type of carbohydrates consumed plays a direct effect upon the levels of blood sugar and subsequently the amount of insulin secreted into the bloodstream.

There are several excellent books, which cover carbohydrate restricted diets in detail. If you are also overweight, you may wish to choose one that also places emphasis upon weight management as well.

A good guideline for determining the amount of sugars and refined carbohydrates often hidden in common foods may be found in the book called *Calories and Carbohydrates* by Barbara Kraus. This book is published by Signet Paperback Books, and the current edition is available in most bookstores.

In your case, you will want to pay attention only to the carbohydrate count of each food, because, for practical purposes, you will not be concerned with calories.

It is important to reduce carbohydrates in your diet, but you must do so slowly. A rapid drop in carbohydrates and hence, available blood sugars, can result in very low blood sugar. By reducing total carbohydrate intake slowly, your body will have the opportunity to adjust insulin production accordingly. Here is a program, which we have been using at our research centers, with great success:

Determine the approximate amount of total carbohydrate you are presently consuming. If in excess of 100 grams per day start following the reduction scale below. If presently less than 100 grams per day, start from where you currently are and lower as per the scale below.

Week 1	100 grams (or less if starting at less)
Week 2	80 grams per day
Week 3	60 grams per day
Week 4	50 grams per day

Stay at 50 grams per day for several weeks as long as you are feeling well and your energy level is good. This should begin to produce a significant weight loss as carbohydrates come down.

If you continue to feel well and your energy levels remain good, drop the carbohydrates to 40 grams per day for an ongoing weight loss and blood sugar management.

The carbohydrates you choose in any week should be made up of complex, whole grains and some fresh fruit such as berries, which are lower in sugars. In all cases, you will want to avoid consuming concentrated sugars and refined starches as these foods will always cause a spike in insulin and subsequently blood sugar.

As your available carbohydrates begin to fall, you will likely experience cravings for sweets, which can sometimes be almost overwhelming. Lingering cravings for sugars can be controlled by specific dietary supplements, which we will discuss later in the program.

If you are a Diabetic, your blood sugar levels will very likely fall steadily as you continue to restrict your carbohydrate intake. For this reason, if you are taking medications, and especially if you are taking insulin, you will need to monitor your blood glucose levels regularly. In the beginning, testing 3 to 4 times per day is not excessive.

As your blood sugar falls, if you are taking medications, you doctor will want to slowly and correctly begin to reduce the amount of medication you are taking since you will not require it in the quantities you were before.

If you add an exercise program to the dietary program, you will achieve results much faster, but you will also need to test your blood sugar more often since it will likely fall even faster.

As your blood sugar normalizes over the next few weeks, you can gradually increase the number of carbohydrates in the diet. Eventually you will get to the point where, if you are a Hypoglycemic, your symptoms will begin to return. If you are a Diabetic, your blood sugar will once again begin to rise. This is called the carbohydrate threshold. It is usually different for each person, so you will have to establish what that number of carbohydrate grams would be for you, each day.

Once you know your threshold for carbohydrate intake, you must simply confine your daily consumption of carbohydrates to an amount approximately 10 to 20 percent below that figure. This will enable you to keep your symptoms and/or blood sugar levels in check.

SPECIAL NOTE FOR UNDERWEIGHT HYPOGLYCEMICS: If you have hypoglycemia and are of normal weight, or especially if you are underweight, you cannot totally restrict your carbohydrate intake. To do so would produce even greater weight loss and subsequent fatigue.

You need to count carbohydrates, but you will have to keep the level above one, which will produce further weight loss. To make this calculation, determine your 'carbohydrate threshold' by using the preceding method. Once you begin reducing your total carbohydrate intake, at some point you will start loosing weight. Then, increase your carbohydrate consumption to 10 percent above the level, which produces the weight loss.

In order to keep your weight up, but still produce a minimal insulin response, you must learn how to choose carbohydrate foods wisely. The faster carbohydrates break down into simple sugars, the quicker and greater the insulin response. For this reason, you must choose complex carbohydrate foods, which take several hours to slowly break down into simple sugars. Examples would be whole grains (such as black wild rice), breads that are truly whole grain, legumes, and certain vegetables.

Foods you need to avoid are those containing sugar, honey, molasses, corn syrup or any other forms of simple sugars. Additionally, you must avoid highly refined starches such as anything made with refined white flour, refined grains and pastas as well as over-cooked root vegetables such as potatoes. All of these foods will convert to glucose too rapidly causing an insulin response, throwing you into a state of low blood sugar.

As you start to control your carbohydrate intake, remember that there can be hidden sugars in many things you eat.

Food	Sugar content in Teaspoonfuls
Soda Pop (12 oz)	3-12
All Cakes & Cookies (4 oz serving)	5-10
Candies (1 piece)	1-5
Canned Fruits (½ cup)	2-4
Ice Cream (3 oz)	3-5
Malted Milk Shake	10-16
Jams & Jellies (1 oz)	1-6

You can see how it adds up. Sugars are hidden in other foods as well, including breakfast cereals, breads, rolls, and anything made from refined white flour.

I will be the first to tell you that it is difficult to abstain from the very foods you not only crave, but are actually addicted to; carbohydrate sensitivity is a genuine addiction. Instead of leaving you to your own frustrations, I will tell you about several specific nutrients and nutrient co-factors, which will both help you win your battle with sugar addiction and make your body function more effectively as you pursue your program of glucose and insulin management.

Dietary Supplementation for Hypoglycemia & Diabetes.

For the person afflicted with insulin-related disorders, one nutrient, a mineral, offers unparalleled promise and is a pivotal element of support. That mineral is Chromium. Yet,

Chromium alone is far less effective than when properly combined with other nutrient cofactors, which provide a complete targeted approach to the problem. Together, they contribute a synergistic and infinitely greater assurance of an appropriate solution.

In addition to Chromium, the mineral Vanadium and alpha lipoic acid, have been shown to be very helpful in assisting the body in the regulation of glucose and insulin. Following are the ratios of these nutrients, which we have used with tremendous success at The Institute. This formula, along with Full Spectrum Nutrition, has helped tens of thousands of people live a normal life, free from Hypoglycemia and Diabetes. Together with the proper diet as outlined earlier, it can ensure that you will not have to progress to further stages of these diseases. Further, you will not have to suffer the numerous and debilitating side effects which arise from excess insulin in the blood.

Components of a Comprehensive Glucose/Insulin Regulating Formula

Chromium	300 mcg
Vanadium	1200mcg
Bitter Melon	50 mg
Gymnema sylvestre leaf	25 mg
Alpha Lipoic Acid	15 mg
Syzgium cumini seed	5 mg
Hydroxycitric Acid	650 mg

This is the exact formula we use at our Clinics and Research Centers around the world. It is available from Phoenix Nutritionals, Inc. (see appendix for resource information)

Managing Stress

As illustrated earlier, stress, especially un-manageable stress, can wreak havoc with the glandular systems of the body. Since both Hypoglycemia and Diabetes are endocrine disorders, stress has a rapid and intense negative impact on these conditions. If we are to gain control over these problems, managing stress is very important.

During periods of stress, the body can consume very high amounts of certain nutrients. When these nutrient levels are depleted, the nerves become irritated and additional stress becomes impossible to manage.

For this reason, we always use a combination of nutrients in higher amounts when working with Hypoglycemics and Diabetics. These nutrients, in the following combinations and ratios, have proven time and time again to stabilize the body's many chemical functions through calming and nourishing the central nervous system.

Stress Management Formula

Vitamin C	1000 mg
Vitamin B1	50 mg
Vitamin B2	50 mg
Vitamin B6	50 mg
Vitamin B12	500 mcg
Pantothenic Acid	1200 mg
Calcium	400 mg
Magnesium	100 mg
Adrenal Substance	200 mg
Valerian Root Extract	200 mg

Once blood sugar, insulin and dietary factors have been considered, over time, you can expect much greater control and management of your glucose disorders. While the degree of success each person will experience is dependent upon many factors, here is just one example of what may be accomplished by following this program:

A Case In Point

Tom M.

Tom, who was referred to us by a third party, first contacted our Institute in April of 1998. When he called, the voice on the other end of the telephone was a desperate one. Tom had been diagnosed with Type II Diabetes about two years before. While taking down his information, we discovered that he was taking 14 different oral medications daily!

Further, his body weight was nearing 300 pounds. Tom was desperate. His doctor told him that his blood sugar was still too high and that if it did not come down in 30 days, he was going to put him on insulin by injection. Tom had done enough reading to know that was not a good recommendation for a Type II Diabetic and he was really scared.

The first thing we did was evaluate his diet. He told us that the diet he was following came from his doctor's office. He said he followed it very strictly. This was our first clue into Tom's dilemma. We asked if he had a copy of his diet handy and sure enough, he faxed it to our office that afternoon. Upon reviewing his diet, one endorsed by the American Diabetes Association, we found that it was 68 percent sugar-forming foods! On this diet, Tom was guaranteed to remain a Diabetic the rest of his short and miserable life!

After reviewing his case, I called Tom and suggested some lifestyle changes, the very ones outlined in this chapter. We put him on a diet that was low in carbohydrates and high in protein and fresh vegetables. We started him on a maintenance program of Full Spectrum nutrition plus targeted nutritional support for his specific needs. We cautioned him to monitor his blood sugar level at least three times daily because we expected it to begin to fall.

To make a long story short, within three months, Tom was medication free. He went from 14 pills to no pills in ninety days! Other exciting changes were occurring for Tom as well. He lost almost 75 pounds. As his bodyweight lessened due to the decrease in the amount of insulin circulating in the bloodstream, his insulin receptor sites began to function better.

Today, Tom remains disease free, as declared by his physician. Sadly, Tom doesn't see that doctor any longer. Upon hearing how Tom achieved his remarkable metamorphosis from disease, his doctor told him never to come back. When Tom questioned why his doctor did not share his excitement over his return from disease, the doctor coldly said, "You did not follow my diet and take my advice."

The reason we say that this is 'sad' is because if Tom's doctor had learned from his patient's case, think how many other patients he might have influenced in a positive way.

Program Summary

DIETARY RESTRICTION. It is imperative that you follow a dietary program that reduces the amount of total sugar-forming foods in the diet.

EXERCISE. A regular exercise program, designed for your age and level of fitness, will accelerate your victory over virtually any phase of hyperinsulinemia.

Dietary Supplements.

FULL SPECTRUM NUTRITION − Provide your body with the 100+ nutrients it needs every day.

GLUCOSE METABOLIZING NUTRIENTS − Use Chromium, vanadium, key herbal extracts, alpha lipoic acid and hydroxycitric acid.

STRESS REDUCING NUTRIENTS - Since stress plays such a direct role in the pathology of carbohydrate intolerance, the addition of stress reducing nutrients is of vital importance. The body's reserves of nutrients such as Vitamin C, Vitamins B1, B2, B6, B12, and Pantothenic Acid are rapidly depleted during times of physical and emotional stress. Carbohydrate Intolerance produces both forms of stress and they exert a negative effect on the entire endocrine system through the action of the adrenal glands. (See Appendix to contact The Institute for Carbohydrate Intolerance Testing)

While this program seems simple enough, it is powerful in the results it can deliver. Thousands have changed their lives with this program and you can too.

Arthritis

What is Arthritis?

It seems like a simple enough question to answer. Everyone knows what arthritis is, don't they? The answer, surprisingly, is NO! Medically, there are no known specific causes of arthritis!

Arthritis is not even a specific disease, but rather the generic name for a group of conditions, likely having individual or multiple different causes. The word 'arthritis', comes from the Greek word which means 'joint'. We have come to interpret the word as meaning inflammation of the joints.

Dr. Francis Pottenger clearly established the relationship between a diet of highly cooked foods and Arthritis in animals. This work was done many decades ago and yet the establishment continues to cling to the concept that diet does not affect this disease. Animals fed diets of raw foods showed no evidence of arthritis. Their counterparts, having been fed a diet of cooked and processed foods, developed a variety of arthritic symptoms at an early age.

One of the worst of all the offending foods for the arthritic patient is processed, pasteurized dairy products such as milk, ice cream and processed cheeses. Every arthritic patient I've ever counseled had been on a diet of over-cooked and over-processed foods for decades.

While no one really knows what causes arthritis, we do know that we can interrupt the disease process and stop the disease from progressing.

There are several types of arthritis. The most common is called Osteo-Arthritis. It concerns the breakdown of the cartilage tissue that cushions and lubricates the joints. Over time, this material is lost over time from a variety of assaults, which may include infections to the joint itself, excessive wear & tear (athletics), and numerous nutritional deficiencies.

Another form of arthritis is called Rheumatoid Arthritis. This is not a degenerative disease in the clinical sense, but rather an autoimmune disorder. It is a condition wherein the body's immune system launches an attack upon the cartilage and connective tissue proteins. Eventually, this abnormality will destroy every joint in the body.

While the cause of Osteo-Arthritis and Rheumatoid Arthritis vary greatly from each other, the end result is the same. Both produce a loss of cartilage and connective tissue through repeated inflammation and irritation of the joint and surrounding physiology.

As the synovial membrane of the joint tissue becomes repeatedly inflamed, the blood supply increases. White blood cells proliferate at these sites, indicating the presence of some form of infection. This increase in cellular activity causes the surrounding tissue and joint to swell. The swelling pushes the bone joints further apart, creating a larger and larger space. As the space between them increases, the risk of further infection and subsequent inflammation occurs.

It is now believed that the acute inflammation and pain experienced by most arthritics is due to damage caused by the proliferation of free radicals. This is why we strongly recommend and include antioxidants in our arthritis management formulas.

Conventional Treatment for Arthritis

Arthritis is usually first diagnosed as a result of patient complaints of pain, stiffness, and loss of motion in specific joints of the body. The physician then customarily recommends taking an over-the-counter pain- killer. Almost all painkillers belong to a family of drugs known as non-steroidal anti-inflammatory drugs. (NSAIDs)

The only popular exception to that group would be Acetaminophen (Tylenol,® Datril® and Liquiprin®) Acetaminophen is not often recommended for arthritis because it contains no anti-inflammatory properties but consumers, unaware of this, take it thinking that it is safer than other over-the-counter pain killers. Unfortunately, it is not.

While NSAIDs are wonderful for occasional aches, pains, or headaches, their constant use renders them increasingly less effective and can produce a variety of potentially serious side effects. The use of NSAIDs is completely out of control. Last year, $2.5 billion worth of these analgesics and anti-inflammatories were sold in the United States alone!

It is estimated that there are at least 100 different NSAIDs either available or in development at any given time. Some of the more popular NSAIDs include: Indocin®, Advil®, Motrin®, Aleve®, Nuprin®, Excedrin®, Midol and Orudis®.

By taking continual high doses of NSAIDs, we interfere with vital bodily functions at a chemical level. Some of the symptoms of NSAID abuse include:

Allergic reactions

Anxiety

Cramps

Diarrhea

Drowsiness

Edema

Headache

Hypertension (high blood pressure)

Indigestion

Kidney problems

Nausea

Nervousness

Sensitivity to sunlight

Ulcers and stomach bleeding

Wounds that heal slowly

The black picture of NSAID misuse doesn't stop here. Many of the deaths that occur each year can be directly linked to excessive NSAID use. Common conditions, which can result in death, involve the kidneys, stomach, and liver, all organs damaged by NSAID abuse.

As the disease of arthritis progresses and the pain and inflammation worsens, doctors resort to using more and more powerful drugs, available by prescription only. Their side effects are the same as we have already discussed with one exception – there are more of them.

Many of the leading anti-inflammatory drugs have been restricted or pulled off the market due to serious side effects. We have developed a new, natural anti-inflammatory formulation that has proven to work as well as these dangerous drugs, but with no side effects at all. Please refer to our natural anti-inflammatory formula below.

The final method of treatment for Arthritis in the 'physician's bag' is, as always, surgery. Joint replacement has become such big business that many hospitals rely upon this type of surgery to stay in business.

The problems with surgery are numerous. The pain, the recovery time, the side effects and the cost must all be considered. Worse yet, just because you have one joint replaced doesn't mean you are out of the hot water. Arthritis is a systemic disease and will, eventually affect all the joints of your body. How many do you want to have replaced?

While the picture of the treatment and prognosis of Arthritis painted is not pretty, the good news is that there is an alternative. Through proper nutrition and subsequent detoxification of the body, even more advanced cases of many types of Arthritis may be successfully improved or reversed.

Nutritional Support for Managing & Reversing Arthritis

Several specific nutrients have repeatedly proven to be of exceptional importance in the prevention, management, and even the reversal of arthritic conditions. Before beginning a discussion of these nutrients, it is important to emphasize the fact that the body works on the principles of synergy and balance.

It requires well over 100 nutrients daily to accomplish the task of not only keeping you alive, but healthy as well. To 'mega-dose' on individual or 'isolated' nutrients, without the simultaneous intake of a Full Spectrum supplement, is unwise. It can lead to drastic biochemical imbalances within the body.

Simply stated, for optimal results in any nutritional support program, use a Full Spectrum dietary supplement as a foundation on a daily basis. Then add the specific nutrients, which have demonstrated their effectiveness in improving the condition at hand.

Following is a listing of select individual nutrients, which have helped many Arthritis sufferers dramatically improve the quality of their lives. Each is accompanied by an explanation as to why that nutrient is of profound value.

ESSENTIAL FATTY ACIDS (EFA): It was heart disease that first drew our attention to the importance of Gamma-linolenic Acid (GLA) and Eicosapentaenoic Acid (EPA) in the prevention and management of chronic disease. Since that time, these Essential Fatty Acids have continued to demonstrate their relevancy in reference to numerous chronic conditions.

In 1985, an article appeared in the publication *Clinical Research* reporting that these Essential Fatty Acids significantly improved Rheumatoid Arthritis in many patients. Further, they are absolutely essential in the management of common or Osteo-Arthritis.

Remember our discussion of prostaglandin's earlier? Well the good varieties are made through the conversion of GLA in the body. In order for this to occur, you must have adequate GLA available. The best sources of essential fatty acids include fish oils, borage oil, flax oil and evening primrose oil.

It is important to note that all of these oils, especially the vegetable sources, are highly subject to rancidity when they come in contact with the oxygen in the air. Rancid oils produce tremendous amounts of free radicals, the very substances we are trying to curtail due to their active role in the Arthritis process.

For this reason, you should be very cautious about the source of the fatty acids you choose. Once exposed to air, they do more harm than good. If you must buy the oils in bottles, they MUST be refrigerated. Much better still would be to purchase the fatty acids which have been extracted from the various oils and then placed in airtight gel capsules.

One further step against free radical formation would be to look for capsules that are opaque in nature. Avoid the clear, see-through capsules. They allow light to penetrate, causing some breakdown of the delicate fatty acids within.

CALCIUM AND MAGNESIUM: Arthritis is caused, in part, by a long term, sub-clinical calcium deficiency. Therefore, taking extra calcium is a logical adjunct to a full spectrum nutritional approach. Calcium requires several co-factor minerals in order to be properly absorbed. Mal-absorption of calcium, due to lack of proper acidity or imbalances in nutrient intake, is the cardinal cause of such problems as kidney and gall stones, bone spurs, and of course, arthritis. The best calcium supplements are comprised of Chelated Calcium and contain supporting mineral co-factors such as Magnesium, Boron, Copper, Manganese, and Zinc.

COPPER: In addition to being an essential co-factor in the absorption and retention of Calcium, Copper has long been associated with the relief of stiff and aching conditions. The practice of wearing copper bracelets for relief of Arthritis pain is an old remedy, but the science behind it is sound. Organic source copper, that which comes from plant sources, is much more absorbable by the body at the cellular level and is therefore the preferred source.

VITAMIN B-6: This is the universal 'transport vitamin'. Virtually every nutrient combined with enough Vitamin B-6 is transported readily to the cellular level. Additionally, Vitamin B-6 plays a direct role in reducing pain from inflammation as well as preventing the nighttime cramps frequently suffered by Arthritis patients. The complete research relating to vitamin B-6 and arthritis may be found in an old book by Dr. John M. Ellis, MD entitled *The Doctor Who Looked At Hands*. This book is, unfortunately, out of print but may still be available in libraries and used bookstores.

GLUCOSAMINE SULFATE: In order for cartilage to maintain its integrity, and not break down because of excessive use, it needs adequate amounts of water. Proteoglycans, structures that bind the collagen within the cartilage, are also the structures that attract the water and keep the joint and surrounding tissues lubricated with moisture.

Glucosamine Sulfate is a major building block of proteoglycans. Glucosamine is, therefore, necessary for making the proteins that bind water in the cartilage matrix. Glucosamine Sulfate not only initiates the production of the key elements of joint and cartilage integrity, but also protects the existing cartilage. Glucosamine can actually help the body repair and replace lost cartilage thereby reversing the disease process!

CHONDROITIN SULFATE: Many of you may be familiar with an age old 'Grandma's Remedy' of eating gelatin if you suffered from stiff joints. It worked because gelatin contains a substance called Chondroitin Sulfate. While Glucosamine Sulfate forms the proteoglycans that fit within the collagen of the cartilage, Chondroitin Sulfate provides a magnetic attraction for water.

Chondroitin's long chain of repeating sugars attracts fluid to the proteoglycan molecules. This accomplishes two things. The fluid acts as the cushion or shock absorber, protecting the cartilage tissue from further assault and breakdown and since joint cartilage has no blood supply, the fluid transports nutrients into the cartilage, keeping them healthy. Without such constant nutrient immersion, the cartilage becomes mal-nourished and dries out.

This results in a thinner, more fragile, cartilage structure. Because gelatin is an incomplete protein, it is very hard to digest for many people. Further, the amount of Chondroitin Sulfate in gelatin is minimal, requiring the need for consuming very large amounts. For this reason we recommend using concentrated Chondroitin Sulfate.

METHYL-SULFONYL-METHANE (MSM): While this nutrient is still relatively new, MSM is effective in the management of many health challenges. For the purpose of our discussion here, MSM is an important adjunct to an overall arthritis support program due to the fact that it relieves both pain and inflammation. MSM has shown benefits for athletes in relieving stress-induced connective tissue injuries. Repeated studies indicate that MSM is as good at relieving pain as many of the over-the-counter NSAID's.

CETYL-MYRISTOLEATE: We have already discussed the benefits of fatty acids in joint health. Cetyl-myristoleate (CMO) is a member of the fatty acid group of nutrients. It is found in the tissues of many animals such as whales and serves to lubricate the joints while suppressing inflammation. It also helps to reduce the autoimmune response in cases of rheumatoid arthritis. Clinical studies continue to support the efficacy of CMO in the management of all types of inflammatory conditions. We are so impressed with this nutrient that I have developed a topical cream, which may be applied to inflamed joints, producing rather rapid, temporary relief from pain. This topical lotion, together with our Joint re-building formula and when needed, our new anti-inflammation formula, have brought relief for thousands of arthritis sufferers.

By combining these specific nutrients with a Full Spectrum foundation, you provide your body with all of its daily nutritional requirements. Remember, at the end of this book, we will provide you with a list of nutrients and the exact potencies and ratios used to successfully achieve positive results.

Other Factors Affecting Arthritis

Whenever we address a chronic degenerative disease of any kind, we must not rule out the possibility of allergic reactions which can contribute significantly to almost any disease process. Such is the case with Arthritis.

There is a group of foods which have been directly linked to the formation and aggravation of Arthritis in many people. These foods all belong to a specific group of foods called the ' nightshades'.

In fact, many members of the nightshade family are so poisonous that they can produce rapid and unpleasant death. Those that do not immediately make you sick are routinely consumed as foods and include: white potatoes (including foods containing potato starch), tomatoes, peppers and eggplants.

All these foods contain a chemical called Solanine, which causes delayed inflammation in some people. If you are having trouble managing your Arthritis after following this program, you may wish to consciously eliminate the nightshades from your diet on a permanent basis.

Other allergies to a wide variety of foods may also play a part the genesis of Arthritis. Therefore, if allergies to foods of any kind are suspected, it is a good idea to have an allergy test and to subsequently avoid all offending foods.

Oxygen: The Universal Cleanser

For many Arthritis sufferers, relief from pain is the first thing on their minds. Pain from Arthritis goes deep into the body and can be severe. In our search for alternatives to drug therapy in the management of Arthritis, we discovered an all natural substance that not only accelerates healing and detoxification of the joint tissues but actually relieves the pain and stiffness connected with all forms of Arthritis.

For over 100 years, we have known about the beneficial effects of super oxygenating the body. In fact, medicine has used super oxygenation in a variety of forms for the treatment of numerous disease conditions.

Hyperbaric Oxygen is often used in accelerating the healing of wounds or burns. Intravenous Oxygen is routinely used by alternative hospitals around the world as part of an overall program of health building rejuvenation, allowing the body to better heal itself from the ravages of virtually all chronic diseases.

While these two forms of oxygenation are effective, they are not readily accessible or affordable to the average person. Because of the work of several pioneers in the field, the use of oxygen for conditions such as Arthritis became somewhat well known. Arthritic people would mix food grade 35% hydrogen peroxide (the only safe form to take internally) with water and drink it. Hydrogen peroxide, in that concentration, has a particularly nauseating taste that is almost impossible to cover up. However, if it is mixed with anything but distilled water, the pathogens and enzymes naturally present in juice and food will cause the oxygen to disassociate. This renders the mixture virtually worthless for oxygenation purposes.

Some time ago, we developed a method whereby the hydrogen peroxide could be buffered, or protected, from disassociation when mixed. Subsequently, we now use our own oral oxygen formula, which contains buffered 35% oxygen along with aloe vera, noni and sterilized natural fruit flavors. (This is available from Phoenix Nutritionals – see Appendix for contact information)

This makes a very palatable drink and may be consumed several times per day. This is especially helpful during the initial stages of the treatment program when the pain and stiffness from Arthritis is most severe.

The Role of Exercise in Recovery from Arthritis

When you are stiff and hurting from the pain of Arthritis, the very last thing you wish to think about is exercise. In fact, some forms of exercise could actually make your Arthritis worse by further damaging compromised cartilage tissue. Yet without exercise, your stiff joints will continue to bind up, even reducing their range of movement and mobility.

The answer is in the proper form of exercise. For those with moderate Arthritis, low impact aerobics on a very cushioned surface are beneficial. Those with more advanced Arthritic conditions should avoid even low impact exercise.

Weight resistance exercises, *together* with stretching exercises, are the best possible combination for the Arthritis sufferer. If you are unfamiliar with exercise and exercise equipment, we suggest that you consult with a physical therapist or exercise physiologist for a program that's right for you. Many of the better gyms and health clubs have personnel who are trained in these areas of specialty. They can get you started on the correct program that will increase your flexibility while ensuring that your delicate joint tissues are not further compromised.

* Special Note for Those Suffering from Gout or Rheumatoid Arthritis

Persons suffering from Gout, a genetic disorder, which prevents the proper excretion of uric acid from the body, can benefit from the basic Arthritis program outlined in this book as well as the following suggestions.

Add Vitamin C to your daily diet until bowel tolerance is reached. To do this, begin with 5000 mg, and increase each day by an additional 5000-mg, until you develop diarrhea. Then reduce your intake to just below that level. (If you are not currently supplementing your diet with Vitamin C, use 2500 mg increments instead of 5000 mg.)

Furthermore, eating cherries or drinking cherry juice is very beneficial for the gout patient. This, along with avoiding purine-forming foods such as red meats, organ meats, sweet breads, shellfish and beer, can help the gout sufferer live a relatively normal life.

For a more targeted approach to the management of Rheumatoid Arthritis those suffering from this condition will benefit greatly by the addition of chicken cartilage to their program.

Fortunately, chicken cartilage is now readily available in capsule form, which saves attacking every chicken in sight! Since potencies for chicken cartilage vary from one manufacturer to another, follow the dosage as outlined on the individual label. Be sure that the product you take is from chicken cartilage, NOT shark cartilage. They are NOT THE SAME! Shark cartilage should ONLY be used in the management of cancer since it prevents the replication of cells.

In our many years of working with thousands of cases of Arthritis, we can assure you that the program outlined in this book is very effective. The fact that the various nutrients are both potent and synergetic makes this program work extremely well.

What follows is the exact protocol we have used at The Institute of Nutritional Science with tremendous success. We suggest that you adopt our program if you wish to have optimal results.

Protocol for the Prevention and Management of Arthritis

DIET: It is important to begin a diet consisting of raw foods. Eat at least one serving of raw cabbage every day as well. Reduce or eliminate the consumption of over processed foods and lifeless foods. Eliminate the consumption of nightshades (discussed earlier in this chapter) and if further problems persist, check for food allergies by having an allergy blood test. If it reveals any severe food allergies, be sure to eliminate those foods from your diet as well.

DETOXIFICATION AND CLEANSING: We cannot stress the importance of properly cleansing the 'organs of elimination' in your plan to treat your Arthritic condition. A Full Spectrum cleansing/detoxification program must address all the organs involved including the liver, kidneys colon and bowel. The following formulation is what we have used successfully on hundreds and hundreds of clients.

Psyllium Husk Powder	400 mg
Aloe Vera Powder	250 mg
Bentonite Powder	250 mg
Celery Powder	150 mg
Cascara Sagrada	125 mg
Irish Moss	100 mg
Peppermint Leaves	100 mg
Senna Leaf	100 mg
Sodium Alginate	100 mg

Bromelain	75 mg
Anise Seed Powder	50 mg
Lactobacillus Acidophilus	50 mg
Ginger Root	50 mg
Turkey Rhubarb Root	25 mg
Chlorophyll	0.5 mg

This formula may be used either with or without a fast. If you are interested in the fasting program we use, you can find it in the appendix section at the end of the book. To use it without a fast, simply use once a day for 14 days. This formula provides both herbal extracts to address all the organs of elimination as well as adequate fiber to assist in the elimination of toxins. (see Appendix for Sources)

After completing the fast or cleanse, it is important to replenish the healthy, good bacteria in the intestinal system. This is best accomplished through the use of a full spectrum acidophilus product, which provides all the various bacterial strains naturally occurring in the gut.

Specific Program For Arthritis Management

EXERCISE: Movement is very important to maintain flexability of joint and connective tissues. If your arthritic condition is moderate to advanced, it would be a good idea to check with your doctor as to recommendations for exercising within your limits. As your arthritis improves, you will be able to increase both the variety and intensity of exercise. Generally speaking, a low impact, lower resistance workout, with emphasis upon stretching and full range of movement is ideal.

DIET: Dietary recommendations have been outlined above.

Supplements:

FULL SPECTRUM NUTRITION (preferably in liquid form) as discussed in Chapter 3.

ESSENTIAL FATTY ACIDS providing primarily omega 3 and 9. (best taken in airtight opaque capsules)

Joint and Connective Tissue Support – To rebuild joint integrity

Vitamin B6	25 mg
Zinc	6 mg
Niacin	40 mg
Evening Primrose Oil	25 mg
N-acetylGlucosamine Sulfate	300 mg
Chondroitin Sulfate	400 mg
CMO	100 mg
MSM	75 mg
Boswellia Extract	100 mg
Nettle Leaf Extract	200 mg

If pain and stiffness is considerable, add liquid oxygen at the rate of one ounce three times per day on an empty stomach (30 minutes before or three hours after a meal), for 30 days.

If you do not get adequate Calcium from your diet, or if you are a female over the age of 45, you need at least 1200 mg of supplemental Calcium daily. It should be taken simultaneously with the mineral co-factors Boron, Copper, Magnesium, Zinc, and Manganese.

Natural Anti-inflammatory Formula

For the millions of people who have or are taking potentially dangerous anti-inflammatory drugs for the management of pain, this formula has proven so effective for pain relief that it is one of the most requested formulas at our Centers:

Curcumin	450 – 650 mg
Boswellia	100 – 200 mg
Natokinase	2.5 – 5 mg
Dl Phenylalanine	450 – 650 mg

Since ratio and absorbability are essential in this formula, we strongly suggest that you use the exact same combination that we do, which is available exclusively from Phoenix Nutritonals, www.phoenixnutritionals.com

Well that's the program. Nothing has been left out and there are no secrets. While some of what we have told you may be familiar, likely, other parts of the program will seem foreign. Nonetheless, it works.

We have literally hundreds of case histories of people whom have benefited immensely from this exact program. You must follow it faithfully and regularly. Arthritis is a chronic condition, meaning that you have it for life. This means that you will have to begin to take a more active role in maintaining and/or regaining your health. If you had known this information years ago, perhaps you would not be in the position you find yourself today. Only you can make the difference by beginning and continuing this program. All of the formulas recommended and as used in The Institute's Centers, are available at many fitness centers and from Phoenix Nutritionals. Their website is www. phoenixnutritionals.com

Candida and Systemic Human Yeast

There is probably more misinformation about this subject, both in medical and nutritional circles, than almost anything I can think of. Books have been written on the subject. Pharmaceuticals have been developed, often with many serious side effects. Yet, in spite of all this effort, little is understood about this annoying and sometimes violent medical problem.

Since this condition is impossible to detect by medical testing, it is often overlooked and even misdiagnosed, creating a 'silent' epidemic. Just how common is this condition? It has been estimated that as many as 60 percent of all women have or have had a problem with yeast infections and localized candida overgrowth at some time in their lives. Roughly 10 to 22 million women have systemic candidiasis and most of them don't even know it. Their symptoms of fatigue, indigestion, muscle weakness, bloating, loss of sexual desire, menstrual irregularities, and mood swings, to name but a few, are accepted as 'part of getting older' or 'just part of life'. Nothing could be further from the truth! And what about men? Can they develop this condition? You bet! In fact, it is often the men, who carry the candida organism, who are re-infecting their wives and girlfriends! Fortunately, we have equal success in treating males, which is often necessary in order to ensure that the women remain free of this condition.

Often women have taken round after round of drugs from their doctors, trying to get some relief. After several attempts, the doctor frequently suggests psychotherapy, thinking that the symptoms must be 'all in her head'. For tens of thousands of others, they turn to the now famous 'candida or yeast diets'. While these eating programs may relieve the symptoms of yeast infection, they certainly do not eliminate it. We have many, many women calling us every month, saying how they have followed the 'yeast diet' for months or even years and yet when they go off the diet for even just one meal, their symptoms return in stealth. This proves that candida diets don't work.

In the past, I have had the privilege of working with some of the leading alternative hospitals in the world. During that time, we developed a method of not only controlling the candida organism, but by completely eliminating the problem! This was incredible news for the many women who suffered, sometimes for years, with ongoing or reoccurring yeast infections.

So, if you suffer from localized yeast infections, candidiasis of the colon and small intestine, or if you have advanced to systemic candidiasis, with all of its potentially debilitating effects, take heart, there is hope!

What is Candida?

Candida albicans is a small budding fungus found naturally in the intestinal tract of all people. When this yeast overgrows, it, along with other yeast-like fungi, account for the major cause of most mycotic infections.

The reason why the candida organism does not proliferate within the body, under healthy conditions, is because it is kept in balance by the friendly bacteria, which also inhabit the intestinal tract. These friendly bacteria are many and are often referred to as the acidophilus family of bacteria. By literally using the candida yeast as food, the acidophilus bacteria maintain a healthy balance within the lower digestive tract of the human body.

What Causes Candida Overgrowth?

As mentioned, it is the friendly acidophilus bacteria that keep the candida in proper balance therefore, anything that damages or destroys the acidophilus in the intestines can lead to candida overgrowth.

The most common cause of acidophilus destruction and candida overgrowth is the improper use of antibiotics. Every time antibiotic therapy is used, the drug is unable to distinguish between the good and bad bacteria, indiscriminately killing them all. Therefore, every time antibiotic therapy is administered, it is essential that the good bacteria be re-implanted into the intestinal tract immediately after the antibiotic therapy is finished. Since most antibiotics are given by mouth, the healthy intestinal bacteria are among the first to be destroyed. Once we have destroyed the natural enemy of the candida yeast, that organism will be allowed to explosively multiply, without control, further unbalancing the delicate synergy necessary for a healthy intestine.

This is the leading cause of vaginal yeast infections so common with women who take antibiotics. You can completely prevent ever having to deal with another yeast infection after antibiotics if you will simply remember to take 10 high potency acidophilus capsules per day for the ten days immediately following the last antibiotic dose.

Other major factors in candidiasis include the use of birth control pills and steroid hormones as found in many pharmaceuticals. Both of these groups of drugs, by means not fully understood, destroy healthy acidophilus, thereby setting up the scenario for candida overgrowth.

Other factors, which can affect the chemistry of the intestines, but to a lesser extent, would be a prolonged diet of over-cooked, over-processed, lifeless foods. In the absence of the natural enzymes present in raw foods, the body must work overtime to produce these enzymes in order to digest foods and keep them from putrefying in the body. Over time, this can cause a depletion of not only enzymes but of acidophilus as well.

How Do I know If I Have Candida Overgrowth?

The only real way to determine if you have candida overgrowth or if it has progressed to systemic candidiasis, is by an analysis of the symptoms present. These, together with the history of antibiotic use/abuse or birth control medication, can frequently establish the presence of a problem. The self-test found later in this section can help you determine if you may have a yeast overgrowth problem and to what extent that problem may exist.

One of the first signs of an overgrowth of the candida yeast organism is gastrointestinal discomfort or disorder. Now, I realize that these problems can be caused by poor diet, lack of nutrition, etc., but, if the problems are not relieved by taking a multi-enzyme product, or if they are severe in nature, it is a good sign that intestinal candida may be out of control. These symptoms may include any combination of bloating, diarrhea, constipation, alternating diarrhea and constipation, feelings of fullness after eating very little, burning stool, lower intestinal gas, cramping, and an itching of the rectum.

Once this overgrowth has begun to take over the chemistry of the digestive tract, it is now in an excellent position to break out of the intestines and invade other parts of the body.

The first of such sites within the body are the moist mucosal tissues surrounding the external anus. One of the reasons why localized yeast infections occur more often in women than men is simple physiology. The vaginal tract, the most common site for localized yeast infections, is but a short journey from the anal opening. Yeast spores have little difficulty traveling that far. Since the vaginal area is also dark, the candida quickly sets up house and starts to grow.

In females, the symptoms of a localized vaginal yeast infection include burning, itching, irritation and often considerable, discomfort. In males, localized yeast infections frequently manifest in what is often called 'jock itch'. As many men can attest, this is often very difficult to eliminate, as the yeast rapidly multiplies in the moist folds of skin, which are rarely exposed to the air.

These conditions can be very annoying and often uncomfortable, but they will not likely threaten your life or cause severe debilitation. This is because, even though the yeast has escaped the gastro-intestinal tract, it is still classified as a localized infection and has not yet become systemic in nature.

As this condition continues uncontrolled, the candida yeast can move up the genitourinary tract and enter the blood stream. Once in the blood, the yeast can take up residence in almost any area of the body wherein moist mucous membranes provide a friendly site. This route into the internal system of the body primarily occurs in the female since their genitourinary tract is much shorter than that of the male. When males develop a yeast infection of their urinary tract it often results in considerable discomfort, even to the point of forming a coating of white yeast on the head of the penis. The most common method for males to contract systemic candidiasis is through oral sex with a female who has a vaginal yeast infection. The male can actually inhale the yeast spores into his lungs or sinuses, the two most common systemic sites found in men. Once this has occurred, even if the woman succeeds in curing her vaginal yeast infection, she frequently becomes re-infected by her male partner.

Another possible route of transmission for yeast to become systemic is through a compromised intestinal lining. Those suffering from colitis, diverticulitis or leaky gut syndrome frequently develop systemic candidiasis as the yeast spores pass through the intestinal lining into the bloodstream.

Once the candida organism sets up house in various sites within the body such as the lungs, sinuses, and even the brain, the fungus can mutate and develop into more virulent strains, making it difficult for the body to manage.

As the yeast continues to grow, it gives off toxins as a result of its metabolism. These toxins form free radicals within the body and it is the free radical proliferation that rapidly advances this condition from merely annoying to debilitating and often life threatening.

Indications of Systemic Candidiasis

An early sign of systemic candidiasis is abnormal or excessive fatigue. Like many of the symptoms of candidiasis, fatigue can be caused by many imbalances within the body. But if you have had a checkup and everything seems okay, candida is a likely suspect. The fatigue produced by systemic candidiasis can start out very slowly and increase slowly over months of time, so much so that you hardly notice or remember when it occurred. If you go to your doctor, he will run a battery of tests and they will all likely come back indicating that you are healthier than even he is! As the condition progresses, you will become more and more fatigued and irritability will set in. This frustration can often lead to difficulties with other family members as your physical condition continues to worsen.

The next marker or indicator for systemic yeast is a feeling of disconnection with your surroundings. Some call it 'spaciness'. Many of the patients we see at our research centers describe this feeling as being detached or 'out of it'. As this worsens, sufferers say that they have difficulty in remembering things and that their ability to concentrate lessens. After time, making decisions become much more difficult as well, and you just want to, sometimes, shut yourself off from the world because everything is too much to deal with.

The third marker that the systemic candidiasis is spreading is the onset of what is often referred to as adult onset allergies. These are distinguished by the fact that you likely never had any allergies before. They can come on rapidly and you will find yourself unable to tolerate smells, chemicals, and some foods. Even everyday household items such as soaps, perfumes and colognes, which you may have used for many years, will become almost intolerable. Sadly, many patients undergo treatment for allergies and see no relief. This is because the symptoms are not actually allergies in the first place, but rather the reaction to the altering of the body chemistry by the proliferation of the candida organism.

The next phase of this process is what researchers call the 'Universal Reactor Phenomenon'. The allergy-like symptoms that bothered you before have now become so severe and so widespread that it seems that everything is bothering you. Most foods now give you indigestion, gas and especially bloating. You cannot wear any cosmetic with a scent and many of your favorite clothes now give you a rash. Upon analysis, you find that you are having less and less good days and more and more bad days.

The last phase of systemic candidiasis is the altering of brain chemistry to the point where mental deterioration takes place. Patients in this advanced state suffer from delusions, anxiety, depression, violent behavior and even thoughts of suicide. Toxic overload and free radical proliferation have now so infested brain tissue that the delicate chemistry of the brain can no longer be maintained.

Now that you better understand the symptoms that can be produced by candida overgrowth, your real problems can begin. Well-meaning friends, doctors and others will try and tell you how they have handled their yeast infections. They will tell you about the 'yeast diets', the drugs – often with serious side effects, and they will tell you that you just may 'have to learn to live with it'. Let's take a look at some of these myths concerning yeast infections and systemic candidiasis so that you may better understand our program for eliminating this problem, not merely controlling it.

Several years ago a medical doctor by the name of Dr Crook, wrote a book based on the work of another physician, Dr. Truss. In this book, he told of the severity of candidiasis, the almost epidemic number of women and many men who were suffering from this condition, and the benefits from using anti-fungal, anti-yeast drugs, together, with a 'yeast free' diet. While the program was only mildly successful, it did make the health care industry aware of the extent of this potentially debilitating condition.

Today we know that the drugs are only effective in very limited circumstances. We know that the so-called candida diet only helps to reduce the severity of the symptoms but does nothing to eliminate the problem. Sadly, through these myths, many women have suffered from candidiasis for years and have never received the relief desired.

The first problem is with the use of drug therapy for candida. Drugs in these categories are often ineffective once the yeast has become systemic. The action of many of the medications takes place only in the intestinal tract. Of the few drugs somewhat effective on systemic yeast, virtually all of them have potentially serious side effects. In consulting the Physician's Desk Reference, we find that these drugs often come with a very strong warning as to their toxicity. Prolonged use of this classification of medications can produce irreversible liver damage and in some cases fatal chemical reactions.

The next issue is that of the so-called 'yeast diets'. We routinely have many, many women consult our Research Institute, seeking help for their ongoing yeast-related problems. Many of these patients have been following the yeast/candida diets, some of them for years. In virtually every case these patients tell of a reduction of some of their symptoms when on such diets, but should they go off the diet for even one meal, their symptoms return with a vengeance. This proves that the diets really don't work. Remember, you don't eat candida. It is a naturally occurring organism found in all humans. What you eat will not cause candida overgrowth and what you avoid will not take the problem away.

In discussing diet it is important to mention that a diet high in sugars or refined carbohydrates can exacerbate the symptoms of candidiasis since, to some extent, the yeast can feed off of these refined sugar foods. This does not mean that a candidiasis sufferer cannot have an occasional sweat treat. Once this condition is under control, they really do not need to limit their intake of these foods any more than anyone else wishing to maintain general good health.

On the subject of diet and candidiasis, please remember: <u>Eating or not eating any food will not cause or eliminate candidiasis!</u>

In an attempt to find natural methods of treating this virulent condition, many women and men have tried the so-called alternative immune-stimulating products. These frequently contain such things as Pau D'Arco, Goldenseal, Echinacea, Garlic and Caprylic Acid. While these substances have proven very useful in increasing immune function, they will not destroy the candida organism and eliminate the excessive overgrowth. We will frequently use an immune enhancement/nourishing combination in our overall management program, but it is essential to completely kill the candida in order to conquer this condition.

Evaluating the Presence of Candidiasis

The following two tests will help you determine if yeast overgrowth is the likely cause of your problems. Further, it will help us determine whether your candidiasis is localized or has progressed to the much more harmful systemic phase.

This first part lists the most probable factors that can cause candida to explode out of control. It was developed at a leading alternative hospital. For every yes answer, circle the number of points given and add up the total number of points at the end of both tests, comparing your total with the conclusions given.

Test One

1. Have you taken a general antibiotic drug, even just once in the last 6 months? 6

2. Have you taken, at any time in your life, antibiotics for respiratory or urinary infections for longer than 2 months, or shorter courses (two weeks) more then three or four times? 35

3. Have you taken specific antibiotics for acne for 1 month or longer? 35

4. Have you ever suffered from vaginitis or prostatitis or suffered from other problems affecting your reproductive organs?   25

5. Have you been pregnant once?   3

   Have you been pregnant more than once? 5

6. Have you ever taken steroid medications such as prednisone or other cortisone-type drugs? 20

7. Does exposure to strong smelling substances provoke or worsen your symptoms?   6

8. Are your symptoms worse on damp, moldy, muggy days or in damp, moldy places? 20

9. Have you ever had athlete's foot, ring worm, 'jock itch' or any other chronic fungus infections of the skin or nails? 20

10. Does Tobacco smoke *really* bother you? 10

TOTAL OF THIS SECTION   _____

Test Two
Part One

In scoring this section of the test if the symptom is occasional or mild give 3 points, if frequent or moderately severe give 6 points, and if the symptom is severe and/or disabling score 9 points. If the symptom does not apply to you at all score a 0.

1. Fatigue or lethargy
2. Feeling of being 'drained'
3. Poor memory
4. Feeling 'spacey' or 'unreal'
5. Depression
6. Numbness, burning or tingling
7. Muscle aches
8. Muscle weakness
9. Pain and/or swelling in joints
10. Abdominal pain

11. Constipation
12. Diarrhea
13. Alternating constipation and diarrhea
14. Bloating
15. Troublesome vaginal discharge
16. Persistent vaginal burning or itching
17. Prostatitis
18. Impotence
19. Loss of sexual desire
20. Endometriosis
21. Cramps or other menstrual irregularities
22. Premenstrual tension
23. Spots in front of eyes
24. Erratic vision

TOTAL SCORE FOR THIS SECTION: _____

Part Two

Score these symptoms as follows; give one point if the symptom is mild or occurs occasionally, 2 points if it is frequent and 3 points if it is severe or disabling to your lifestyle. As before, score 0 if it does not apply at all.

1. Drowsiness
2. Irritability or jitteriness
3. Incoordination
4. Inability to concentrate
5. Frequent mood swings
6. Headache
7. Dizziness/loss of balance
8. Pressure above ears or tingling sensation
9. Itching
10. Skin rashes
11. Heartburn
12. Indigestion

13. Belching and intestinal gas
14. Mucus in stools
15. Hemorrhoids
16. Dry mouth
17. Rash or blisters in mouth
18. Bad breath
19. Joint swelling or arthritis
20. Nasal congestion or discharge
21. Postnasal drip
22. Nasal itching
23. Sore or dry throat
24. Cough
25. Pain or tightness in chest
26. Wheezing or shortness of breath
27. Urgency or urinary frequency
28. Burning on urination
29. Failing vision
30. Burning or tearing of eyes
31. Recurrent infections or fluid in ears
32. Ear pain or deafness

SCORE FOR THIS SECTION: _____

Add up the grand total of all three tests and compare with the results below.

Scores of over 180 in women or 140 in men: Yeast-connected heath problems, likely systemic in nature are almost certainly present.

Scores of over 120 in women or 90 in men: Localized candidiasis is very likely.

Scores of over 60 in women or 40 in men: Yeast related problems are possibly, contributing to your overall problem

Scores of less than 60 in women or 40 in men: Yeast problems are less likely to be at the cause of your symptoms.

Armed with the results of this very accurate test, you can determine the degree of yeast involvement in your health concerns. With that in mind, let's discuss how you can rid yourself of candidiasis and even systemic candidiasis once and for all.

Controlling and Eliminating Candidiasis & Systemic Candidiasis

The following program, which we have been successfully using at our Institute Centers around the world, for over 10 years, will control the symptoms of candida overgrowth while actually destroy the candida, thereby eliminating the problem completely. The program consists of a two- phase approach beginning by safely destroying the candida organism. The second phase consists of re-implanting the healthy bacteria to ensure a sound and balanced environment in the intestinal tract once again.

In observing the candida organism and in fact, all yeast and fungus, we find that they are anaerobic in nature. This means that they do not survive in the presence of concentrated oxygen. Hydrogen peroxide, the local antiseptic, can kill fungus and yeast on contact by bombarding the spores with concentrated oxygen as the hydrogen peroxide releases into oxygen and water.

It stood to reason that if oxygen were that effective locally, it would do just as good a job internally as well. The problem, initially, was how to deliver the oxygen safely. The common 3% hydrogen peroxide, which you buy in drug stores, contains many potentially harmful contaminants and cannot be taken internally. Our search continued and eventually we discovered 35% food grade hydrogen peroxide – a pharmaceutical grade product that is completely pure.

Early attempts to use 35 percent hydrogen peroxide for medical purposes proved to be safe but somewhat annoying for patients. Even though hydrogen peroxide has been used safely for various medical conditions back as far as the late 1800's, the taste of hydrogen peroxide is almost unbearable, especially if you have to take it several times per day for a prolonged period of time, such as in the management of various chronic conditions.

Note: On your own, you cannot mix pure hydrogen peroxide with anything except water. To do so will release the oxygen and render the product virtually ineffective. Our special oxygen liquid suspension is accomplished via a proprietary procedure, which preserves the integrity of the oxygen content. Information regarding obtaining this product may be obtained by contacting our Institute. (see appendix)

Since oxygen kills the candida organism and since oxygen can permeate every cell of the body, hydrogen peroxide is not only safe but very effective in both localized candidiasis and cases of wide spread systemic candidiasis. In fact, liquid oxygen is the only substance effective on candidiasis of the brain, since oxygen easily crosses the blood/ brain barrier.

Is the use of hydrogen peroxide safe? The answer is a resounding yes, if you do it right. Concentrated hydrogen peroxide, such as found in food grade 35%, MUST be diluted in order to be safely ingested. Further, oral oxygen MUST be taken on an empty stomach, 30 minutes before or 3 hours after a meal. To consume liquid oxygen with food in the stomach causes the oxygen to disassociate too rapidly, most of the oxygen being exhaled before it has a chance to absorb through the stomach wall. Further, the presence of natural bacteria in foods accelerates the foaming of the hydrogen peroxide, which can cause nausea and other stomach upsets. Virtually all of these problems are eliminated when you take the formula on an empty stomach. We do NOT recommend the use of pure 35% hydrogen peroxide in any dilution on your own. The only safe formula we know of is offered by Phoenix Nutritionals and is the same one we use at all of our clinics and Centers around the world.

In order to effectively kill the candida overgrowth, we need to bombard the body with concentrated oxygen for a period of between 6 and 7 weeks. The following consumption chart represents the protocol as we are currently using here at our Institute.

The Oxy Flush Program

Begin by taking one ounce of the Premixed Liquid Oxygen formula, on an empty stomach, three times per day. (an ideal time would be upon arising in the morning, before lunch and again either before your evening meal or just before bed.) You must wait 30 minutes or longer after taking the Oxy formula before eating or drinking anything but water. (Use only Oxy Aloe from Phoenix Nutritionals!)

After two weeks, increase the dosage of the Liquid Oxygen formula to 2 ounces three times per day, on an empty stomach, for a total of 6 ounces of the premixed formula per day. Maintain the 6-ounce per day dose for a period of 4 to 5 weeks.

This ends the cleansing cycle and the killing of the candida organism.

Next it is important to re-implant the healthy acidophilus back into the intestines as follows.

Obtain a bottle of high quality multi-source acidophilus capsules, preferably the highest potency you can find. Take 10 of these capsules all at once, on an empty stomach, once per day. Do this for 10 days. This will restore the natural bacterial balance to your intestinal tract.

For some systemic candida sufferers, the prolonged yeast has compromised their immune system. A classic indication of this is the fact that you catch every cold, flu and other opportunistic infection that comes along. The following program is designed to rebuild, boost and nurture your immune system. These nutrients not only stimulate the immune system into better function but also nourishe the system, ensuring that your immunity is in a healthy state of readiness next time it's needed.

We use a combination of the following immune-enhancing factors:

Colostrum Concentrate

Mycelium Mushroom Extracts

Echinacea

Astragallus Extract

Panax Ginseng

Pau D'Arco Extract

Vitamin C

Vitamin A

Zinc

You must remember that you are not alone and this is not some kind of experimental program. We have been using this exact protocol on women and men just like you for over a decade and with excellent results.

Ladies, if you suspect your husband or significant other may also be contaminated with candida overgrowth, it is essential that they too, go through the program outlined here. If not, you may find yourself being re-infected again after you have been cleaned up by this program.

Preventing Candida Overgrowth from Re-occurring

Now that you are once again enjoying a healthier state of being and the synergistic balance of bacteria has been restored to your intestinal tract, it is important to understand what you need to do to ensure that you don't become affected by this problem again in the future.

If you need to take antibiotics again, for any reason, do so if needed, but always, always, always, re-implant the healthy bacteria back into the intestines by taking high potency acidophilus capsules for 10 days after the last day of antibiotic use.

If you are female and taking birth control pills, be sure and either consume bacterial foods such as yogurt, buttermilk, or take 2 to 4 capsules of multi-source acidophilus every day.

If you should develop a localized vaginal yeast infection, use three ounces of our premixed oxygen liquid together with 3 ounces of warm water and douche, holding the fluid for 5 to 10 minutes, three times per week. This will likely, catch the problem before it has the chance to spread and once again become systemic in nature.

Males, if you should develop 'jock itch', or other fungal type of skin condition. Wash the genital area with a three percent hydrogen peroxide solution, available at drug stores, before and after every intercourse.

Lastly, everyone, regardless of your age or health concerns, should be taking a Full Spectrum Nutrition product, which provides the body with at least the 100+ known nutrients the body needs to maintain health and internal chemical balance.

For optimal absorption and retention consider using a liquid delivery system for your Full Spectrum Product. This will enable your body to better utilize the nutrients at the cellular level.

Protocol Summary

Destroy Candida overgrowth with Buffered Liquid Oxygen

Week One & Two: 1ounce three times per day on empty stomach
Week Three – Six: 2 ounces three times per day on empty stomach

Re-implant healthy bacteria

Use a multi-source acidophilus product @ 10 capsules per day for ten days.
Begin this the first day after the last day of liquid oxygen.

If Your Immune System Has Been Compromised, Nourish & Rebuild With:

Colostrum Concentrate 100 mg

Beta 1, 3 D Glucan 25 mg

Echinacea Purpurea Leaf 25 mg

Pau D'Arco Extract 50 mg

Mycelial Mushroom Biomass 200 mg

Take this combination three times per day for 30 days

Yeast infections, candida overgrowth and even systemic candidiasis, are common occurrences in our environment. Because they produce symptoms that may also be caused by many other conditions, it is important to eliminate the obvious symptomatic causes first. If you have a majority of the symptoms listed previously and your doctor has not been able to find a cause, you might consider trying this protocol. It cannot harm you in any way, even if you don't actually have a candida problem. It may still be of benefit as a cleansing and detoxifying program, helping to eliminate any of a wide variety of low grade virus or bacteria.

If you are suffering from this condition in any degree, take heart, there is hope. Thousands and thousands of women and men before you have followed this protocol and succeeded in conquering their candida problems – you certainly can too.

Controlling Cholesterol & Triglycerides

According to the American Heart Association, more than 100 million people in the United States alone, have high levels of Cholesterol. In spite of this fact or perhaps because of it, Cholesterol, one of the most misunderstood of all substances in the human body, has been the center of both attention and controversy for several decades. Regardless of the amount of discussion concerning this essential substance, there remains, many myths concerning Cholesterol and its role in both health and disease.

Much of what you will read here will be in direct contradiction to almost everything else you have read or heard about Cholesterol. This is because I have looked at this problem as a biochemist rather than as a medical doctor. Doctors look at Cholesterol and see it as the sticky fatty substance that clogs arteries and leads to occlusions and heart attacks. I see Cholesterol as an essential substance, manufactured by the body, to meet daily needs. I agree with medicine wholeheartedly, that excess Cholesterol in the bloodstream can greatly complicate an existing cardiovascular problem, but Cholesterol has NEVER CAUSED the problem. I also agree that excess Serum Cholesterol is not a healthy situation, but I totally disagree as to how to manage and eliminate this problem.

Cholesterol is a normal and essential substance. Why then, does it build up in the blood stream to dangerously high concentrations in some people but not others? The answer to this question will be found, I believe, in the pages that follow. We will not only outline the cause of this problem, but a safe, and simple way to lower Cholesterol, increase HDL and lower LDL as well as manage another type of blood fat far more dangerous to your health and even your life than excess Cholesterol and they're called the Triglycerides.

In the last 25 years, people have been taught to fear Cholesterol as some kind of evil foreign substance that gets into your blood vessels and plugs up arteries leading to heart disease, this, in spite of the fact that there has never been one, single, clinical study to prove that Cholesterol is the cause of ANY form of cardiovascular disease.

Because of this hysterical paranoid attitude towards Cholesterol, millions have gone on low Cholesterol, low fat diets, in a desperate attempt to lower Serum Cholesterol. For the majority of people, these rigid dietary restrictions have only lowered Cholesterol by a few meager percentage points. The end result is that they are placed on one or more of a group of drugs called Statin drugs. While these are often quite effective in lowering Serum Cholesterol levels, their side effects are just beginning to be realized, the worst of which is liver failure. There just has to be a better and safer way.

There will be no boring and bland low fat, low Cholesterol diets; there will be no drugs, many of which are so dangerous that regular monitoring is required with blood tests. Instead, there will be a program that everyone can follow, with very little impact on their present lifestyle.

Once you understand the WHY of something, managing the problem automatically becomes easier. We have freed thousands of people from the stress of desperately trying to 'diet' their Cholesterol levels back to normal. We have freed thousands of people from the risks and dangers of the leading anti-cholesterol drugs, replacing them instead, with safe and healthy nutrients. This can happen for you also.

How Did We Get In This Mess?

For decades medical science has both believed and taught that blood fats, namely Cholesterol were at the cause of what had become the number one cause of death – the myocardial infarction or 'Heart Attack'. Coronary Thrombosis, or blood clots seemed to most often occur at sites in the coronary arteries where lesions and fatty deposits had reduced or cut off blood flow.

In 1974, the actual cause of Heart Disease, the leading cause of death, was finally determined. In the years afterward, numerous clinical studies would confirm the validity and accuracy of this cause.

Many of you will be surprised and shocked to hear that Dietary Cholesterol was NOT found to be the cause at all. It is now established that the studies conducted by Dr. Earl P. Benditt of the University of Washington, School of Medicine in Seattle, which illustrated that Cholesterol deposits on the artery walls were the END result of the mutated cellular deterioration of the artery wall, not the cause of it. In other words, Cholesterol doesn't stick to healthy arteries!

How did this myth start? Well, autopsies on thousands of bodies, mostly male at the time, revealed thick deposits of a yellowish sticky substance adhering to the walls of the arteries in key junctions along the cardiovascular tree. Upon analysis, this substance was found to be Cholesterol. Unfortunately no one bothered to ask the question *why* was this substance there.

There are many, well established risk factors for the development of Heart Disease such as cigarette smoking, lack of exercise, obesity, excess stress and a lack of proper nutrients. Cholesterol should NOT be part of this list. Excess Cholesterol only becomes an increased risk factor after 90 percent of the arterial damage has already been done!

Coronary Thrombosis, the leading cause of Heart Disease is a relatively new medical condition. While today, it accounts for more premature deaths than any other cause, there were no cases of this problem before 1890. Between 1900 and the present time, coronary disease has struck down higher numbers of people, and at younger and younger ages in each succeeding decade.

These statistics are important because we are told that it is the excess fat and cholesterol-rich foods in the 'modern' diet that has lead to this sorry situation. Not so, because our ancestors, certainly before 1890, consumed a diet much richer in fat and cholesterol-contributing foods than in our era of low fat fanaticism, yet heart disease was virtually unknown at that time!

In 1914 the four most common forms of Heart Disease were Rheumatic, Hypertensive, Enlargement, and Syphilitic. By 1930 the four most prevalent forms of this disease were Hypertensive, Coronary, Rheumatic and Syphilitic. By 1950 Coronary Heart Disease had taken the number one position over all other forms of heart disease and has steadily risen to epidemic proportions ever since. In fact, in the last 25 or 30 years – the period of the low fat/low cholesterol craze, Coronary Heart Disease has doubled several times!

Since we can establish that Heart Attacks have been the leading cause of death for only the last 50 years, presently they are killing more than 800,000 people every year, and Cholesterol and the High Cholesterol Diet has been around for eons of time, Cholesterol is not the likely villain.

The Cholesterol Myth

While avoiding Cholesterol is one of the worst forms of food-faddism to ever be conceived, it continues to receive the blessing of the American Heart Association and the American Dietetic Association.

In the 1970's a plethora of clinical studies clearly showed that Cholesterol was not the bad guy we had been led to believe. Dr H. Newland, published in the Annals of Internal Medicine in 1976 stated, *"The lipid hypothesis – which lipids cause arterial disease and that lowering lipids will decrease arterial disease – is no longer viable and should be recognized as such"*.

Since the 1950's hundreds millions of dollars have been spent on study after study, attempting to prove that Dietary Cholesterol can induce Heart Disease in humans. Much of the funding for these studies has come from companies, which manufacture cereals and polyunsaturated fat products.

The fact of the matter is that you don't have to eat Cholesterol for Cholesterol to be present in excess quantities in the body. The body produces Cholesterol from a variety of substances including protein, fats or carbohydrates. Further, the majority of total Cholesterol in the human body at any given time, is manufactured by the body, in the liver.

Cholesterol is absolutely essential to the health and well being of the human body. In fact, excessively low levels of Cholesterol are far more dangerous than elevated levels, leading to a rapid increase in the risk of stroke and gallbladder disease. In 1980 French researchers, studying over 7,000 male workers found that the risk of several types of cancers rose exponentially as total Serum Cholesterol levels fell below 200 mg/dl, the level the Heart Institute calls 'normal'!

Not accepting the findings of the French study, the National Cancer Institute conducted a much bigger study on 12,488 men and women. The results again indicated that the participants with the lowest Cholesterol levels were more than twice as likely to be diagnosed with cancer than those with the highest Cholesterol levels.

Cholesterol is essential to physical health. Some of the functions of this important substance include:

- Keep the membranes of our cells functioning properly. Too little Cholesterol can cause the membrane to become too fluid and fall apart
- Compensates for changes in membrane fluidity, maintaining it within the narrow limits that assure optimal membrane function.
- Manufactures sex hormones, which maintain the differences between the genders.
- Manufactures adrenal corticosteroid hormones, which regulate many metabolic functions within the body, and maintains water and electrolyte balance.

- It is necessary for normal growth and development of the brain and nervous system.

- Vitamin D is manufactured in the body from Cholesterol.

- Bile acids, which emulsify fats, are derived from Cholesterol. Through bile acids, Cholesterol performs vital functions in the entire digestion and absorption of fats, oils, and fat-soluble vitamins.

- It is secreted by glands in the skin, which cover and protect the skin from dehydration, cracking and wear and tear.

The point we need to remember is that Cholesterol levels in the blood are regulated naturally in healthy individuals. In a radical study way back in 1953, it was proven that even if you force-fed exceedingly high amounts of Dietary Cholesterol to people, you could only raise the Serum Cholesterol for a very short period of time, after which the body would make the necessary adjustments, and bring the levels back to normal. Another study, published in the Journal of Mt. Sinai Hospital, in that same year, showed that blood Cholesterol will rise after a person eats a large quantity of Cholesterol, but within a few hours will return to the level maintained before eating.

Remember the egg scare? Every so often the news media bombards us regarding the dangerous practice of eating too many eggs. After all eggs contain Cholesterol and 'we don't want to get heart disease now do we?'. If we examine total egg consumption from 1950 to 1990, something curious is revealed. From 1950 forward egg consumption steadily declined, due to the Cholesterol scare, with a rapid cessation of egg consumption between 1960 and 1970, and again between 1982 and 1994. If we lay a graph of the incidence of heart disease over one of egg consumption, we find that as egg consumption declined, heart disease rose in equal proportions. Why? Well, the egg does contain Cholesterol, but it also contains other factors that help the body regulate Cholesterol from all sources. With this nutrient now missing from the diet, the body could less effectively regulate Cholesterol from all sources. This, combined with other heart protective factors naturally found in eggs, we saw an increase in heart disease. There are numerous studies that show that the consumption of eggs does not raise Cholesterol levels in healthy people.

Another dangerous side effect of consuming excess amounts of these oils is their effect on the liver. As we will soon see, the liver is the organ responsible for regulating Cholesterol in the blood stream. When the liver becomes congested, most often because of toxins or Free Radicals from rancid vegetable oils, it cannot carry out many of its vital functions, one of which is the regulation of blood fats.

Cholesterol Lowering Drugs Are Dangerous

The majority of medications currently in use to lower Cholesterol are of a family called Statin drugs. These include popular drugs such as Zocor, Mevacor, Lipitor, and Pravachol. One of the primary concerns with these drugs is their ability to interfere with, or to deplete key essential nutrients.

While there may be many other concerns, we already know that the Statin drugs interfere with the absorption of fat-soluble vitamins A, D, E and K. This is due to the loss of bile acids, which are needed for proper absorption of these vitamins. Statin drugs may also impair calcium absorption and increase its excretion. This would not be a good thing for older people, especially women, who need to be aware of calcium loss and adequate calcium intake. Iron deficiency, caused by this family of drugs can lead to decreased energy, anemia and impaired immune function. Folate deficiency may also occur with Statin drugs, resulting in fatigue, anemia, elevated homcystiene levels, (a high risk factor in heart disease) anorexia, insomnia, diarrhea, and increased risk of infection.

Another nutrient, which cannot be synthesized in the body when taking Statin drugs is CoQ10. Statin drugs block Cholesterol production in the body by inhibiting the enzyme called HMG–CoA reductase in the early stages of its synthesis in the mevalonate pathway. This same pathway is also shared in the manufacture of CoQ10. In the long run a CoQ10 deficiency can predispose individuals to many Free Radical induced conditions as well as a significant increase in the risk of heart disease, the very condition that these drugs are intended to prevent.

There are further health risks for women using Statin drugs. According to a study published in the Journal of the American College of Cardiology, in 1998, 500 postmenopausal women with Heart Disease were given either a leading Statin drug, or a placebo. The results of the study indicated that those receiving the Statin drug had a much greater incidence of breast cancer, compared with the placebo group.

Of course the biggest concern over the use of Statin drugs is their potential toxicity to the liver. This is why most patients taking these drugs must have routine blood tests to monitor their liver function.

All of this risk with often little benefit. The December 12, 2001 issue of the Journal of the American Medical Association reviews a study, which found that 66 percent of the patients using Statin drugs had far less LDL Cholesterol reduction than expected, and 18 percent experienced no reduction, or even had an increase in their LDL Cholesterol levels. (This is the 'bad' cholesterol)

If you are currently taking a Statin drug, you may want to discuss these issues with your doctor. Certainly, at the very least, you will want to supplement your diet with a good Full Spectrum dietary supplement and perhaps extra CoQ10.

Shortly, we will discuss the many alternatives to Statin drug therapy for controlling Cholesterol levels, but first let's look at what those Cholesterol test numbers mean.

How To Read A Cholesterol Blood Test

Total Cholesterol is usually a measure of HDL and LDL. HDL or High Density Lipoproteins are the 'good' Cholesterol and tend to protect the heart and blood vessels, while LDL, or Low Density Lipoproteins are considered the 'bad' Cholesterol as they are easily subject to oxidation and free radical formation.

Normal levels of Cholesterol should be between 150 and 220 total. 220 to 240 would be considered borderline high and above 240 is considered high and a risk factor for complicating arterial problems. Note that recently, the American Heart Association has endorsed a lowering of the safe levels of cholesterol from 220 to 200. This has done relatively little to change the situation other than the fact that now, millions more of us would qualify for statin drugs!

Another lipid group often measured in routine blood tests are the Triglycerides. Elevated Triglycerides are often a result of poor insulin utilization, excess carbohydrate consumption and lack of exercise. The normal range is 35-130. It is not impossible to have levels as high as 3,000 or above as seen in many diabetics.

Other Factors Involved in Elevated Cholesterol

Since we know that it is the job of the liver to regulate Cholesterol production in relationship to dietary intake, when these lipid levels rise, it is an obvious indication that the liver is having some problems with this regulation mechanism. This can have many possible causes.

Toxicity of the liver is a common problem. Our environment is filled with tens of thousands of chemicals not known to the human biochemistry just a few decades ago. When ingested, it is the liver's responsibility to denature these chemicals and eventually remove them from the living system of the body. For reasons not fully understood, some people are able to do this with greater efficiency than others. For those not so lucky, toxins can build up in the liver, eventually causing complications that can negatively affect the liver's ability to carry out its many thousands of functions, one of which is regulating Cholesterol.

Some time ago, medical doctors and research scientists began noticing a strange connection between those suffering from insulin resistant disorders such as Carbohydrate Intolerance, which leads to Obesity, Hypoglycemia and of course Type II Diabetes, and an increase incidence of elevated Cholesterol. It seems that the percentage of those people with insulin related conditions had a much higher risk for very elevated Cholesterol levels, frequently above 300. We now understand the role of insulin on liver function and when insulin levels are kept under control with diet, exercise and key nutrients to enhance insulin receptor site function, we see Cholesterol levels in these individuals coming down all by themselves.

Lastly, a major factor negatively affecting Cholesterol regulation by the liver is the excess consumption of vegetable oils. As we mentioned earlier the abuse of polyunsaturated oils, which oxidize rapidly when exposed to the air or heat, produce exceedingly high levels of Free Radicals, among them the very ones that have been identified in the degradation of the artery walls, leading to Atherosclerosis. By keeping the use and consumption of these oils to a minimum, we can go far in not only preventing the formation of these Free Radicals, but also in keeping the liver healthy and better able to do its job of lipid regulation.

What About Triglycerides?

If we consider the physiology of the body, as the arteries, damaged from Atherosclerosis, continue to narrow, the larger the particles in the blood, the greater risk of a potential blockage. Consider then, that the Triglycerides are the largest physical objects free floating in the bloodstream. Therefore, their regulation is just as important as that of excess Cholesterol.

Triglycerides are formed from the excess presence of glucose in the body. When carbohydrates are ingested they are all, eventually, converted to the sugar of the body, which is glucose. As glucose levels rise, insulin is secreted from the pancreas in order to lower blood sugar levels. Insulin converts the excess glucose into glycogen, which is the stored form of glucose and places it in the liver or the muscle cell. The body's storage capacity for glycogen is extremely limited. Once these storehouses are full and the diet continues to provide excess carbohydrate, insulin converts the glucose one step further into Triglycerides and stores them as body fat in the fat cells.

Individuals with excess insulin disorders such as Carbohydrate Intolerance, Syndrome X, Hypoglycemia and Type II Diabetes, often have enormously high levels of Triglycerides in their blood. The excess insulin, being produced in response to the excess carbohydrate intake or the failure of the insulin receptor sites, is converting all the available glucose into Triglycerides and increasing the storehouse of fat. This is why those suffering from these disorders are frequently very overweight, while at the same time always tired and run down. Their blood sugar is often low and the insulin levels high.

In order to best regulate Triglycerides levels, a reduction of carbohydrates, especially refined carbohydrates, is necessary. Further, increasing exercise causes the conversion of stored Triglycerides back to glucose for energy. If you suffer from one of the complications of an excess insulin condition, controlling insulin levels through diet, exercise and key targeted nutrition is essential. (Refer to our discussion of diabetes and hypoglycemia previously.)

Normalizing Blood Fats - Safely

If low Cholesterol diets fail to lower total Cholesterol in most people and Statin drugs are riddled with potentially serious side effects, what is the answer to the Cholesterol problem?

There are many nutrients that may be used in a multi-faceted approach to Cholesterol Management. Firstly, factors that will aid the liver in cleansing and detoxifying would be helpful, for as the liver is cleansed, it can better do its job. Secondly, there are key nutrients such as Fatty Acids, Phospho-lipids, Phytosterols, Fiber and specific nutrients, which have shown to both support liver function and aid in directly lowering or removing excess Cholesterol from the body.

By combining these nutrients together with specific dietary modifications such as slightly reducing the amount of saturated fat, eliminating virtually all polyunsaturated oils and increasing dietary fiber, thousands and thousands of people have been able to lower their total Cholesterol levels to within the accepted normal range without the need for potentially dangerous drugs. Let's take a detailed look at the program.

Detoxification

Since Cholesterol regulation is largely a responsibility of the liver, ensuring that the organ is cleansed and free from excess toxic buildup would be pivotal in the process of Cholesterol management. The Fast we have developed, together with key herbal extracts, designed to help the organs of elimination dump toxins into the waste matter of the body for eventual elimination, has been used, with great success, by our Institute for many, many years. We find it often is essential in helping individuals on the road to natural Cholesterol Management. Details of this fasting program may be found in the appendix section in the back of this book.

NOTE: I have used this Fast in many different types of disease conditions over the years. Recently people have been contacting The Institute saying that they cannot find the particular combination of herbs and fiber, which we recommend. You can obtain this exact formulation, sold as **ToxiCleanse**™ from Phoenix Nutritionals, Inc. at 1-800-440-2390.

<u>A SPECIAL NOTE FOR DIABETICS:</u> If you are currently taking oral medications for your diabetes, or insulin by injection, consult with your physician before undertaking this or any other fast as it may rapidly alter your blood sugar. You can also obtain excellent results by using our detoxification formula in conjunction with regular diet. Details for this modified program may be found in the appendix section of this book.

Nutrients That Help Regulate Cholesterol

Once again, nutritional science has come to the rescue for those suffering from elevated Cholesterol. Since this is primarily a liver problem, our program revolves around using natural substances that help the liver do its job. We also use key nutrients, which are responsible for carbohydrate metabolism, which is indirectly related to our problem. Lastly, we use fiber from a variety of sources to help remove excess Cholesterol from the body. Let's take a closer look at these beneficial factors.

Chromium

When excess carbohydrates are consumed, such as provided by the Standard American Diet, they are quickly converted to Triglycerides and stored as body fat. This not only provides the primary causative factor for obesity, but creates an elevation of Triglycerides in the blood stream.

Guggulipids

As we have stated repeatedly in this text, the liver is responsible for producing and regulating Cholesterol in the body, but can do so only if it is functioning properly.

Nutrients that can contribute to assisting the liver in this task are going to ultimately, go a long way in regulating blood fats. Such is the case with the Guggulipids.

Guggulipid is extracted from the gum of the Commiphora Mukul tree that is native to India. There are two primary active Guggulipids. Z-guggulsterone and E-guggulsterone. These compounds work by increasing the liver's ability to metabolize Cholesterol, especially the LDL or 'lousy' cholesterol. This ingredient is very important for those individuals whose HDL to LDL Cholesterol ratios are going in the wrong direction.

These compounds are not new. They have been recognized and used for centuries in the ancient Indian medical tradition of Ayurvedic. In clinical studies, Guggulipids have been proved to lower Serum Cholesterol and Triglycerides as well as lower the LDL and raise the HDL.

One of the many studies performed on humans using Guggulipids alone showed that they could drop Cholesterol levels anywhere from 14 to 35 percent in as little as 90 days. Levels of good Cholesterol

(HDL), increased in these participants by 16 to 20 percent. Overall, Guggulipids were seen to work as effectively as prescription drugs, but without any side effects. In fact the use of Guggulipids at doses 10 times higher than necessary for a positive effect, showed no toxic effects whatsoever.

Pantothine

Pantothine is a molecularly altered form of the B vitamin Pantothenic Acid. This structure change makes Pantothine much more active within the chemistry of the human body and as such, is used in a variety of clinical and therapeutic applications.

One of these is in the regulation of Cholesterol. A pivotal study, published in Minerva Med. in 1990, involved targeting women of perimenopausal age. Since Cardiovascular Disease is the leading cause of death in women, this study is of particular importance. After 16 weeks of treatment with Pantethine, significant reductions of total Cholesterol, LDL Cholesterol and LDL and HDL ratio were observed. Overall efficacy percentage of the treatment was close to 80 percent. Other studies confirm the benefits of Pantothine in blood lipid regulation and have shown its ability to inhibit Cholesterol synthesis.

Since Pantothine prevents the peroxidation of fats, it provides yet another key benefit in the prevention of cardiovascular disease pathology. The current consensus among researchers is that Atherosclerosis, the condition that leads to closing down the blood flow in the arteries, is caused by free radical damage to the inner wall of the artery. These free radicals are believed to be generated, primarily, from the oxidation of vegetable oils either before or after ingestion. Pantothine provides protection from this oxidation process and as such, inhibits the production of Free Radicals at the arterial sites.

Inositol

Another member of the B vitamin family, Inositol or more specifically, a particular type of Inositol called Inositol Hexanicotinate, has shown itself to be another super star in the arena of liver support and hence Cholesterol regulation.

For many years the medical profession has recognized and utilized the Cholesterol lowering effects of the B vitamin Niacin (Nicotinic Acid). The one major drawback to this method of treatment is that very high doses of Niacin are often needed to provide a positive response and at that dose, the flushing properties of Niacin can often become annoying and uncomfortable. Inositol Hexanicotinate combines the blood fat lowering effects of Niacin with the fat burning effect of inositol. By using this nutrient, we get a double benefit without the flushing side effect of pure Niacin alone.

Phytosterols: Beta Sitosterol

Scientists have been searching for reasons why vegetarians, while often being deficient in protein, seem to have a much lower risk for Cardiovascular Disease than others. One of the main reasons seems to be the ingestion of a group of plant alcohols, found in all vegetables, called the Phytosterols.

The average individual consumes only about 200 to 400 mg of these compounds from the diet due to a lack of consumption of fresh fruits and vegetables. Vegetarians, on the other hand, due to larger consumption of these food groups, get almost twice that amount daily. Of all the many Phytosterols, Beta Sitosterol is the most active. There are over 50 published studies using Beta Sitosterol. These studies have shown that Beta Sitosterol substantially lowers blood lipid levels even if there are no major changes in the diet!

Beta Sitosterol works by decreasing the absorption of Cholesterol in the digestive system *and* by decreasing the amount of Cholesterol in the liver. Beta Sitosterol works by locking to the fat molecules consumed and by blocking the fat molecule absorption gates in the intestines. The fats and Cholesterol are then excreted rather than absorbed. Since the liver manufactures more Cholesterol than anyone could possibly get from diet, Beta Sitosterol is an ingredient of choice since it also exercises a positive effect in helping the liver to regulate the total Cholesterol it produces.

By combining Beta Sitosterol with Guggulipids, the benefit is much greater than through the use of either one alone. When used in combined effort, we can expect to see such responses as the binding and excretion of excess free Cholesterol, the blocking of absorption sites in the intestinal walls, an enzymatic change in the liver, causing it to better regulate Cholesterol production and an increase in liver enzymes, which act on the complete breakdown of fats.

Fiber: Oat bran, Apple Pectin and Psyllium Husk

Fiber serves as a carrying agent in the intestines, helping the body to remove waste more efficiently. Such is the case with Cholesterol. Fiber, the bulking agent in the diet, can help remove unwanted Cholesterol from the digestive system before it gets the chance to be fully absorbed into the bloodstream. Recent studies now show that specific types of fiber, namely Oat Bran, Apple Pectin and Psyllium Husk, have an even greater benefit on Cholesterol Management due to a key ingredient found inside them.

Clinical studies have established that not only is the fiber itself beneficial in helping the body mobilize Cholesterol but a powerful ingredient found in some forms of fiber called Beta Glucan, actually exercises a direct lowering effect on free Cholesterol! So once again, we see that not all nutrients are the same. Certain types of fiber are preferred over others for key compounds they contain, which the body can, and does, readily make use of.

Lecithin

I have been in the nutrition field for over 30 years, and during that time, the standard 'holistic' treatment for elevated Cholesterol has always been Lecithin. Available in any health food store, Lecithin often works alone, in lowering Cholesterol significantly. This is because it contains Inositol (see above) as well as Choline, a fat metabolizer, and the amino acid Methionine. Together, their action upon the liver is profound.

For many however, Lecithin alone was not enough to exercise a long-term effect on liver function and hence Cholesterol Management. Today we use a combination of all the active compounds and nutrients listed above. For most people, this provides their bodies with the support they need to safely regulate Cholesterol levels without the dangerous side effects of the popular prescription drugs.

In cases of severely elevated Cholesterol, we often use the above formulation in a double therapeutic dose *together* with Lecithin granules for the first 90 days. Once Cholesterol numbers begin to come down and the ratio of HDL to LDL has improved, we can begin to lower the dose of the formula and eventually stop the use of the Lecithin altogether.

My Protocol For Managing Cholesterol and Triglycerides

By now you should understand that much of the information you have read or heard about Cholesterol and Triglycerides has likely been inaccurate. Cholesterol is not the evil enemy as portrayed by dieticians, many medical doctors and the media. In fact, just the opposite is true, Cholesterol is vital to your life and Cholesterol levels, which are too low, are far more dangerous to your health and life than those, which are too high.

We feel that prescription drugs, namely the Statin drugs, have too many side effects to be considered as the first line of treatment and should only be considered when all other methods of management have failed.

Dietary change can make a difference for many with elevated Cholesterol, but these changes often need to be drastic and hence are difficult to follow for long periods of time. For many, dietary changes provide little or no benefit in lowering blood fats.

The following protocol is the *exact* program we have tested and used on thousands of people, just like you, with very satisfying results. We will outline exactly how we recommend you to undertake this program for the fastest response.

Phase I: The Therapeutic Program

If your total Cholesterol levels are above 220 and certainly if they are above 250, you will want to be very aggressive in managing this problem up front. Unlike most pharmaceuticals, which are started at low doses and slowly increased, the nutritional approach is the opposite. We start with a therapeutic dose, which is quite aggressive, and as the body chemistry slowly changes, we then can lower the dose to a maintenance level that's right for each person's body.

If you fall into this category with Cholesterol levels in the range above, begin with the following program for at least 90 full days. After 90 days have your Cholesterol levels checked again and monitor your progress.

1. Cleanse the liver with the liver, with key herbs and fiber as indicated earlier in this booklet. The formula we use at our research centers is called **ToxiCleanse™** and is available from Phoenix Nutritionals by calling 1-800-440-2390.

2. Begin at once, to take a combination of the key ingredients we outlined. This exact formulation is available from Phoenix Nutritionals, and is sold under the name **Cholest-Eze™**. The therapeutic dose for the initial 90 days would be as follows:

Chromium	400 mg
Guggulipids	400 mg
Inositol Hexanicotinate	600 mg
Pantethine	200 mg
Phytosterols (Beta Sitosterol)	700 mg
Oat, Apple Psyllium Fiber	1800 mg

3. Add Lecithin Granules, from your health food store to give the liver an extra boost. Use the granules rather than the capsules as they have shown to work both better and faster than the liquid. Use one heaping tablespoon of Lecithin granules twice per day. You may mix these in either, juice, a protein shake, or sprinkle on foods such as salads. They will not dissolve as they are a fatty substance so in a drink you must stir and then drink down quickly.

4. Take a Full Spectrum Nutrition formula every day, as outlined in chapter 3. One of the biggest causes of disease and disorder of any kind, within the human body, is chemical imbalance. The body requires at least 100 nutrients every day, including vitamins, minerals, amino acids, fatty acids, phytonutrients from plants and key powerful antioxidants to protect us from Free Radical damage to the DNA of our cells.

5. Exercise. This is often called one of the longest four letter words in the language. It seems that people would rather do almost anything than get a little exercise. Remember that the body was meant to be active, not just with one finger on the television remote control either, but really active. Exercise will help cleanse the liver, which is responsible for Cholesterol regulation and millions of other chemical functions within the body. Further, exercise and a reduction of refined carbohydrates, are key in normalizing Triglyceride levels (see below).

Maintenance Program

Once your Cholesterol numbers start to come down to about 200 or lower, or if you are starting this program with levels in this range and want to prevent problems in the future, the maintenance program will be for you. We suggest that you begin to lower the amount of nutrients in the therapeutic program above, slowly. The body doesn't like radical changes and we must understand that while we are often anxious to reverse our health problems, we didn't get them overnight and they do take time to reverse.

The maintenance dose of the key nutrients, are as follows:

Chromium	200 mg
Guggulipids	200 mg
Inositol Hexanicotinate	300 mg
Pantethine	100 mg
Phytosterols (Beta Sitosterol)	350 mg
Oat, Apple Psyllium Fiber	900 mg

You should be able to get along very nicely on this maintenance dose providing you do not have a genetic predisposition to Cholesterol problems. If so, a higher dose may be needed to maintain proper control.

A Special Note for Triglyceride Control

If you also are dealing with elevated Triglycerides, it is essential that you also make two lifestyle changes in addition to the program above. Firstly, you must increase your level of exercise. Be sure you are doing some form of exercise for a minimum of 30 minutes, three or four times per week. Also, you can bring Triglyceride levels down rapidly by greatly reducing total carbohydrate consumption and eliminating all refined carbohydrates and sugars from your daily diet. Remember, it is excess sugar, in the form of glucose, which is converted into Triglycerides by the action of insulin.

This program has proven to be very effective for thousands and thousands of people. Through new- found knowledge and the uncovering of information locked away in dusty, boring medical journals, we now have a program for the management of blood fats that targets the *cause* rather than the innocent effects. Once the liver is properly cleansed, detoxified and nourished, it can do a far better job of regulating Cholesterol than any man made drug will ever be able to accomplish.

Menopause

Menopause and *'the change of life'* are terms used to describe the transition from a period of reproductive function to one of expanding horizons. The last half of a woman's life should never be perceived as 'the end' or as a loss of 'womanhood', but as an opportunity for her to modify her role in life.

Usually by the time menopause has set in, a woman has raised children and is now ready to experience the many joys and opportunities that the future holds. The time that follows can be joyous years filled with travel, leisure, grandchildren, and time to enjoy all the best life has to offer. Sadly many women face this period with considerable worry and even fear. They have heard the horror stories of the complications both during and after passing through menopause.

Unfortunately, many of these fears are often justified, since innumerable women do indeed suffer from both the physiological and psychological phenomena, which can make this period less than pleasant for some, and down right miserable for others.

If this were an inevitable part of aging, and nothing could be done about it, we would somehow bear up under the load and endure. But thankfully, unlike many issues over which we have little or no control, that is NOT the case here. If we are properly informed and advised, we will discover that there is much we can do to make the transition a smooth and pleasant one.

While many menopausal women exhibit symptoms typically associated with menopause, many others pass through this phase of life virtually unaffected. Therefore, we must deduce that these unpleasant manifestations are not inevitable.

Taking this viewpoint, this section will serve to explain the process of menopause and to offer safe and highly effective solutions to those who need them.

What happens during Menopause?

The average age in which the menopause process begins to occur is usually somewhere between forty and fifty, the most common period being from 45 to 48. Interestingly, research has shown that there is some connection between the onset of puberty and the onset of menopause. If you began to menstruate early, you will have a greater chance of entering the menopause later in life than those who went through puberty at a later age. Further, there appears to be a connection between late menopause and women who have had multiple children.

At some point, as the body nears the end of its reproductive period, the ovaries are supposed to gradually become inactive. This process should be slow and virtually undetectable in the healthy woman, provided her diet is adequate and she is using Full Spectrum dietary supplementation on a regular basis. Even women whose ovaries cease producing hormones rapidly can still be relatively symptom free, providing their health has been maintained.

There are literally thousands of women who go through this process with little or no ill effects. Sadly, there are an equal number of women who do not. For them, this period of glandular change produces distressing or overwhelming side effects.

The most frequent symptom experienced during and post menopause is called the 'hot flash'. This vaso-motor event can occur many times during the day and night and most often involves the face, neck, and upper chest area. The skin becomes bright red and very hot, often producing profuse perspiration and a feeling of suffocation. If the attack is severe, the woman can experience feelings of anxiety and panic, having to 'get up and move around', or 'go out for a breath of fresh air'.

As these hot flashes proceed, they not only become more intense, but the periods of sweating also become more profuse, often requiring a complete change of clothing. Women suffering from these uncomfortable episodes are forever trying to open windows and doors to get some air, while others are cool or uncomfortably cold.

Some of the other symptoms frequently associated with the menopause include dizziness, headache, difficulty in breathing, shortness of breath, and heart palpitations. In more severe cases, mental depression, mood swings, insomnia, and erratic behavior begin to develop. This combination of both physiological and psychological side effects can act as a 'double whammy', taking their toll not only on the unfortunate female, but her entire family and circle of friends.

Sadly, many women go untreated for these devastating side effects either because their doctors do not fully understand the severity of the problem, or they genuinely do not understand how to address the condition.

Of all the possible problems associated with the menopause, the psychological or mental side effects can be the most devastating. The depression, agitation, insecurities, anxiety, and inability to concentrate frequently result in the women entering a destructive downward spiral of loss of self-esteem. In turn, this leads to her feeling that she is 'no longer a woman', or that she has lost her appeal to the opposite sex.

Many women become fixated upon the idea that they have lost their beauty and that it is just a matter of time before they will age, their skin will wrinkle, they will lose their sex drive, and they will become a saggy, flabby, bag of flesh.

This does not have to be the case however. With a proper diet, a regular exercise program, emphasizing strength training, and a daily Full Spectrum dietary supplement program, any woman can maintain her attractiveness and her physical attributes. There is no reason why a woman who makes the decision to properly take care of herself cannot enjoy an active sex life to a very advanced age. Frequently, healthy women remain sexually active longer than most men do.

Of the numerous myths associated with a woman's 'change of life', many may stem from the fact that estrogen is the predominate hormone giving women their feminine attributes. When estrogen is no longer being produced by the ovaries, the assumption is that her femininity is over.

The female body has an excellent backup system called the adrenal glands. They are supposed to take over, producing a hormone similar to estrogen, when the ovaries cease their work. This hormone provides enough chemical support to carry out all of the functions that estrogen would normally perform, except for those which prepare the body for conception.

When women have difficulties and unpleasant physiological and psychological symptoms during and after menopause, the blame can be directly attributed to a failure of the adrenal glands to function properly while serving as a 'back-up' system.

The Cause of the Problem

As indicated before, the adrenal glands, two very important glands situated just above the kidneys, play a major role in the transformation from metabolic regulation by ovarian estrogens to metabolic regulation by 'estrogen-like' hormones. It is the adrenal glands that are responsible for taking over the job of producing these hormones to carry out all of your important biochemical activities, except the menstrual cycle.

The problem with this pretty picture is that many women suffer from moderate to severe adrenal hypo-activity. This is because the adrenals have many responsibilities within the body chemistry, and they often become overworked and undernourished.

One of the biggest jobs of the adrenal glands is to engage the *'fight or flight'* state during periods of danger of perceived danger. We say perceived danger because most of the time when the adrenals are stimulated to secrete these powerful *'fight or flight'* hormones, it is a false alarm and no real immediate danger is actually present.

This over-stimulation of the adrenal glands, by perceived dangers, causes these glands to become exhausted. Repeated stimuli from our environment leads to further and further exhaustion, and subsequent greater inability for the adrenal glands to produce the vital 'estrogen-like' hormones needed after menopause.

If you suffer from moderate to severe symptoms of menopause, your adrenal glands are not functioning properly. This is generally due to the fact that they are continually being over-stimulated by external stresses, which you are not able to mentally or emotionally cope with.

The constant stress produced by a variety circumstances keeps the adrenal glands stimulated. Because of this, they are almost continually in a state of fatigue. During these perceived threatening situations, the adrenal glands prepare the body to either fight for survival or run for its life. Yet, virtually all of these situations are emotional or psychological stresses, requiring no 'fight or flight' response.

These 'false alarms', which trigger a constant adrenal response, keep the body in a state of emotional tension leading to many of the psychological side effects of menopause. There are, however, some physical chemical situations that can further exhaust the adrenal glands.

The Curse of the SAD Diet

Over the past few decades, the American diet has deteriorated into one of mostly sugar, the wrong type of fats, and little protein. This eating pattern has come to be known as the Standard American Diet (SAD). Abbreviated SAD, this eating regimen is truly worthy of its acronym.

The Standard American Diet consists mostly of highly refined carbohydrates and sugars, all of which raise the blood glucose levels in the body, causing insulin to be secreted from the pancreas. This process, in and of itself, does not adversely affect the adrenal glands, but what follows does.

The mechanisms involved in regulating blood sugar include the pancreas and the insulin receptor sites upon which insulin acts. Over time, they become exhausted, causing fluctuations in blood sugar levels. As the irregularities worsen, the individual develops what is known as hypoglycemia, or clinical low blood sugar.

Every time the body's blood sugar dips below normal, the adrenal glands are called upon to produce a hormone called cortisol, which will convert sugar stored in the body (glycogen) back into active glucose, which is useable for energy. This constant demand upon the adrenals further overworks them, reducing their ability to meet estrogen hormone needs.

At the time when the ovaries cease to produce estrogens and the adrenal glands must take over, the stresses and the diet of many women prevent these all-important glands from doing their much-needed job.

When the adrenals are so overworked that they can produce only a fraction of the estrogen-like hormones needed, symptoms of menopause are the result. What are the symptoms of over-exhausted adrenals?

Dry mouth

Circulatory system stimulation – hot flashes and/or chills

Elevated blood pressure

Lowered blood pressure

Hypoglycemia – low blood sugar

Excessive perspiration

Nervousness and shakiness

Anxiety

Mood Swings

Depression

If you take a close look at these typical symptoms of adrenal exhaustion, you will see that they are virtually the same as those of menopause!

Most of these symptoms are the result of an overactive sympathetic nervous system. Estrogen, and later on in life, the estrogen-like hormones from the adrenal glands, are responsible for modulating the sympathetic nervous system. If these are deficient or missing, the problem can accelerate out of control. One example of this sympathetic nervous system response is to force the blood, normally pooled in the interior of the body, to the surface, causing the common hot flashes.

There is virtually no way to control the symptoms of menopause without addressing the needs of the adrenal glands. If you are under an excessive amount of stress or if you are a high strung type of personality, it will be impossible for you to manage your menopausal symptoms and regulate your body without first addressing these issues.

Helping the Body to Transform Gracefully

Since the adrenals are at the heart of the menopause problem, and stress is at the heart of the adrenal problem, we must begin with a discussion of stress management if we wish to achieve optimal results.

Learning to relax is something we all talk about but very few actually practice. Our society, for some strange and perverse reason, almost worships stress. We honor and reward those who can seem to withstand high doses of stress and survive. If we really understood the detrimental effects of stress upon the body, we would reward and recognize those who have learned to manage the stress in their lives rather than those who have not.

All stress is cyclic in nature. Once stress is produced, it alters the body chemistry, causing more physical stress, which in turn causes more emotional stress. Menopause is no different. It is stress, which further weakens the adrenals. If this condition is left untreated, the cycle repeats itself ad infinitum.

Hopefully, you can see the picture. In order to break this cycle, we must approach the problem from two separate angles. First of all, we must manage emotional stress through relaxation techniques and time management. Secondly, physical stress must be managed by adding to our diet specific nutrients, which have been shown to calm the sympathetic nervous system and nourish the adrenal glands.

Managing Emotional Stress

If we sit down a few minutes and take stock of our lifestyle, we can all find ways in which, through a little forward planning, we could reduce the amount of daily stress in our lives.

So often, people try and cram 90 minutes into every hour of the day. Then they cannot understand why they are constantly under pressure and always behind schedule by the end of everyday. Time management is a very important skill to develop.

Another enormous source of internal emotional stress comes from the formation of, and stubborn attachment to, opinions. These opinions are usually about things we see or hear, and our reactions to them. In most cases the opinions we form serve little purpose except to excite our emotional nerve centers, putting more and more stress on our adrenal glands.

If you sit back a moment and analyze just how the many opinions you form, and desperately cling to, affect life, you will have to admit that they do not really serve much purpose. Opinions have never changed anything for the better, only positive actions have. Incidentally, positive activity rarely produces stress because it sets up a free flow of human energy, which can actually energize and rejuvenate the body.

Diet and Nutrition to the Rescue

Any nutritional program that seeks to address and improve the symptoms of menopause must place strong emphasis upon the nutrients involved in stress. Since the adrenal glands are the stress glands, these nutrients can be effectively used to provide adrenal support.

When we think of the stress nutrients, the B-complex must come to mind first. While all of the B-complex nutrients are not directly involved in the stress cycle, those that are directly involved will be consumed in great volume during periods of high stress.

Pantothenic acid, a B-complex nutrient, is the chief stress-relieving nutrient. In the absence of Pantothenic acid, the adrenal glands begin to shrivel up and become filled with dead, inactive cells. Under this condition, the adrenals cannot produce cortisone or the estrogen-like hormones.

So important is Pantothenic acid that even a slight deficiency reduces adrenal function. The more stress you find yourself under, the greater the consumption of Pantothenic acid will take place. It is not uncommon, under periods of severe stress, for the body to consume in excess of 2000-mg of Pantothenic acid per 24-hour period!

The twin stress relief nutrient to Pantothenic acid is vitamin B-12. This essential nutrient is also consumed in much higher amounts during stress. By taking extra vitamin B-12, it not only replaces this loss, but also feeds the nervous system and helps to prevent the sympathetic nervous response so common in uncontrolled menopause.

While adrenal hormones are produced without the aid of vitamin C, the need for this antioxidant nutrient rises during the menopause. When the adrenal glands are over-worked, they are subject to internal hemorrhage. Vitamin C prevents this breakdown of the integrity of the cardiovascular system. One obvious sign of a vitamin C deficiency is the breaking of the small capillaries in the legs and on the face.

We must also consider vitamin B-6 in any approach to menopause. Vitamin B-6 is the universal carrier nutrient, helping all other nutrients in its presence to be better absorbed where specifically needed.

Herbology, the science of plants for health and healing, has made some powerful contributions to the management of menopause. There are many herbs and herbal extracts, which have been used for hundreds of years and remain today, some of the best sources for re-balancing the body chemistry of the menopausal woman.

Black Cohosh is the first herb that deserves our attention. Used widely by native Americans, and indigenous peoples of Central America, Black Cohosh has long been a favorite in the relief of menstrual cramps and symptoms of menopause. Studies show that the use of Black Cohosh, as part of a total program, can increase the estrogenic effect of other herbs.

The next herb of mention is Dong Quai. In Asia, Dong Quai is regarded as the 'female' tonic of choice. Clinical studies conducted on this herb support the efficacy of Dong Quai in reducing and eliminating hot flashes, so often occurring during the menopausal years.

Licorice Root is an ancient herb used for its positive effect upon the adrenal glands. Since the adrenals are at the heart of the solution, Licorice Root should always be included in the management program.

One of the most annoying complaints from women of menopausal years is the drying out of the vaginal tract. This uncomfortable condition frequently leads to a decreased libido and all the self-esteem issues connected with that problem. Red Raspberry, has been used by the ancients to encourage easy labor. Why is this important during menopause? It is because Raspberry exercises a relaxing, lubricating effect on the longitudinal muscles of the uterus, helping the body to reduce the symptoms of vaginal irritations.

Mexican Wild Yam is probably the best-known herb for managing menopause. Creams made from this herb have been shown to increase progesterone, an important hormone group, in post-menopausal women. Many excellent preparations are available.

Although not a vitamin, Lecithin is another important nutrient. This fatty substance, along with fatty acids such as Omega 3 and Omega 6, is essential. It provides the sterols, which are the raw materials, or building blocks needed by the adrenals when making hormones.

Many who suffer from menopause have trouble sleeping at night. This lack of satisfying rest further contributes to the central nervous system irritation and subsequent symptomology. If sleeping is a problem, it can be addressed in several ways through the use of specific herbs.

Firstly, natural calming herbs such as Kava Kava, are highly recommended if you find yourself high strung and anxious. Secondly, if you take Valerian Root an hour or so before bed, along with some calcium, you will fall asleep more easily.

Finally, I recommend the herbs Damiana, Suma, and Schizandra for their long-standing female properties, which include vaginal support and increased libido.

Another factor often greatly affecting the menopause is a lack of protein. All hormones in the body are constituents of protein and a lack of this body building substance can result in overall hormone deficiencies. Everyone needs a minimum of 80 grams of high quality protein every day; you will require more if you are active.

Enter the Phytoestrogens

Absolutely essential to hormone regulation during menopause is another group of nutrients called Phytoestrogens. These substances, which come from plants, are capable of producing mild estrogenic effects. These effects can be greatly enhanced by using a Phytoestrogen product composed from a variety of sources. By providing these estrogen effects, symptoms of menopause can be greatly reduced.

Dietary phytoestrogens and other phytoestrogen-containing herbs, some of which we have already discussed, offer other significant advantages as well.

What About Estrogen Therapy?

I am sure most women have heard about the potential health problems associated with the use of either synthetic or even natural estrogen replacement. The significant health risks associated with this therapy include an increase in cancer, gallbladder disease and the thrombo-embolic diseases, such as strokes and heart attacks.

If your physician determines your need for hormone replacement therapy, seek another opinion. If you discover that you must have this treatment, always insist upon receiving bio-identical hormones, which match human hormones rather than being extracted from horse urine! This will greatly reduce the risks involved with this type of treatment.

The good news is that the plant derived Phytoestrogens we discussed do not carry any of these increased health risks. Therefore, they should be used as the first treatment of choice. Remember, as with nutrients and supplements, Phytoestrogens work best when in proper combinations rather than separately or individually. Currently, we are successfully using Phytoestrogens from flavones, flavonols, flavanones, isoflavones, saponins, and ligans.

Progesterone is another hormone most deficient in women of menopausal years. In fact, it was the late John Lee, MD, who brought the awareness of the power of topical progesterone to millions of women. At our Clinics, we use a topical progesterone cream very similar to that recommended by Dr. Lee. We have improved our formula by adding a carrying agent, which allows for the deeper penetration of the active progesterone to the sub-dermal layers of the skin.

A Word About Hysterectomy

The hysterectomy can bring about all the same symptoms of menopause with additional problems and increased nutritional needs.

There are several different types of hysterectomy procedures. Those having a 'full' or complete hysterectomy enter what could be called 'instant menopause' because the ovaries have been removed. This means that your body has not had the chance to gradually adjust to the hormone and glandular changes.

In this situation, we can further help support the body by increasing the potencies of some of the nutrients and compounds previously discussed. We can also add other nutrients to help mitigate some of the short-term side effects of the surgery. Itemized later in this chapter is an excellent protocol, listing ingredients and potencies recommended for an initial program.

After a complete hysterectomy, two of the big problems are fluid retention and electrolyte imbalance. Potassium can be very helpful in this situation since it will help accelerate the sodium/potassium pump and rid the body of excess fluid and built-up toxins. By using a supplement that provides not only potassium but calcium and magnesium as well, all the major electrolytes are addressed and any deficiencies can be eliminated.

Women who undergo a total hysterectomy, and hence enter 'instant menopause', can be very sensitive to glucose metabolism. When blood sugar levels rise and fall erratically, the typical result is frequent mood swings, anxiety and loss of energy. This being the case, special attention should be given to the amount of sugar and sugar-forming foods in the diet.

A diet consisting of high amounts of these foods should be eliminated. If these dietary changes do not solve the blood sugar level problems, supplementing with aspartic acid, bilberry extract, and the minerals chromium and vanadium, should prove to be extremely helpful.

Osteoporosis

Another serious menopause related condition is osteoporosis. This condition is caused by the lack of calcium in the diet and/or the body's inability to properly digest, absorb, and assimilate calcium. This results in the loss of bone density.

Several myths are associated with osteoporosis. Firstly, we are always told it is a woman's disease. It is not. Men also get osteoporosis; it is just more common in women. Secondly, we are told it is a hormone problem. That is not exactly accurate. However, severe hormone imbalances can accelerate osteoporosis and should be addressed by the methods outlined in this book.

If you do not have severe imbalances and related symptoms, you do not need hormone replacement therapy, or anything else, to prevent osteoporosis. This disease usually begins at a much younger age and by the time you are middle age, the stage for this debilitating disease is already in place.

There are two major causes leading to the development of osteoporosis. First and foremost it is a calcium deficiency. Calcium is the most difficult mineral for the body to absorb and hence many people, especially women, can be more or less constantly in a deficient state. The most common form of calcium sold as a dietary supplement, is Calcium Carbonate. Sold under a variety of brand names, Calcium Carbonate is composed primarily of egg shell and dolomite calcium.

This form of calcium is very inexpensive and therefore very popular. The problem with this form of calcium is that it is also very alkaline, making it nearly impossible to absorb.

In order for calcium to be absorbed into the body tissues and thereby returned to the bone, it must be acidic. Having a pH of 6.0 or lower is ideal. Calcium carbonate has a pH around 11, making it very alkaline. The only way the body can absorb and utilize this calcium is by acidifying it down to a much lower level. Natural hydrochloric acid, produced in a healthy stomach, serves this purpose nicely. The problem is that most people, after the age of 40, no longer produce adequate amounts of hydrochloric acid. This is due to the over consumption of dead, lifeless foods that have been over-cooked, canned, frozen, or otherwise adulterated from their natural state.

This dietary abuse, for years or decades, leaves the body deficient in hydrochloric acid and enzymes. If you suffer from indigestion, heartburn, gas, bloating or belching after meals, you can rest assured that you are not absorbing calcium either.

The second major cause of osteoporosis is the lack of natural stomach acids. If you take calcium carbonate, for example, and you have a hydrochloric acid deficiency, your absorption of this form of calcium will be only about 10 percent. This means that if you are taking a 1000-mg tablet of calcium, you are actually getting only about 100-mg of useable calcium. That is nowhere near enough to prevent osteoporosis.

Therefore, in addressing osteoporosis from a nutritional standpoint, we first use a form of calcium that has been pre-acidified. The combination of calcium we use successfully at The Institute is a 50/50 blend of Calcium Citrate and Calcium Malate. This is the only combination proven in double blind, placebo-controlled studies, to both prevent further bone loss and to increase bone density in post-menopausal women!

To this combination, we add the six co-factor nutrients necessary to carry the calcium back to the bone and increase absorption. They include Vitamin D, Magnesium, Boron, Manganese, Copper and Zinc. Since these nutrients must be present at the same time as the Calcium, we have combined them into one single capsule to ensure absorption.

If we suspect a pH imbalance in the body, we know it would be impossible to achieve adequate calcium uptake. For those individuals, we conduct a pH test to determine acid and alkaline ratios. If the individual is indeed too alkaline, we use a preparation consisting of Betaine hydrochloride (natural hydrochloric acid), and a variety of precursor substances used by the body to build enzymes.

Lastly, we use a synthetic version of a plant compound called Ipriflavone. This nutrient has demonstrated an enormous role in preventing and treating osteoporosis, especially in women.

Ipriflavone prevents bone breakdown, while enhancing the bone-building process. Over 150 studies have examined the effects of Ipriflavone and most all were very positive. In one study, 79 post-menopausal women were given either Ipriflavone or a placebo. After the one year period, the results showed that Ipriflavone was just as effective as estrogen!

The great thing about Ipriflavone is that it doesn't have any estrogen effects, so it will not contribute to the side effects often seen with that therapy.

The Menopause Protocol

In summarizing the many factors, which can positively improve symptoms of the menopause, we offer the following protocol. We start with the basic, or foundation program, and offer suggestions on how to proceed if adequate control is not achieved.

Step 1: The Foundation.

Before beginning any dietary supplement program aimed at mega-dose amounts of specific nutrients, the foundation of the internal biochemistry must be addressed. We do this through a concept developed at The Institute. It is called Full Spectrum Nutrition and it addresses the complete daily nutritional needs of the human body.

Every day of your life you need at least 100 nutrients in order to maintain bio-chemical activities within your body. These nutrients include amino acids, fatty acids, vitamins, major minerals, trace minerals, phytonutrient chemicals from plants and extra-strength, heavy hitting antioxidants to protect the body from free radical damage caused by toxins in the environment. Regardless of lifestyle or physical condition, everyone needs this combination of daily baseline nutrients.

Once this has been attained, we then add the following nutrients for specific menopausal support.

Vitamin B6	25 – 50 mg
Pantothenic Acid	250-500 mg

Zinc	5 – 10 mg
Pregnenolone USP	25 – 50 mg
Lecithin	100-200 mg
Ipriflavones	200-300 mg
Red Raspberry	25 mg
Black Cohosh Root	30 mg
Damiana Leaf	25 mg
Don Quai Root (4.1)	75 mg
Mexican Yam Root	200 - 400 mg
Suma Root	25 mg
Schizandra Berries	25 mg
White Peony Root	100 mg
Hesperidin	50 mg

Phytoestrogen Compound including:

Flavons – bioflavinoids

Saponins – Sarsaparilla, Muira Puama and Wild Yam

Phytosterols

Isoflavons

Ligans

Progesterone Cream Applied topically if needed

This formula is exactly the same as used in all of our Centers. See the Appendix for information on how you can obtain this combination. The formula is called MenoEze.

Step 2: Adjunct Nutrients for Specific Support.

If considerable stress, mood swings, and/or anxiety is involved, we add another high potency stress formula, providing more B-complex with a continued emphasis upon Vitamin B12 and Pantothenic Acid.

This high potency stress formula is one of the founding formulas for many protocols designed at our Institute. This is simply because stress is at the heart of so many health concerns. This very effective stress formula is called StressEze.

The 'golden years' are supposed to be the best years of life. They should be filled with time to expand your horizons, take on projects, and fulfill interests that had to be postponed earlier in life due to other commitments.

In order for you to be able to really 'live' these years to the fullest, they cannot be filled with the annoying and often debilitating symptoms and side effects of the menopause.

By following the guidelines set forth herein, every woman can look forward to enjoying the post-menopausal years and reap the rewards, which they deserve for a lifetime of hard work.

In closing this section, I must remind you that the protocols given here are only as good as how faithfully you follow them. Since they are based upon natural nutrients and nutrient co-factors, they will not, suddenly and instantly, transform your body chemistry overnight. Conversely, they will not put your body and your health at risk, as do many forms of hormone therapy.

You can truly have the quality of life and experience the joy you have waited for. Take responsibility for your health by caring for the only real house you will ever have - the body in which you live.

Addressing the Needs of Men

Some of the problems men routinely face later in life include a diminished libido or sex drive, prostate problems, which include benign prostatic hypertrophy (BPH) – an inflammation of the prostate gland, prostate infection, and of course, prostate cancer. Well guys, take heart; there are solutions for these problems.

Impotence: Rekindling the Fire in the Furnace

The age of the magic pill seems to be upon us. What a great time for an aging man to be alive! The new 'sex pill', sold under many different names, is the greatest – or is it?

With every wonder drug there is often a dark side. The sex drugs are no exception. Sadly, many people who are taking these drugs often should not be doing so. Further, many of the side effects can go from merely annoying to fatal in the presence of other medications. Is there a safer way? Oh yes!

As a man ages there are several factors that can adversely affect both his sex drive as well as his physiology. For example, about 85% of Erectile Dysfunction is caused by organic or physical circumstances while 15% are caused by psychological problems such as depression, performance anxiety, and stress.

Factors Leading to Impotence

Drugs:

Alcohol

Antihistamines (allergy medicine)

Antihypertensives (blood pressure medicine)

Antidepressants

Antipsychotics

Tobacco

Tranquilizers

Endocrine Disorders:

Diabetes

Hypothyroidism

Decreased male sex hormone production

Elevated prolactin

Elevated estrogen

Other Disorders:

Cardiovascular Disease (atherosclerosis)

Depression

Hypertension

These obvious, and not so obvious, factors should be ruled out and/or eliminated before further steps are considered. Once these have been addressed, there are several nutrients, mostly herbs, which can assist in both increasing sex drive as well as improving physiological performance.

Building a Safe and Effective 'Sexual Potency' Formula

Nutrients, specifically herbs, are not only generally safe but in most cases, very effective as well. Following is a list of ingredients you should consider if you are suffering from impotence and lack of sexual drive.

VITAMIN E: You should ensure that you are taking at least 400 IU daily.

VITAMIN B3 (NIACIN): This nutrient will cause dilation of the capillaries, helping to increase blood flow to the penis.

ZINC: Long associated with sexual prowess, zinc is the main constituent of all male hormones. The seminal fluid contains the highest amount of concentrated zinc in the male body.

PABA (PARA-AMINOBENZOIC ACID): This B-complex nutrient also increases specific hormone production.

Helpful Herbs
Fo Ti Root

Gotu Kola Nuts

Aveena Sativa Leaves

Damiana Leaves

Ginseng Root

Rubi Fructus Leaves

Muira Puama Extract

If erectile dysfunction is caused by circulatory problems consider the following…

Dimethylglycine – a potent oxygenater

Octacosanol

Gamma Oryzanol

Ginkgo Biloba

The use of these herbs and nutrients is exceedingly safer than the pharmaceutical choices. These alternatives should be considered BEFORE resorting to more invasive treatments. You can find out more about our very successful formula for this problem by contacting The Institute. (See Appendix)

Another thing to remember is that natural products don't work quite as fast as drugs. You can't expect to take a natural product and be ready, willing, and able in an hour. If you have an ongoing problem, consider taking these nutrients and herbs on a daily basis, right along with the rest of your health-building program.

The Prostate

Every man dreads the pain, annoyance, and embarrassment caused by the problems that surface when the Prostate Gland no longer functions properly. We are all too aware of those annoying problems such as painful burning upon urination, or having to get up three or four times a night, disturbing what otherwise might have been a restful sleep.

Left unchecked, prostate problems and related symptoms continue to increase. Other annoying conditions can develop, such as being unable to sit through a movie or business meeting without excusing yourself to make a trip to the bathroom.

Another area that strikes terror by the mere mention of the word is Prostate Cancer. You need to recognize the early warning signs of this potentially fatal form of cancer as well as your options for both preventing and controlling this condition in your life.

If you have a prostate condition, read this section carefully BEFORE you elect a more invasive procedure. If you have already begun pharmaceutical treatment and it has proven less than effective or the side effects of the medication are less than desirable, consider the protocols outlined in the pages ahead. They have been well researched and clinically tested on thousands of men with excellent results.

Facts about Your Prostate

Your prostate consists of both gland and muscle tissues, covered with a fibrous outer coating. Its glandular function is primarily to produce semen, the lubricating and transport fluid, which carries your sperm from the testicles out through the urethra. The muscular action of the prostate provides power for the seminal fluid, increasing the force of the ejaculation. Another part of its muscular action includes assisting the bladder in the flow of urine.

Anatomically, the prostate gland is located right under your bladder. It surrounds a portion of the urethra, a tube which carries both urine and semen through the penis.

As we age our prostate naturally grows. This is due to the muscular tissue, since all muscles grow with age and use. Prior to puberty your prostate is quite small, about the size of a small marble. After puberty it goes through a rather rapid growth spurt. During young and middle adulthood the prostate is roughly the size of a golf ball. Under healthy conditions, it should remain about this size for many, many years.

Then after about age 50, it begins to grow again. How much it grows and if it becomes inflamed depends upon a variety of factors.

Prostate Enlargement

This condition is the most common prostate problem, making it the number one reason why men over 50 visit their doctor. Medically the condition is called either Benign Prostatic Hyperplasia (BPH) or Benign Prostate Hypertrophy. The use of the term Benign in the name means that it is a condition which is not cancerous. But that's the only good news about it.

BPH can be very distressing and painful. In some rare instances it can lead to a life-threatening situation.

The symptoms of prostate enlargement or BPH, are inconvenient, painful and often debilitating.

Warning Signs of Benign Prostatic Hyperplasia

1. **A weak stream of urine - even though the urgency is there.**
2. **Dribbling after the initial urine stream subsides.**
3. **Frequent nocturnal urination. (getting up two, three, or more times per night)**
4. **Feeling of fullness in the bladder**
5. **Total inability to urinate due to blockage of the urethra.**
6. **Inability to empty the bladder.**
7. **Stopping and starting during urination**
8. **Painful orgasm**
9. **Impotence or diminished libido**
10. **Fatigue**

As we mentioned earlier, BPH is one of the most common complaints of men from middle age forward. In the United States alone, 2 million men visit their doctors every year for this condition. These visits result in hundreds of thousands of prescriptions to be written for medications that not only have a fair amount of side effects, but have been shown to be only about 20 percent effective in the long-term management of the problem.

A Simple Test For Early BPH

Respond to each statement with either a yes or no answer. We will only be concerned with the yes responses.

1.   **Urination has become more difficult than it used to be.**
2.   **Many times I have to 'push' to start the flow of urine.**
3.   **I awake two or more times each night to urinate.**
4.   **When urinating, the stream stops and starts again several times.**
5.   **I have a feeling that after urination, my bladder is not fully empty.**
6.   **It is harder to wait, when I have to relieve myself, than it used to be.**
7.   **My urinary stream is weaker and less forceful than before.**

If you answered yes to just one question on this test, you should pay close attention to signs of additional complications. If you answered yes to two or more statements you likely have early BPH.

This is not a cause for concern. Most all these are early warning signs and you are still in an excellent position of managing and even reversing this problem through the use of completely natural methods.

The Role of Hormones.

When your prostate naturally begins to grow again around the age of 45 or 50, hormones are essentially responsible for this problem. Testosterone, the male sex hormone, reaches its peak between the ages of 16 and 20. After age 20, it slowly begins to decline while the production of other hormones such as Prolactin, Estradiol and Follicle related hormones increase.

Once we reach middle age, production of an enzyme, which has been labeled 5-Alpha-Reductase, increases, oftentimes dramatically. This enzyme converts Testosterone into another hormone called Dehydrotestosterone, a relative.

During our younger years, this hormone is essential. It is responsible for our sex drive and sexual development. Later in life however, an excess of this hormone produces a variety of negative manifestations including excessive body hair, a loss of hair on the head, Adult Onset Acne and excessive growth of the Prostate Gland.

Studies continue to show that those men with higher amounts of Dihydrotestosterone during middle age will have a much greater chance of developing all of the above symptomology, including prostate enlargement.

Medicine to the Rescue but...
Is Life Really Better Through Chemistry???

As soon as the apparent cause of BPH had been identified, the drug companies wasted little time in coming up with a chemical, which could be sold to the many millions of men suffering with this problem. It seemed simple, just find a drug that inhibits the formation of 5-Alpha-Reductase, and everybody will be happy - and rich!

The drug companies never mentioned the tremendously high incidence of impotence and decreased libido as well as numerous ejaculatory disorders in men taking the drug.

To make matters worse, none of these drugs do one single thing to help your body reverse BPH. They may help alleviate some of the annoying symptoms, but the cause of the disease remains and the progression continues unabated.

The Natural Way to Prevent & Reverse BPH

In the protocol for BPH, we find benefit from vitamins, minerals, and especially selected herbs. Let's talk about some of the major players in the natural fight against BPH. Then we'll give you the complete protocol.

Enter the Herbs

Herbology is mankind's oldest form of medicine. In our desperate search for answers to many devastating diseases, we are once again returning to nature, seeking plant derived chemicals for the management of sickness. I often wonder what the state of human health might be today if we had not strayed so far away from nature and a natural way of life.

The first herb that must be considered in any prostate program is known as Serenoa Repens. You may be familiar with it as Saw Palmetto.

We actually use the berry produced by this plant for the magical effects it has upon prostate health. If you remember our discussion of the role hormones play in the evolving process of BPH, then you know that Testosterone alone is not a bad thing, but when it is converted to Dihydrotestosterone we have a problem.

Concentrations of extracts from the Serenoa repens berry actually block the conversion of Testosterone into Dihydrotestosterone! The herb is not only all-natural but it is safe and inexpensive as well. The pharmaceutical industry produces chemicals to try and block the production of the enzyme 5-Alpha-Reductase, causing terrible side effects; nature has given us a natural method of accomplishing the exact same thing with absolutely no side effects whatsoever!

How long has this plant been used for health? Longer than the drug companies have even been in existence! American Indians routinely used the berries from the Saw Palmetto plant to help with genitourinary tract problems.

In recent years, at least 16 scientific double blind, placebo controlled clinical studies have been conducted on the extract of this ancient plant. Every single study has shown that it improves urination, urine flow, reduces pain, and reduces prostate size.

Serenoa repens has been in use in many countries of Europe for at least 15 years. Yet despite this lengthy track record of results and satisfaction, drug companies still suppress this information in the United States. According to clinical studies conducted by Merck themselves, less than 50 percent of the men taking the drug Proscar® evaluated it as effective. By the same token, similar evaluation studies conducted with Serenoa Repens indicated that 90 percent of the men taking it were completely satisfied with the results!

Nature comes to the prostate rescue once again in the form of another plant called Pygeum africanum. A native of Africa, it too has been used for decades in many places around the world to successfully treat and reverse BPH.

One clinical study involving Pygeum africanum showed that 80 percent of the participants reported significant improvement in their symptoms after just 30 days into the study.

The amino acids Glycine, Leanne, and Glutamic Acid have shown to help relieve prostate symptoms such as getting up at night, frequency and urgency of urination, and impaired urine flow. In one clinical study, men using these three amino acids alone, with no other treatment, observed that they had an 80 percent reduction in night time awakenings and over 70 percent of them reported a reduction in the urgency to urinate.

Although we earlier introduced you to several specific nutrients paramount to the treatment of BPH, they are worth reviewing. The vitamins B-6, C, and E are crucial for several reasons. Vitamins C and E are powerful antioxidants, important in the prevention and mitigation of most chronic disease conditions. Vitamin B-6, the universal catalyst or carrier, helps all other nutrients to work better.

Additionally, Vitamin B-6 has a direct effect upon Prolactin levels, reducing them safely and naturally. A reduction of Prolactin prevents the conversion of Testosterone to Dihydrotestosterone.

Lastly, we have a single mineral, but a very important mineral. Zinc has long been associated with male sexual health. This is because Zinc is an integral part of hormone structures and a major constituent of seminal fluid and is involved in the production of sperm.

As we age, a zinc deficiency can lead to impotence and prostate enlargement because the prostate tissue requires Zinc to maintain its health and integrity. Further, adequate Zinc also prevents the formation of Dihydrotestosterone, making it a multi-purpose mineral for total prostate health.

PROTOCOL FOR THE PREVENTION, MANAGEMENT, AND REVERSAL OF BENIGN PROSTATIC HYPERPLASIA:

We have been using the following formula in the management of a variety of prostate problems and it has proven to be very successful:

Vitamin E	150 IU
Vitamin B6	25 mg
Zinc	20 mg
Glycine	200 mg
Glutamic Acid	200 mg
Alanine	200 mg
Lysine	100 mg
Serenoa repens	500 mg
Pygeum africanum	100 mg
Stinging nettle	100 mg
Pumpkin seed	100 mg
Lycopene	20 mg

We all have the ability to return to a healthier and more balanced life. It is an undeniable fact of nature. The decision to make positive lifestyle changes will initiate a metamorphosis within our bodies, enabling us to maintain or regain our optimal health. If you suffer from impotence or prostate problems, know that there are natural protocols available that can help you prevent or reverse these concerns of aging.

Caring For The Mind As Well As The Body

As an ever-increasing number of baby boomers age, society is having to face greater challenges with age-related disorders. Chronic degenerative diseases are on the epidemic rise, each caused, at least in part, by changes in the delicate biochemistry of the human body, from years of abuse and neglect. Poor diet, lack of exercise, toxins and poisons in our environment, and age itself, all begin to take the toll of decades of assault.

When we consider the deterioration of the aging human body, we must realize that this process is taking place in the brain as well as in the body itself. Brain chemistry, the ability of the brain to function rapidly, to recall information quickly, and other cognitive functions, slow with aging.

As brain chemistry changes, the brain's ability to perform in a optimal manner begins to break down. Other, outside factors, can also contribute to the deterioration of the brain. Inactivity, not using the brain, is a big contributing factor. It is often said 'use it or lose it.' This often applies to brain function. As we age, we all too often lose interest in the world around us. Staying interested in life around us is essential to being able to remember what happens.

Stress is another key factor in memory. Excess stress can so alter the ratios of key brain chemicals that the brain can almost shut down. How many times have you been under excess stress, only to find out, after a time, that you just can't remember anything anymore. Fortunately, the body has built in mechanisms to protect the delicate circuitry of the brain from overloading. Managing stress is key in the pursuit of optimal health, both physical and mental.

In the last decade alone, we have learned more about brain chemistry and age-related memory loss than in all the decades past. Once again, nutrition and natural substances come to the rescue in helping to prevent and even reverse these conditions of brain function, just as they have proven themselves to be the optimal approach for the prevention and even reversal of dozens of other chronic diseases.

While, no doubt, there is still much we can and will learn about the human brain, there is enough well established, documented information that everyone can now take positive steps to preserve and reverse the effects of aging on their brain function.

What is Memory?

In an obvious sense, memory is the ability to recall information from events and experiences in our past. In a more complex sense however, that ability to recall information requires a complex and intricate process, involving many chemicals. The brain stores memories in short-term and longer-term locations.

When memory begins to slow or fail, it is most often noticed in the short-term department. When we are over-tired, over-stress etc., it is also the short-term memory that seems to suffer first. How many times have you struggled to remember a telephone number, or someone's name you met just a few days ago? You just know you know the number or the name, but you just can't quite remember it. This happens to all of us, at one time, or another, but when it begins to be frequent or consistent, then it's time to do something about it.

Short-term memory relies often on the element of concentration. If you call the information operator and ask for a telephone number, we often concentrate on each numeral in the number in order to get the order straight when redialing. When we study for tests and exams, we cram the information, concentrating and trying to repeat the information in our heads, over and over again in the hopes of committing it to memory. For many, this process works, for others it is less effective.

The brain can be compared to a large office filing cabinet or if you will, the hard drive on your computer. Virtually everything that has happened to you, everything that you experienced, learned, and committed to memory, is stored somewhere in the seemingly infinite storehouses of the human brain. To illustrate why we can remember some things for long periods of time and not others, you might say that if, at the time of the experience, it was perceived as important by the brain, it labels the file the information is in, making retrieval easier later on. Much of the information we intake, we view as relatively unimportant past its present moments use, hence we don't bother to label it, but it is simply filed away unmarked. This, makes it much more difficult to find later on, should we try and remember or recall the information.

Memory works throughout our brains, by a very complex process involving billions of neurons, which exchange information and transport that information from one portion of the brain to the other. This process involves many key brain chemicals, which must concentrate and then break down in order to complete the information transport. Each neuron has small projections, called dendrites, which act like miniature antennae, receiving impulses from other neurons. Extending from one end of each neuron is a large axon, which is responsible for conducting nerve impulses to the dendrites of other neurons. These axons can be short or can extend for three feet or more. Each axon is protected by a layer of insulation called myelin, or the myelin sheath.

In order for information to be stored or retrieved, a microscopic gap is necessary to control and change the information or the impulses. This gap is called the synapse. The Messages or information traveling in to or being retrieved from, storehouses, travel down the axon until they reach the point of synapse, where they need specific chemicals, called neurotransmitters, to build a bridge over the gap or synapse, allowing the information to be transferred to the next neuron.

It is at this point of synapse that memory can either be rapid, sluggish, or fail altogether. The speed with which memories are retrieved is largely dependent upon the amount of available neurotransmitters, or chemicals needed to build the bridge or gap between neurons. As we age, our bodies often are unable to make adequate amounts of specific neurotransmitter chemicals and memory and even the thought process itself begins to slow down.

Reasons Why We Can't Remember

Short-term memory can fail us intermittently, at almost any time in our lives. Factors that can impair the brains ability to recall information can play a part in our lives without respect to age. The reason why we seem to notice a loss of memory more often later in life is due to the additional factors that accompany the aging physical body, which are not present at a younger age.

Stress, for example, can be a detrimental factor at any age. Even small children can be over-stressed to the point where it affects their cognition and memory patterns temporarily. Other factors, such as inactivity, chemical changes in the brain, and simple aging itself, compound matters as we grow older. Let's take a look at some of these key points and see how they can affect the way your brain functions.

Age

As we grow older, the body is unable to carry out repairs and replacements as effectively as in earlier years. The body can be likened to an automobile, in that, as the car gets older, it not only requires more maintenance to keep it running, but it doesn't perform as well as when it was newer.

We are living in an age where more people are becoming health conscious than ever before, we exercise, try and watch what we eat, at least much of the time, and now, for the first time in history, over 50 percent of the population takes some form of dietary supplement! In spite of these positive trends, very little is done to help preserve and protect the functioning of the brain. Just as with the body, the delicate biochemistry of the brain needs to be nourished. Today, thanks to great strides in the bio-medical field, we have isolated not only the active chemicals responsible for the synapse process, but also the nutrient precursors necessary for the body to manufacture these important chemicals in adequate amounts.

Inactivity

There is an old saying, 'what you don't use nature will take away'. We usually think of this in physical strength, meaning that if you don't exercise your muscles, they will atrophy. Well, the same can hold true with the brain. It wants to think and be active! Sadly, as many of us age, we become increasingly disinterested in the world around us, often living in the past, fondly referring to it as the 'good ol' days'. This lack of mental stimulus causes the brain to shut down many of the neurological pathways, simply because they are not being used. If this goes on for prolonged periods of time, many of these pathways are permanently lost.

I have a good friend who is a retired physician and every day he rides his stationary bike for 45 minutes to exercise his body. He adds one further element however to the workout. While he rides the bike he works crossword puzzles! He says that in this way he can work his mind as well as the body – pretty good thinking.

Sadly, for most people, especially as we grow older, the biggest and often the only source of stimulation is the television set. The TV does not require us to think or even respond, we simply turn it on and sit there while it entertains us. This leads to less and less use of the brain neurons, deepening the problem of a lack of mental acuity.

Everyone should make an effort to be interested in something, a combination of hobbies and an interest in current affairs in some manner. Staying in touch with reality or the current affairs is important to help us remain in the present moment, which brings me to our next point.

Not Being in the Now

There is an interesting concept in life that many of us never really think about, that being the fact that everything that ever happens, to us or someone else, only occurs in the now – the present moment.

Initially, one might think about taking issue with that statement, citing examples of things that took place in the past or plans and appointments that will take place in the future. The fact is, that past and future are really figments of our imagination. Everything that happens to you, in fact everything that ever happens, happens in the NOW.

As an example, I was giving a lecture to a group recently, and when I made that statement, a man raised his and said that he disagreed because tomorrow was garbage day and he will have to take the trash cans out tomorrow morning. I told him to be patient and wait until tomorrow and just as he was wheeling the trash to the curb, take note of when he is doing that. He will find that he is doing it NOW. We can't do anything tomorrow or at any other time in the future because when tomorrow, or next week or next year arrives and we actually do whatever it is we had planned, it will be now again!

Stop and take a few moments to think about how often we are thinking and being either in the past or anticipating the future, and how little time we spend being in the present moment. Well, if we are somewhere other than the present moment and everything happens in that moment, is it any wonder we can't remember what happened! We simply weren't present when it happened.

It is no secret that emotional disorders make up the majority of human ills today. This is evidenced by the fact that of the top 10 drugs sold in civilized nations, 8 of them are either anti-anxiety, anti-depressants or sleeping medications. The fact remains that depression, regrets and remorse come from living in the past. Anxiety, fear, and apprehension come from obsessing over the future that hasn't arrived yet.

Unmanaged Stress

Remember our discussion of the chemicals of the brain called neurotransmitters? These chemicals are greatly affected by chronic stress and the response cycle it can produce. Excess stress can slow or shut down the transport of glucose to the brain, without which, brain cells cannot function. Stress depletes nor epinephrine, a key and essential brain neurotransmitter, responsible for storing memories.

Stress increases the body's need for proteins. Stress depletes key nutrients, especially vitamin C and the mineral zinc. And if that was not enough, stress produces hormones that accelerate the overall aging process, including that of the brain.

Chemical Changes

When we speak of accelerating aging, reductions in the production of neurotransmitters, etc., we are talking about the chemistry of the brain. Every one of the factors affecting memory that we have discussed so far, such as aging, stress, inactivity, etc., in their own way, disturb, or alter brain chemistry. In addition to these there are many outside influences, which can alter both the chemistry of the body as well as the brain or mind.

One of the biggest factors affecting our overall health, including brain health is what we ingest. A diet of dead lifeless foods filled with over-refined nutrient deficient calories robs the body of dozens of key nutrients that it needs to maintain biochemical balance. Excess alcohol consumption can literally fry brain cells. Cigarette smoking produces so many chemicals that enter the body through the lungs and if the liver cannot rapidly filter them out, stay in the body causing everything from genetic mutation to cancers of many types.

Prescription Medications

Many groups of drugs, routinely prescribed, can make you feel unfocused, slowing down recall time and making both concentration and paying attention difficult. Over time, some of these medications can have lasting negative affects on the brain and our ability to rapidly recall short and medium term memories.

Typical groups of drugs that can cause cognitive difficulties would be drugs for sleep, anxiety and depression such as the benzodiazepines. Other classes of drugs of concern would be antihypertensive agents, sedating drugs, antipsychotic drugs, opioids, digitalis, anti-Parkinsonian drugs, antidepressants, and corticosteroids.

If you are taking any medications from one of these groups and you feel your ability to think and remember is being compromised, discuss this concern with your doctor as soon as possible. You can't in many cases, simply stop the medications abruptly yourself. Be sure you work with your doctor in this matter.

We can now see that there are many factors both internal and external that can affect our brain chemistry and our ability to reason and remember. Let's summarize these points:

MONITOR YOUR ALCOHOL INTAKE – one cocktail or two glasses of wine, preferably red is healthy

DON'T SMOKE CIGARETTES! – give up if you are already smoking.

STRENGTHEN YOUR IMMUNE SYSTEM – a diet of whole foods and regular exercise will help

NEVER STOP LEARNING – learning and experiencing newness keeps the brain producing new dendritic spines

LEARN THE SIDE EFFECTS OF YOUR MEDICATIONS – if your medications can affect brain chemistry and you notice symptoms, discuss this matter with your doctor right away.

Since the area of biochemistry and nutrition are specialties of mine, we will be discussing some of the most promising nutrients for brain function support and memory recall in just a bit, but first, let's take a little self-test and see how you score.

Self-Test For Cognitive Function and Memory

Answer each of the following questions with either yes or no.

1. Do you walk into a room and forget why you are there?
2. Do you forget the names of your friends if you haven't seen them for awhile?
3. Do you often misplace your glasses, keys, pens, etc.?
4. Do you forget telephone numbers, often before you can hang up from information and dial the number?
5. Do you forget important appointments?
6. Do you find it difficult to concentrate for even an hour?
7. Do you have problems remember things that happened as recently as yesterday?
8. Do you have difficulty remembering if you have performed routine tasks such as locking doors, shutting windows or turning off appliances?
9. Do you forget birthdays and anniversaries of people you know rather well?
10. Do you frequently repeat yourself?
11. Do you frequently forget the point you are trying to make in a conversation?
12. In order to feel mentally sharp and alert, do you need to rely on caffeine?

If you scored 3 to5 yes answers, it is likely that you have some short to medium term memory problems

If you scored 6 or more yes answers, it is very likely that you are suffering from memory deprivation caused by one or a variety of influencing factors.

Now, let's test your ability to think and concentrate:

1. Do you have trouble completing sentences?
2. Do you spend a lot of time going through documents or books looking for things?
3. Are you becoming more disorganized and less efficient?
4. Do you often have trouble spelling familiar words?

5. Do you have trouble learning new things or find learning frustrating?

6. Are you less coordinated than before?

7. Do you easily get lost when driving to a new location?

8. Do you find yourself having to re-read sentences and paragraphs to get the meaning?

9. Do you find it increasingly more difficult to do more than one thing at a time?

10. Do you have trouble concentrating if there are even moderate distractions around?

11. Do you get lost, even when you are driving somewhere you have been before?

12. Do you feel it takes you longer to learn and grasp new things that it did before?

If you scored 3 to5 yes answers you may have mild problems with cognition and concentration.

If you scored 6 or more yes answers, you very likely have problems with cognition and concentration.

Now What?

What if you scored higher than you would have like on our little quizzes? Does that mean that you are becoming senile? Does that mean you are a candidate for Alzheimer's? Probably not.

The vast majority of people who suffer from the little annoyances pinpointed in our quizzes, have nothing more than an imbalance of brain chemistry, usually the neurotransmitters, depleted by one or more of the many possible causes discussed earlier.

The good news is that nutrition can come to the rescue and in most cases, completely reverse short to medium term memory problems. Even as recently as the past decade, science has made tremendous strides in identifying the key neurotransmitters in the brain responsible for memory and cognitive function and isolated the natural nutrients that the brain needs to manufacture and maintain the delicate balance of the essential brain chemicals. Let's look at some of the more promising nutrients.

Nutrients to Support Brain Function and Memory

KEY AMINO ACIDS – While there are several amino acids involved in the formation of neurotransmitters in the brain, two stand out as being important to memory. Firstly

Glutamine, which is the precursor of a key neurotransmitter called GABA, can improve the clarity of thought and increase mental alertness. GABA is the calming neurotransmitter, so those who are also troubled with agitation and stress, will benefit from this amino acid. The next amino acid is Tyrosine. Tyrosine is needed for the brain to manufacture the neurotransmitter dopamine. Dopamine deficiency in the brain can lead to such symptoms as obesity, food cravings, depression, mood swings, diabetes, binge eating, and an inability to effectively handle stress. You can now see that increasing dopamine levels in the brain can help with more than memory, it can improve your mood and make weight loss easier! To ensure maximum absorption and uptake across the blood/brain barrier, amino acids should always be taken with a little vitamin B6, which is the carrier nutrient for amino acids.

GINKGO BILOBA – This herbal extract from the ginkgo tree is one of the most important natural substances for increasing circulation and oxygenation to the brain. The use of ginkgo is well established with over two hundred medical studies having been published in peer reviewed medical journals. Many of these studies have been able to establish an increase in cognitive abilities and short-term memory recall. Another plus for ginkgo is that it tends to work very rapidly, often in as little as a few days. Mega doses of ginkgo have produced increases in short-term memory in as little as an hour! Of all the nutrients we have for brain function, ginkgo shows some of the greatest possibilities for the management and prevention of Alzheimer's.

LECITHIN – This fatty substance, derived from soy, provides many supportive substances for healthy brain function, in fact, it is often called the 'brain food'. Lecithin contains high concentrations of a substance called phosphatidyl choline, which is the material the brain uses to manufacture acetyl-choline, the primary neurotransmitter of thought and memory. In early stages of memory decline, lecithin can be of significant benefit. In addition to supporting brain function and memory, lecithin is also very beneficial to the liver, helping it to detox and to regulate the production of other essential fats such as cholesterol. In order to obtain maximum benefits from lecithin, we use a concentrate, which isolates the active components in the lecithin, which are key to memory recall. In order to ensure that these co-factors are absorbed and utilized, it is important to take the nutrient DMAE (dimethylamine ethanol) together, at the same time.

DMAE – A rather recent player in the brain nutrient arena, DMAE helps to absorb and produce acetylcholine when it is combined with phosphatidyl choline, derived from lecithin. DMAE has a direct effect on memory, especially supporting short-term memory function and recall. In numerous clinical studies, DMAE was found to be as effective for improving short-term memory as any of the common pharmaceuticals. Additional benefits of DMAE are improved moods, greater energy and a heightened sense of well-being. Since DMAE can be stimulating, it is often used in children with hyperactivity disorders as it is much safer than most of the medications in current use.

VINPOCETINE – The major benefits of this nutrient is its ability to increase brain oxygen levels, glucose metabolism in brain cells and to protect against free radical damage generated by toxins in the brain. Another exciting function of this herbal extract is its ability to enhance the communication between neurons within the brain. The result of this is faster recall of stored information in the brain, which improves the short-term memory of the user. In several studies, vinpocetine has demonstrated its ability to improve memory. Within a very short period of time, those in the study noticed a significant improvement in their memory and their ability to recall information accurately.

HUPERZINE A – Another herbal extract, huperzine A comes from a rare moss, which has been used by Far East healers for many centuries. The active ingredient in the moss plant, huperzine A has the ability to sharpen both cognitive function and memory. Researchers believe that it can also help to prevent the onset of Alzheimer's in the early stages. The mental benefits associated with huperzine A appear to stem from the extracts ability to prevent the breakdown of acetylcholine, the chemical essential to memory function.

BACOPA – Another herbal extract, this time originating in India, may be found in the ancient books of Ayurvedic medicine as a treatment for memory loss, epilepsy and as an antioxidant. Bacopa has been used for centuries to support clear thinking and enhance memory function. Clinical studies on this herb support its ability to improve brain function, increase concentration, and to protect the delicate synaptic functions of the nerves in the hippocampus, the seat of memory in the brain.

CHOLINE – A B complex vitamin, choline is the precursor for many brain chemicals, the most important of which is acetylcholine, which is essential for proper transmission of impulses from one cell in the bran to another. Choline improves the transmission of memory impulses from one neuron to another. Since our brain is unable to manufacture this essential raw material, it is imperative that we get adequate supplies from either diet or supplementation. The Standard American or industrialized Diet (SAD) rarely provides adequate supplies of any nutrient, choline included. This makes supplementation of this key precursor very important.

BORON- Simply put, boron is responsible for maintaining the electrical activity of the brain. A deficiency of this trace mineral causes sluggishness and you react slower and are less alert. A deficiency of boron also causes poor performance of tasks involving eye-hand coordination, manual dexterity, attention, and short-term memory. Each of these abilities is governed by the bio-electrical system of the body and the heart of this bioelectrical activity may be found in the brain and nervous system.

GABA – GABA (gamma-aminobutyric acid) is one of the few neurotransmitters that can be manufactured and taken orally with benefit. GABA exercises the calming, stabilizing effect on brain function. It is essential for the 'high strung' person who finds it difficult to relax and settle their brain function. GABA controls the brain's rhythm so that you can function at a steady moderate pace, rather than live in extremes of over-stimulation or lethargy. This balancing is essential to optimal brain function in many ways. It creates and receives electrical impulses in a smooth flow across membranes. The end result of the imbalance of electrical impulses, which can come in short sudden bursts when GABA is deficient, is the negative impact on your emotional well-being.

PHOSPHATIDYLSERINE – In some ways, we have saved the best for last. Of all the memory, brain enhancing nutrients currently known, phosphatidylserine is probably the single most powerful agent there is. There are, presently, dozens of clinical studies supporting the effectiveness of phosphatidylserine in a wide variety of supportive brain functions. College students have long used phosphatidylserine when cramming for exams in school as it improves the ability to learn and recall lists of words and pages of textual information. One study showed that phosphatidylserine improved attention, memory and mood. Another study, using patients with varying degrees of dementia, living in nursing homes, all showed a significant improvement in memory. Further, it was noted that this nutrient may make elderly people more receptive to environmental stimuli, which in and of itself would not only increase recall, but help them to adapt to their environment easier. Currently, there is ongoing research into the effects phosphatidylserine may have on both preventing and managing Alzheimer's disease. While there is still no evidence that even mega doses of the nutrient can actually cure the disease, prevention still remains our best route of approaching the condition.

Our Program for Improving Memory and Cognitive Brain Function

In addition to the areas previously discussed, you can also use Targeted Nutrition to help sharpen and improve your memory.

The current formula we are using at our Centers around the world is as follows:

FULL SPECTRUM NUTRITION – Designed to provide the body with all the 100+ nutrients it needs on a daily basis. If your multiple does not contain at least 100 nutrients you are not getting the maximum benefit from your supplementation program.

TARGETED NUTRITION FORMULA – This formula provides all of the known key nutrients and herbal extracts for proper brain function and memory enhancement.

Vitamin B 6	10 – 20 mg
Vitamin B 12	200 mcg
Pantothenic Acid	25 mg
Huperzine A	400 - 800 mg
Choline	150 – 300 mg
Vinpocetine	15 – 30 mg
DMAE	100 – 200 mg
Ginkgo Biloba	50 –100 mg
Lecithin Concentrate	300 – 600 mg
Bacopa	15 – 30 mg
Glutamine	200 – 400 mg
Tyrosine	100 – 200 mg
GABA	250 – 500 mg
Phosphatidylserine	20 –40 mg

The above formula, as used in our Centers, is available in many fitness centers and from individual nutrition advisors. If you should have trouble finding this formula, please feel free to contact our offices at 1-888-454-8464 for a referral.

In closing, it is said that a ' mind is a terrible thing to waste' and I couldn't agree more! I could also add that 'a mind is a terrible thing to lose'! As we age, functions of body and mind tend to decline, but we live in a great time wherein we can take positive steps to preserve and protect both.

The key of course, is that you have to actually do something about it, it will not come to you by itself. If you find you have trouble remembering to do the things in your life that are good for you, all I can say is that is the first sign that you need a memory formula! Take care of what you have today and you will likely still have it tomorrow.

I have highlighted several of the key health challenges of greatest concern to most people. It is my hope that this information leads you to taking the steps necessary to prevent, manage or even reverse these conditions. Many thousands have successfully done so before you.

In the next chapter we will provide you with a virtual encyclopedia of health problems and offer you a protocol of natural substances, which have been proven, by numerous clinical studies, to be both safe and effective in the management of these concerns.

The Nutritional Protocols

CHAPTER 5: NOW THAT YOU HAVE A GOOD UNDERSTANDING of how simple lifestyle changes in your diet, a little exercise and a Full Spectrum dietary supplement can dramatically increase both the quality and quantity of your life ahead, this chapter will focus on targeted nutrients for specific health challenges.

We have applied the concept of the Trilogy of Good Health, made easy, to each of these health conditions and offer you suggestions on how diet, exercise and key supplements can prevent, improve, manage or even reverse these problems.

What follows, is one of the most current and complete Nutraceutical Pharmacopoeia currently available. The recommendations given for each condition have been carefully researched and are, in many cases, the result of years of personal successful application with individuals just like you.

When reading through specific conditions, you may wonder why certain recommendations you may have read about are missing.

In many cases, it is because I could not find sufficient clinical data to support their use. I have tried to include only those recommendations for which there are clinical studies, trials or usage. By so doing, I can assure you that the suggestions made are both safe and effective.

Over time of course, as science progresses, there will be legitimate additions to these protocols and they will appear in subsequent editions of this book.

The protocols that follow are in alphabetical order, making them easy to access and refer to.

Interpreting the Protocols

The protocols that follow MUST be taken with a Full Spectrum nutrition program as outlined in previous chapters. The supplementary recommendations are to be taken *in addition* to a base-line Full Spectrum nutritional program.

Reference Range

In many instances, you will see a range of potency for a specific nutrient (i.e. Vitamin C- 2 to 4 grams). This represents the range of dosage used in clinical studies for a specific condition.

I have provided this reference range so that you will know what the minimum effective level is as well as the maximum safe upper dose.

The Trilogy of Good Health In Application

Since diet and exercise also often play a pivotal role in both the prevention and management of health conditions, in each case, I have provided dietary recommendations and exercise suggestions, if any, which have shown to benefit the particular condition.

Abscess

An abscess is a localized infection that has become encapsulated. They are frequently treated with antibiotics and occasionally they need to be opened or removed surgically. The use of antibiotics destroys B Vitamins and the natural bacteria in the gut. These bacteria must be replaced to maintain digestive system health. Emphasis should also be placed upon immune enhancement to ensure that these localized infections are minimized in the future.

Full Spectrum Nutrition Plus:

Immune Enhancing Factors

Collostrum Concentrate	100mg
Mushroom Mycelial Biomass	200 mg
Beta- 1,3-D Glucan	50 mg
Echinacea Purpurea Leaf Ext.	25 mg
Astragalus Ext.	50 mg
Pau D'Arco Ext.	50 mg

The Immune Enhancing combination may be given every two hours for several days during acute infection.

Zinc Gluconate	60 mg per day
Vitamin C	1-3 grams per day

If antibiotics are used add multi-acidophilus capsules in order to replenish the 'good' bacteria throughout the digestive system:

Multi-acidophilus	10 capsules per day for 10 days

EXERCISE: Aerobic or endurance exercise detoxifies the body of poisons

DIET: A diet of whole foods with emphasis upon fresh fruits and vegetables

Acidosis

A condition of excess acidity in the body, Acidosis may be caused by the presence of kidney, liver, or adrenal disorders. Improper diet, obesity, stress, fever, and excess acidic vitamins can cause a temporary state of Acidosis. Diabetics are also at risk if they are uncontrolled.

To determine if your acid/alkaline range, consider taking the pH test offered by The Institute of Nutritional Science. Our contact information may be found in the Appendix section at the end of this book.

Acidosis is not nearly as common as a condition of excess alkalinity, if you have this problem, it needs to be addressed quickly.

Full Spectrum Nutrition Plus:

Kelp	10 tablets daily
Potassium	100 mg/ twice daily
B-Complex	100 mg/ twice daily

Increase consumption of raw fruits and vegetables and reduce consumption of protein foods temporarily until your pH has been balanced.

Acne

Labeled the curse of youth, Acne strikes over 80 percent of those between the ages of 12 and 25. During this period of time, hormone acceleration depletes the body of much of its zinc supply. This mineral is essential in preventing the bacterial infection, which develops in the sebaceous glands in hair follicles.

The extra rush of hormones accelerates the production of oils, especially on the face, chest, and back. This situation, combined with multiple nutrient deficiencies, leads to skin infection. Other factors that can cause Acne, or make it worse, include heredity, excessively oily skin, allergies, oral contraceptives, stress, and high amounts of junk foods containing unnatural fats.

This condition is addressed both topically and through supplementation internally. It is important to keep the skin clean. Use an alcohol-free cleanser and apply a hypo-allergenic cream containing Zinc Stearate to promote healing.

Full Spectrum Nutrition Plus:

Zinc Stearate Cream (15%)	Use topically twice daily
Zinc Gluconate/chelate	20 mg 2-3 times per day
Chromium Chelate	200 mcg per day
Vitamin A (natural only)	50,000 – 100, 000 IU per day
Reduce vitamin A once improvement is seen to 25,000 IU per day	
Essential Fatty Acids	4-6 capsules per day
Lecithin Granules	1 tablespoon per day

EXERCISE: Endurance exercise will help detoxify the body and cleanse the skin

DIET: Avoid chocolate, concentrated sweets and too much dairy. Drink plenty of water, consume whole foods, and consider doing a detoxification fast.

Acne Rosacea

Follow the above outlined program but add the following…

Niacin (as Niacinamide)	200 mg 3 times per day
High potency Stress Formula	
B-Complex	as directed
Multi-Enzyme with Hydrochloric acid	2-4 per meal

Acquired Immune Deficiency Syndrome (AIDS)

{See also Immunodepression)

A devastating destruction of the immune system, believed to be caused by a virus, AIDS rarely kills anyone in and of itself. The secondary infections within the body develop as a result of severe immune suppression and rampant free radical formation and subsequent damage.

Combine the protocols under immunodepression while adding high amounts of the antioxidant N-Acetyl Cysteine.

Addison's Disease - See Adrenal Disorders

Adrenal Disorders

The Adrenal Glands are responsible for producing powerful hormones, many of which are involved in the stress response. Through increased stress and tension these glands can become exhausted, leading to the over-production of the hormones responsible for the 'fight or flight' syndrome. This can result in exhaustion, anxiety, mood swings, and even depression.

Long-term use of drugs such as Cortisone can cause the Adrenal Glands to atrophy. Diseases such as Pituitary disorders and Tuberculosis can cause outright adrenal failure.

Stress management is an all-important factor in restoring good adrenal function. Fortunately, there are several nutrients which nourish the Adrenal Glands, thereby helping to prevent excessive exhaustion.

Full Spectrum Nutrition Plus:

High potency Stress Supplement	4-8 capsules per day
Pantothenic Acid	500 – 1000 mg /2-3 times per day
Vitamin B12	200 mcg/ 2 times per day
Raw Adrenal Extract	6-12 per day

| Vitamin C | To bowel tolerance |
| L-Tyrosine | 500 –1000 mg once per day on Empty stomach. |

EXERCISE: Important for stress management, but don't overdo as this will further exhaust adrenal glands

DIET: Use fresh fruits and veggies, consume fatty fishes such as salmon, and avoid alcohol, caffeine and tobacco.

Consider Stress Management techniques

Age Spots

Those flat brown spots, sometimes called 'liver spots' are most often caused by radiation damage to the skin from free radicals. While the spots themselves are benign, they do indicate that the body is overloaded with internal toxins. This waste is steadily destroying living cells within the body, including brain and liver cells. These spots are most often caused by excess sun exposure, the consumption of vegetable oils, lack of exercise, or a toxic liver.

Full Spectrum Nutrition Plus:

Follow the systemic liver, kidney, bowel, bladder, and colon cleanse found in the Appendix.

Multi- Antioxidants	400-800 mg per day
Bioflavonoids	2,000 mg per day
Vitamin A (natural only)	10,000 IU

AIDS – See Acquired Immune Deficiency Syndrome

Alcoholism

Alcohol is a classic example of a substance that can have beneficial effects in moderation but can become a relentless executioner when taken in excess. Alcoholism is a chronic disease wherein the victim must have alcohol on a regular basis. It is not necessarily based upon quantity, although with time, more and more usually is needed. Excess alcohol causes massive destruction within the body. It is an immune suppressant and generates massive amounts of free radicals. Prolonged misuse results in damage to virtually every cell of the body.

While abstinence is essential with most alcoholics, achieving this goal may be impossible without the help and support of a professional clinic or organization equipped to deal with addiction. During recovery, the following nutrients will prove helpful by both protecting the body from the ravages of alcohol and easing the cravings.

Full Spectrum Nutrition Plus:

B-Complex Stress Nutrients	4-8 capsules per day
Vitamin B1	200 mg 3 times per day
Fatty Acids	3 grams per day
Pantethine	300 mg 2-3 times per day
Selenium	100 mcg
L-Glutamine	1 gram 2 times daily

Heavy Hitting Antioxidants including N-acetyl, L- Cysteine, Milk Thistle, Coenzyme Q10, Grape Seed Extract, and Quercetin	400 –1200 mg per day

To lesson the cravings for alcohol:

Evening Primrose Oil	1 gram 3 times per day
Taurine	1 gram 3 times per day

EXERCISE: Helps to detoxify the body from free radicals formed from excess alcohol

DIET: Avoid vegetable oils and foods cooked in them as these fats can further damage the liver. Reduce or eliminate refined sugars as they are metabolized very similar to alcohols and can trigger cravings. Consume a diet of whole foods with emphasis on fresh fruits.

Alkalosis

The opposite of Acidosis, and far more common in its mild form, Alkalosis occurs when too many alkaline forming foods are ingested or when the natural production of the stomach's hydrochloric acid is depleted.

Symptoms of Alkalosis include poor digestion, heartburn, sore muscles, creaking joints, bone spurs, drowsiness, hypertension, hypothermia (or being cold all the time), edema, night cramps, asthma, constipation, and burning, itching skin.

Emphasis must be placed on fixing first the Hydrochloric Acid levels in the stomach. In addition to the specific supplements listed below, the diet should be adjusted to include more protein foods such as meat, fish, and fowl. You can test your acid and alkaline balance quite easily by obtaining a pH test kit from The Institute of Nutritional Science. (See the Appendix at the end of this book.)

Full Spectrum Nutrition Plus:

Betaine Hydrochloric Acid	2-4 capsules with each meal
Multi purpose enzyme formula	2-4 capsules with each meal
Apple Cider Vinegar	2 Tbl 2 or 3 times per day

Allergic Rhinitis – See Hay Fever

Allergies

All allergies are an autoimmune response to either food or environmental factors, which are normally innocuous to the human body. These hyper-sensitivities can be genetic in origin, like most autoimmune disorders, or they can be the outcome of excess toxicity within the body for prolonged periods of time.

Food allergies are best dealt with by either avoiding the offending foods, or rotating them, so they are not consumed more than once in every five days.

Airborne allergies are much more difficult to deal with, since they cannot be avoided. Mold, pollen, dust, animal dander, and chemical sensitivities present the greatest challenges.

While avoidance, as much as possible, is still the best way to deal with multiple allergies, the following nutrients may lesson the symptoms.

Full Spectrum Nutrition Plus:

High potency Stress Formula	4-8 capsules per day
Pantethine	600 – 900 mg per day

Quercetin	1000 mg per day
Vitamin C	3-5 grams per day
Fatty Acids	1000 mg daily
Licorice extract	1-3 capsules
Niacin (a natural antihistamine)	50-100 mg 2 or 3 times daily

EXERCISE: Avoid over-exercising if in the acute stage of allergic reaction as this will increase the release of histamines. Once allergies are under control, regular exercise is helpful

DIET: Avoid all foods that you are allergic to.

Alopecia – See Hair Loss

Aluminum Toxicity – See Heavy Metal Poisoning

Alzheimer's Disease (See also Memory Improvement)

This debilitating disease is estimated to affect over 2.5 million people. As the mean population exceeds age 50, this condition will likely become more and more prevalent. Simple forgetfulness should not be confused with Alzheimer's Disease. (see memory improvement)

Dementia, a symptom of Alzheimer's, is also a symptom of many disorders and can be induced by the presence of many diseases and nutritional deficiencies.

True Alzheimer's is difficult to diagnose, but we approach it nutritionally from many angles, which include modalities for Dementia and other memory-related conditions.

Antioxidants are likely to be our biggest natural weapon against these types of disorders.

Full Spectrum Nutrition Plus:

High Potency Antioxidants:

Coenzyme Q10, Superoxide Dismutase, Grape Seed Extract, Quercetin and N-Acetyl Cysteine	400 mg 3 times per day
Ginkgo biloba	50 mg 3 times per day

DIET: Increase fiber and consume high amounts of fresh foods. Do not drink tap water due to the possibility of heavy metals such as aluminum.

EXERCISE: Regular exercise can reduce or prevent the onset of this condition, according to several studies. Activities studied included biking, walking and golf.

Amyotrophic Lateral Sclerosis – See Neuromuscular Degeneration

---

Anemia

Anemia is a condition that reduces the amount of oxygen that the blood is able to transport. This reduces the amount of red blood cells resulting in weakness, dizziness, irritability, depression, pale complextion, and loss of menstruation. Early symptoms of anemia include loss of appetite, headaches, constipation, irritability, and lack of concentration.

Iron Deficiency is the most common cause of Anemia. Any condition that causes regular or prolonged loss of blood can induce temporary Anemia.

NOTE: Iron deficiency can be caused by a lack of Copper in the diet, which prevents available Iron from being absorbed into the cells.

Full Spectrum Nutrition Plus:

Folic Acid	800 mcg twice daily
High Potency B-Complex	As indicated on label
Iron Gluconate	As determined by doctor
Raw Liver Extract	500 mg 2 or 3 times per day
Copper Chelate	2-6 mg daily
Zinc	20 mg daily
Raw Spleen Extract	100 mg 2 –3 times daily
Vitamin C	1000mg twice per day
Vitamin B12	100 mcg for 30 days
Digestive Enzymes w/ Hcl	2-4 per meal
Selenium	500 mcg per day

DIET: To increase the absorption of iron, consume foods such as broccoli, eggs, greens, plums grapes, raisins, and yams. Avoid foods such as chocolate, rhubarb, spinach, and most nuts and beans as they contain high amounts of oxalic acid, which can retard iron absorption.

Angina

Excessive pain in the upper torso, specifically the center of the chest to the left shoulder and arm. There are many causes, but generally it is a lack of oxygen to the heart muscle, which is most often caused by the narrowing of the arteries around the heart.

Full Spectrum Nutrition Plus:

Oral Chelation Formula	6-9 per day
Bio-electrical Trace Minerals	1 ounce twice per day
Calcium/Magnesium	1500 mg per day
Essential Fatty Acids	3 grams per day
Arginine	4-8 grams per day
L-Carnitine	2 – 3 grams per day
CoQ10	100 – 200 mg per day

In severe, acute cases, consider the immediate use of Intravenous Chelation treatments from a trained Chelation Therapist or Doctor. Follow up this treatment with a tested Oral Chelation Formula for prevention. Contact The Institute for information on this special formula for oral chelation. (see appendix)

Ankylosing Spondylitis

Exercise is very important in reducing the degree of permanent damage that can result from this condition. Emphasis should be upon flexibility exercises. A program of exercise done under water, in an exercise pool, is frequently tolerated best especially in the beginning.

Full Spectrum Nutrition Plus:

Vitamin B6	50 mg per day
Chondroiton Sulfate	200 – 400 mg per day

Glucosamine Sulfate	200- 400 mg per day
MSM	100 mg per day

Natural Pain Relief

dl-Phenylalanine*	250 mg 2 or 3 times per day

*Note: do not take if you have uncontrolled high blood pressure.

Anorexia

This eating disorder, which primarily affects females, was often thought to be solely psychological. While there is no doubt that emotional ties exist, nutrition may be very helpful for those suffering from this condition. Of special importance would be liquid nutritional products, since their absorption rate is much higher than capsules or tablets.

Even though the individuals are frequently of ideal weight or even underweight, they become obsessed with the concept that they are fat. This results in such dangerous practices as vomiting up meals, taking laxatives, or simply starving. While this condition should not be addressed without including psychological counseling, the following nutrients will help to keep the body nourished and replace those specific nutrients lost through the use of laxatives or the practice of regular vomiting.

Full Spectrum Liquid Nutrition Plus:

Calcium	1000mg per day
Magnesium	500 mg per day
Potassium	100 mg twice per day
Zinc	50 mg per day
Additional Liquid Trace Minerals	1 ounce per day
Acidophilus	5 capsules per day on empty stomach
Multi Enzyme Product	2-4 with each meal
B-Complex Stress Formula	As indicated on product label

DIET: Avoid sugars and concentrated white flour products. Avoid processed foods with additives. Be sure to consume at least 80 to 100 grams of protein daily.

EXERCISE: Regular exercise will help reduce stress levels. Do not over do it however, as this can exhaust the adrenal glands.

Anxiety

Stress has become a way of life in our society. With everyone trying to fit 90 minutes of work into every hour, it's no wonder than stress-related health problems are escalating.

Of all the leading prescription drugs, over half of them are for either Anxiety or Depression. Prolonged unmanaged stress overworks the Adrenal Glands, which are the 'fight or flight' system of the body.

This results in Anxiety due to the constant presence of powerful adrenal hormones in the blood stream. Following are nutrient recommendations for helping your body to deal with stress by nourishing the adrenal response system. Also listed is my all-natural tranquilizer replacement formula, which may be used for short periods of excess stress.

Full Spectrum Nutrition Plus:

Calcium	800 mg per day
Magnesium	400 mg per day
Essential Fatty Acids	500 mg extra per day
B-Complex Stress Formula	As per label directions
Valerian Root Extract	2 Capsules at bedtime
Kava Root Extract	100 mg 2 or 3 times per day

Natural Tranquilizer Replacement

Take the following combination every four hours:

Calcium	400 mg
Magnesium	100 mg
Vitamin B6	50 mg
5- Hydroxy Tryptophan (5-HTP)	200 mg
Kava Root Extract	100 mg
B-Complex Stress Formula	1 capsule
Vitamin B12	500 mcg

DIET: Consume fresh fruits and veggies. Avoid stimulants such as coffee, colas, black tea and chocolate.

EXERCISE: Exercise is one of the greatest stress relieving activities we can do. Try and get at least 30 minutes of resistance and endurance exercise three or four times every week.

Appetite Problems

Many health challenges can result in a compromised appetite. Chronic diseases, infections, and digestive disorders can lead to poor eating habits. This is especially true with older people, because as we age our digestive processes become less and less effective. The following program may help in correcting digestive problems and may improve appetite.

Full Spectrum Nutrition Plus:

Multi-Enzyme Formula with Hcl	2-4 per meal
Acidophilus	5 per day on empty stomach
B-Complex Stress Formula	as indicated until appetite returns
Zinc Gluconate	50 mg per day

DIET: If underweight, consider using concentrated weight gain shakes, which provide high calories with minimal intake.

EXERCISE: Concentrate on resistance exercise, which often stimulates the appetite center.

Aphthous Stomatitus (Canker Sores)

Ulcerations inside the mouth, the Canker Sore manifests itself as a small white ulcer like sore. These sores can take as long as two weeks or more to heal. There are several factors that contribute to the Canker Sore such as acid/alkaline imbalance, allergies to chocolate, stress, immune suppression, and a bacterial imbalance in the mouth. Diabetics often have problems with this condition due to Metabolic Acidosis.

Full Spectrum Nutrition Plus:

Multi-Acidophilus	3-6 capsules per day
Betaine Hydrochloride (Hcl)	1 –3 capsules per meal
Zinc Gluconate	50 –100 mg per day (short term)
Folic Acid	1 mg per day
Vitamin B12	1000 mcg twice per day
Licorice Root Gargle	3 –4 times per day
Acidophilus	3-5 capsules per day

Arrhythmia - See Cardiac Arrhythmia

Arteriosclerosis (Atherosclerosis)

These conditions are really one and the same. Arteriosclerosis is the thickening of the artery wall due to Calcium deposits and is also referred to as Calcification of the arteries.

Atherosclerosis, a similar condition, is when fatty deposits also line the interior of the artery wall. Both these conditions have the same basic cause, which is free radical damage to the muscle wall of the artery, primarily through the over–consumption of vegetable oils in the diet. (See Chapter 4 for a complete discussion of this condition.)

Full Spectrum Nutrition Plus:

Oral Chelation Formula	as directed on product label
Liquid Plant Derived Minerals	1 ounce twice per day
Vitamin E	400 –800 IU per day
Lecithin Granules	2 Tbl per day
Garlic Concentrate	4 –8 capsules per day
Multi-Digestive Enzymes	2 – 4 with each meal
Folic Acid	1 mg 3 times per day
Niacin	100 mg 3 times per day
Taurine	1000 mg per day
Essential Fatty Acids	4-6 grams per day

Multi-Antioxidant Compound containing
Coenzyme Q10, Grape Seed Extract,
Bilberry Extract, Quercetin,
Silybum Marianum and N-Acetyl Cysteine   400 –800 mg per day

NOTE: If the condition is acute, the above protocol will work too slowly for you to benefit from. Consider taking Intravenous Chelation Therapy from a professional trained in this procedure. After the initial crisis has passed, follow up with this protocol for prevention and maintenance.

Contact The Institute for information on this specialized oral chelation formula. (see appendix)

DIET: Avoid all vegetable oils except olive oil.

EXERCISE: Regular moderate exercise such as walking daily.

Arthralgia – See Rheumatism

Arthritis (See also Rheumatoid Arthritis)

There are several forms of arthritis. The most common is Osteo–arthritis, which is characterized by inflammation and pain in a joint or several joints.

Arthritis is a condition caused by the proliferation of free radicals within the body. Once developed, arthritis produces multiple toxins, which increase both the inflammation and pain as well as the actual progression of the disease.

Therefore, any program addressing Arthritis, must also address detoxification of the body. (See Appendix for our detoxification program.)

Full Spectrum Nutrition Plus:

Essential Fatty Acids	4-6 grams per day
Liquid Organic Trace Minerals	1-2 ounces per day
Calcium/ Magnesium/ trace minerals	4-8 capsules per day
Vitamin C	2- 4 grams per day
B-Complex Stress Formula	as indicated on label for 30 days

Arthritis Combination Including:

Vitamin B6	25-50 mg/day
Evening Primrose Oil	50 mg/day
Glucosamine Sulfate	500 mg/day
Chondroitin Sulfate	500 mg/day
Cetylmyristoleate	150 mg/day
Nettle Leaf Extract	400 mg/day
MSM	75-100 mg/day
Boswella Extract	100-200 mg/day

Detoxification Program   **(see Appendix)**

Multi Enzymes with Hydrochloric Acid   2 –4 with each meal

NOTE: The Institute uses a Targeted Formula, which contains the right balance of all these nutrient factors. Contact them for further information. (see Appendix)

If pain is considerable, consider the following:

dl-Phenylalanine*   500 mg twice per day

     *Note: do not take if you have uncontrolled high blood pressure

Curcumin	As Directed
Liquid Oxygen	1 ounce three times per day

DIET: Cherries, pineapple, eggs, garlic and asparagus contain factors that can improve arthritis.

EXERCISE: Regular exercise, to your own tolerance, is essential for restoring flexibility and reducing pain. Low impact resistance and cardio exercise is best.

Asthma

A severe form of allergic response, Asthma is a series of spasms in the muscles surrounding the small air passages in the lungs. Symptoms of Asthma include coughing, wheezing, tight constricting feeling in the chest, and difficulty in breathing.

Asthma can be a very acute, life threatening condition and must be handled aggressively. When Histamine forms as a result of the allergic response mucus fills the lungs and bronchi.

Full Spectrum Nutrition Plus:

Vitamin A (natural only)	25,000 IU per day
B-Complex Stress formula	as indicated on product label
Multi-Digestive Enzymes	2-4 with each meal
Essential Fatty Acids	2 grams per day
Pantethine	600 – 1000 mg/day
Antioxidant Combination Including:	
Coenzyme Q10, Quercetin and especially N-Acetyl Cysteine	800 mg per day
Calcium	1000 mg per day
Magnesium	600 mg per day
Vitamin C	2 grams daily
DHEA	25 – 50 mg per day
Ginkgo biloba	40 mg per day

DIET: Increase consumption of fresh fruits and veggies. Get tested for food allergies and eliminate any offending foods, which may make you asthma worse.

EXERCISE: Light exercise is best. If exercise aggravates asthma, consider using 3,000 mg of vitamin C about an hour before your workout or 1 oz of Liquid Oxygen. (See Sources in Appendix)

Atopic Dermatitis – See Eczema

Atherosclerosis – See Arteriosclerosis

Athlete's Foot

This fungal infection can be very virulent and difficult to control once it sets in. The environment of the feet is ideal for the proliferation of fungal growth. Like most fungus in the body, this is also controlled by the presence of healthy bacteria in the gut. When these bacteria are destroyed, the fungus is free to spread very rapidly.

Full Spectrum Nutrition Plus:

Multi-Acidophilus	5 Capsules twice per day
Garlic Extract	5 capsules per day
Liquid Oxygen	1 ounce three times per day

You may soak your feet in a solution of 35 percent Food Grade Hydrogen Peroxide and water. Make this by adding one ounce of pure 35 percent hydrogen peroxide to a gallon of water. Soak feet twice a day for 20 minutes.

Atrial Fibrillaton – See Cardiac Arrhythmia

Attention Deficit Disorder (ADD)

Severe learning disabilities can lead to the inability to focus and concentrate and are becoming more common. The theory is that it is caused by a combination of genetic mutation from the parents and exposure to toxic chemicals in the children.

Research done at The Institute of Nutritional Science, has proven that radical treatment with powerful drugs are not only unnecessary for this condition but may cause more harm than good in the long run. Nutrient deficiency is most assuredly at the heart of these problems.

There are also several adjunct factors, which if present, can contribute to the overall **problem.**

Full Spectrum Liquid Nutrition	*1 tsp. per 20 pounds of bodyweight*
Or for children age 10 and older	*1 ounce per one hundred lbs. bodyweight*
Essential Fatty Acids	2 –3 capsules per day
Calcium Citrate/Malate	

| Ages 2 –5 | 200 mg per day |
| Ages 6 + | 500 – 1000 mg per day |

Stress-Related Nutrients

Children under 45 pounds:

| Niacin (as Niacinamide) | 25 mg up to 100 mg max per day |
| Vitamin C | 50 mg up to bowel tolerance |

Children over 45 pounds:

Niacin (as Niacinamide)	50 – 200 mg
Vitamin C	to bowel tolerance
Pyridoxine	50 – 400 mg
Riboflavin	50 – 200 mg
Calcium Pantothenate	100 – 800 mg
Magnesium	50-200 mg
Zinc	5 – 30 mg

If excessive hyperactivity is a factor, test for heavy metal poisoning such as mercury, lead or cadmium and add:

| Caffeine | 100 mg per day |

If the child craves sweets, suspect carbohydrate intolerance, and add:

Chromium	100 mcg
Vanadium	500 mcg
Aspartic Acid	300 mg
Bilberry Extract	20 mg

If short-term memory is affected consider adding the following:

| Phosphatidylserine | 100-200 mg per day |
| Phosphatidylcholine | 100-200 mg per day |

Finally, many individuals displaying attention deficit symptoms suffer from multiple allergies. I suggest you take the RAST test (a blood test) which will determine all airborne and food allergies. If food allergies are detected, it will be necessary to either eliminate those foods or rotate them, eating them no more often than once every five days.

Those dealing with Attention Deficits may want more information. I suggest my booklet entitled, ***Drug Free Answers to Correcting Learning Disabilities***, available from The Institute of Nutritional Science.

DIET: Consume fatty fishes such as salmon. Ensure diet is high enough in protein – 80 to 100 grams daily. Avoid refined carbohydrates, replacing instead with fruits and whole grains. Eliminate any possible food allergies.

Autism – See Attention Deficit Disorders

Auto-Immune Disorders

Auto-immune conditions come about due to a genetic mutation, which causes the immune system to view harmless substances as toxic.

Allergies, Crohn's Disease, and Rheumatoid Arthritis are typical examples. The body sees substances such as dust, mold, pollens, and certain foods as toxins and builds antibodies against them. This produces Histamine and the classic allergic response. In the case of Rheumatoid Arthritis, the body sees its own cartilage and connective tissue as foreign and builds antibodies to attack and destroy it.

Anyone suffering from any Auto-Immune condition should NOT take immune stimulating substances without the express supervision of the trained professional. In many cases these ingredients accelerate the activity of the immune system and can accelerate the Auto-Immune Disorder thereby making it much worse.

Full Spectrum Nutrition Plus:

Vitamin C	To Bowel Tolerance
Vitamin E	400 IU Extra per day
Selenium	100 mcg per day
Essential Fatty Acids	500 – 1000 mg extra per day
High Potency Antioxidants	400-800 mg per day

Backache

Most aches and pains in the lower back are due to weak muscles, which can no longer hold the spine in proper alignment. Exercises to strengthen these muscles are often essential. Calcium and Magnesium deficiencies can contribute to low back pain as well.

Full Spectrum Nutrition Plus:

Calcium/Magnesium/ trace minerals	4 –8 capsules per day
Horsetail Extract	As indicated on product label

If Arthritis is the cause of the lower back pain, see the Arthritis protocol.

Baldness – See Hair Loss

Bed Wetting

While the cause of this condition is unknown, it is believed to be a combination of psychological and nutritional factors. Factors that can contribute to this problem physically include, food allergies, small or weak bladders, and urinary tract infections. It is believed that protein deficiency can also cause this problem.

Full Spectrum Nutrition Plus:

Protein Powder Drink	10 –25 grams protein per day
Calcium	500 mg per day
Magnesium	250 mg per day
Zinc	10 mg per day

Take the RAST blood test to determine possible allergies.

Bee Sting

For the most part, Bee Stings are annoying and a little uncomfortable, but for some they can be life-threatening. If you have a severe allergy to Bee Stings, you must carry the appropriate medications to avoid possible Anaphylactic Shock.

If you don't have an allergy to the venom, simply remove the stinger carefully with tweezers and apply liquid minerals to the bite two or three times per day.

Full Spectrum Nutrition Plus:

Pantothenic Acid (natural Antihistamine)   500 mg per day

Drink Yellow Dock Tea and apply topically to sting area

Bells Palsy

This is a neurological condition, usually of the face, which can come on quite suddenly and last for several days or even weeks. It causes a drooping of one side of the face due to an inflammation of the nerves.

Full Spectrum Nutrition Plus:

Vitamin B-12	1000 mcg per day
Calcium	1000 mg per day
Magnesium	500 mg per day
Essential Fatty Acids	1000 mg per day
Valerian Root Extract	As indicated on product label

Benign Breast Cysts

While this is a relatively harmless condition, it can be frightening to a woman who feels lumps in her breasts. Naturally, she will assume the worst and think it is evidence of Cancer. Most of the time these lumps are blocked ducts, or in some cases, Benign Cysts, which form as a result of fat metabolism irregularities stemming from the liver. By cleansing the liver and providing nutrients to help the liver process fats, we can virtually eliminate the occurrence of these Benign Cysts in breast tissue.

Full Spectrum Nutrition Plus:

Lipotropics

Choline/Inositol/Methionine   1000 mg 2 to 3 times per day

Vitamin A	10,000 – 25,000 IU per day
Vitamin E	400 IU per day
Kelp (iodine)	6-10 tablets per day
Essential Fatty Acids	1500 mg 2 times per day

Benign Prostatic Hyperplasia

The most common reason why men over age 50 visit a doctor, Chronic Prostate Inflammation is not only annoying but potentially problematic too. When the inflammation is sufficient to prevent the voiding of the bladder, waste material remains for prolonged periods, greatly increasing the risk of urinary tract and bladder infections. (See chapter 4 for a complete discussion of this condition.)

Full Spectrum Nutrition Plus:

Serenoa Repens (Saw Palmetto)	500-1000 mg per day
Pygeum Africanum (70:1)	100 – 200 mg per day
Glycine	200-400 mg per day
L-Glutamic Acid	200-400 mg per day
Alanine	200 – 300 mg per day
L-Lysine	200mg per day
Pumpkin Seed Powder	100-200 mg per day
Stinging Nettle Leaf (Urtica dioica)	100 mg per day
Lycopene	20-40 mg per day
Zinc	25 mg per day extra
Essential Fatty Acids	1000 mg per day

NOTE: It is important to rule out Cadmium Toxicity, which can produce the same prostate symptoms. A hair mineral analysis will reveal the presence of any heavy metals in soft tissues.

Beriberi

This is a nutrient deficiency disease caused by a gross deficiency of the B-Complex vitamins, especially B1 (thiamin).

Full Spectrum Nutrition Plus:

High potency B-Complex 50 mg	1 twice daily
Vitamin C	2-4 grams daily

Bitot's Spots – See Eye Problems

Bladder Infection (Cystitis)

This is caused by a bacterial infection, and inflammation of the organ responsible for holding urine until voiding. If left unchecked, this condition can result in Cystitis. Oftentimes, antibiotic therapy is necessary to arrest a long-term infection, however the following protocol can prevent reoccurrence.

Full Spectrum Nutrition Plus:

Cranberry Juice	12 ounces 4 or 5 times per day
Vitamin C	4 –5 grams per day
Multi-Acidophilus	3 capsules three times per day
L-Cysteine	500 mg twice per day until infection subsides
Zinc Gluconate	25 mg extra per day

DIET: Drink plenty of fluids, especially water and cranberry juice. Foods like celery and watermelon are natural diuretics. Avoid citrus fruits, which are alkaline and can contribute to bacterial growth. Avoid alcohol, caffeine and carbonated beverages.

Bleeding Gums

This condition is frequently the result of multiple nutrient deficiencies or the presence of Bacterial Gum Disease. In either case, the following protocol has been instrumental in saving the teeth of many thousand of clients who have visited The Institute over the years.

Full Spectrum Nutrition Plus:

Vitamin C	To Bowel Tolerance
Calcium	1000 – 1500 mg per day
Magnesium	500-800 mg per day
Vitamin E	800 IU per day
Hydrogen Peroxide	
Mouthwash and Tooth paste	use twice daily

Blood Lipid Elevations

While it is my position that Elevated Lipids play only a very small role in the progression of Cardiovascular Disease, I do not believe that Elevated or Unbalanced Lipids are a healthy situation either.

When we discuss Lipids in the blood, we are referring to three basic things, Cholesterol/ Cholesterol Ratio, Triglycerides, and Elevated Lipoproteins. Elevated Cholesterol is caused by the Liver's inability to effectively regulate the body's production of Cholesterol. Elevated Triglyceride is a result of excess carbohydrate and refined sugar consumption.

Cholesterol Regulation

Full Spectrum Nutrition Plus:

Pantethine	600 – 1200 mg per day
Lipotropics	
(Choline, Inositol & Methionine)	1000 mg twice daily
Lecithin Granules	2-3 tablespoons daily
Essential Fatty Acids	1000 – 2000 mg per day
Vitamin C	To Bowel Tolerance
Garlic	2 – 4 grams per day
Guggulipids	200-400 mg per day
Phytosterol Complex	250-500 mg per day

Consider adding more fiber to your diet – up to 10 grams per day.

High Triglycerides

Full Spectrum Nutrition Plus:

L-Carnitine	2 – 3 grams per day
Essential Oils from Fish	
(EPA/DHA)	1 – 2 grams per day
Chromium	400-800 mcg per day
Vanadium	500 mcg per day

Reduce consumption of refined carbohydrates and sugars and increase exercise level.

High Lipoprotein (a)

Full Spectrum Nutrition Plus:

N-Acetyl Cysteine	2 –4 grams per day
Vitamin C	4-8 grams per day
Lipotropic Formula	
(Choline, Inositol & Methionine)	1000 mg twice per day
Gamma Oryzanol	500 – 1000 mg per day
Lysine	500 mg per day
Proline	500 – 1000 mg per day

Boils

Localized infections on the skin, which are usually filled with pus. Boils are a result of excessive toxicity in the system, especially the blood. This situation may be brought on by excessive consumption of junk foods, oxidized vegetable oils, food allergies, stress, poor hygiene, toxic bowels, or bloodstream. Emphasis must be ultimately placed upon removing the cause of the toxins and cleansing the blood and the organs of elimination.

Full Spectrum Nutrition Plus:

Chlorophyll	1 tbsp. 3 times per day
Garlic extract	2 capsules 3 times per day
Vitamin C	To bowel tolerance

Detoxification Fast	**(see appendix)**
Liquid Oxygen	1 ounce twice per day

EXERCISE: Regular exercise will improve immune function and help to eliminate toxins through the skin

---

Bone Spur – See Heal Spur

Breast Cancer – See Cancer

Breast Cysts – See Benign Breast Cysts

Breastfeeding Difficulty

Frequently, a mother wishing to breastfeed a newborn may have problems either producing milk or producing an adequate supply of milk for baby's needs. These problems are often caused by stress or a protein deficiency.

Full Spectrum Nutrition (1/2 dose) Plus:

Protein Powder Drink	25 – 50 grams protein per day
Multi-Acidophilus	2 – 4 capsules per day
Calcium	1500 mg per day
Magnesium	500 mg per day

Bright's Disease – See Kidney & Bladder Problems

Broken Bones

The healing time for broken bones can be reduced considerably through the use of aggressive nutrition, especially from plant derived liquid bio-electrical trace minerals. These minerals accelerate the positive/negative knitting of bone tissue and reduce the healing time.

Full Spectrum Nutrition Plus:

Calcium	1200 mg per day
Magnesium	600 mg per day
Bio-electrical organic trace Minerals	1 ounce 3 or 4 times per day
Vitamin C	3 –5 grams per day

Bronchial Asthma – See Asthma

Bronchitis – See Asthma

Bruises

A condition where the small blood vessels under the skin rupture and fill the surrounding tissue with blood, bruises can be very painful and quite unattractive. While it is normal to bruise after a blow to the skin, when bruising occurs on only slight contact, it is usually a sign of bioflavonoid deficiency.

Full Spectrum Nutrition Plus:

Vitamin C	2 –4 grams per day
Citrus Bioflavonoids	3 –6 grams per day
Alfalfa tablets	5 – 10 tablets per day
Vitamin E	200 IU extra per day
Zinc Gluconate	15-30 mg per day

DIET: Consume fresh, uncooked fruits and vegetables.

Bruxism

The clinical name for tooth grinding, bruxism is usually the result of un-managed stress, which manifests itself during sleep as the grinding of teeth. The best way to approach this matter is through managing the underlying stress. Elevating specific nutrients to reduce stress may also be helpful.

Full Spectrum Nutrition Plus:

Calcium	1500 mg per day
Magnesium	750 mg per day
Stress B-Complex formula	As per the label instructions
Vitamin C	3 grams per day
Zinc	25 mg per day

Consider Stress management techniques

Bulimia – See Anorexia

Burns

The following protocol will help heal any degree of burn and reduce the scaring.

Full Spectrum Nutrition Plus:

Potassium	100 mg twice per day
Protein Powder Drink	25 – 50 mg extra protein per day
Vitamin C	2 – 4 grams per day
Vitamin E	400 IU extra
Vitamin E Cream	Apply topically to healing wound
Liquid bio-electrical	
Trace Minerals	Apply topically to healing wound
Bromelain Cream	Apply topically after burn has healed to prevent scaring

Bursitis

This painful condition is the result of an inflammation of the Bursae, the small fluid sacs around joints, muscles, tendons, and bones. While the most common cause is over-straining and injury, this condition can also be caused by allergies or calcium deposits from an over-alkaline system.

Full Spectrum Nutrition Plus:

Calcium	1500 mg per day
Magnesium	750 mg per day
Multi-Enzyme	2 –4 capsules per meal
Hydrochloric Acid (Betaine)	2-4 capsules per meal
Vitamin C	2 grams per day
Bioflavinoids	2 – 4 grams per day
Quercetin & N-Acetyl Cysteine	400 mg per day

ANTI-INFLAMMATORY HERBS: Bilberry, Curcumen, Feverfew, and Devil's Claw. (Contact The Institute for information on the best natural anti-inflammatory formula)

DIET: Consider a short-term fasting program (see appendix) to detoxify the body.

EXERCISE: This is important to maintain flexibility, but in the short term, you may need to abstain from exercise until the acute phase of the condition passes.

Cadmium Poisoning – See Heavy Metal Poisoning

Cancer

The treatment modalities for Cancer are almost as extensive as the number of cases. There are certain specific treatments for specific types of cancer.

Sadly, many of the most effective alternative treatments for Cancer are not available in the United States. The following nutrient recommendations are divided into two groups, the prevention of Cancer and the more aggressive program for those with existing Cancer.

Since Cancer, of all types, is the result of a faulty immune response, it is imperative that stress in your life either be eliminated or effectively managed.

Full Spectrum Nutrition Plus:

Bio-electric Organic Trace Minerals	2 oz extra per day
High B-Complex Stress formula	Per the label instructions
Antioxidants: Coenzyme Q10, Lycopene Quercetin, Milk Thistle and	
N-Acetyl Cysteine	800 – 1200 mg per day
Essential Fatty Acids	2000 mg per day
Folic Acid	1 – 3 mg per day
Zinc	25 mg per day
Mushroom Extract	300 mg per day

Existing Cancer: In addition to all of the above add:

Shark Cartilage 750 mg capsules	10 per day
Liquid Oxygen	1 ounce 3 times per day
Increase Folic Acid	10 mg per day

EXERCISE: A combination of resistance and aerobic exercise to your own tolerance will keep the strength up as well as improve immune function.

DIET: Consume fresh fruits and vegetables, especially cruciferous vegetables such as broccoli, Brussels sprouts, cabbage and cauliflower. Consume garlic as it helps with immune function. Consume almonds as they contain natural laetrile, which is an anticancer chemical.

Candidiasis

The Candida Albicans organism is a naturally occurring entity within our gastrointestinal tract and has important function. It is kept in balance by the presence of Acidophilus.

When Acidophilus is destroyed by poor diet, antibiotics, birth control medications, or disease, the Candida Albicans can explosively multiply.

If left unchecked, it can become systemic, taking up residence in various sites of the body, including the brain. The most common site for systemic Candidiasis proliferation in males is in the lungs. (See Chapter 4, for a complete discussion of this condition)

Full Spectrum Nutrition Plus:

Liquid Oxygen Flush	(see appendix)
Multi-Acidophilus	10 capsules per day for 10 days After the above oxygen flush.
Multi – enzymes	2-4 per meal
Betain Hydrochloride (Hcl)	1 – 3 per meal
Essential Fatty Acids	500 mg per day

DIET: It is not necessary to follow a strict yeast diet as these diets do not control or eliminate this problem. You should however, consume a healthy diet and reduce or eliminate refined sugars until the problem is eliminated with liquid oxygen.

Canker Sores – See Apthous Stomatitis

Capillary Fragility

When the walls of the capillaries become thin due to nutrient deficiencies, they can rupture (see bruises) and produce unattractive spider-like veins. This is primarily due to a Citrus Bioflavinoid Deficiency.

Full Spectrum Nutrition Plus:

Vitamin C	2-4 grams per day
Citrus Bioflavinoids	2-4 grams per day
Vitamin E	400 IU extra
Zinc	25 mg extra

Capillary Hyperpermeability – See Edema

Cardiac Arrhythmia

Cardiac Arrhythmias are electrical disturbances, which cause the heart to beat out of natural rhythm. While there are potentially many causes, the most recent research shows that most all Arrhythmias are linked to an imbalance of electrolytes, especially Magnesium.

Full Spectrum Nutrition Plus

Magnesium Chelate	1000 mg per day
L-Carnitine	1000 mg per day
CoEnzyme Q10	100 – 200 mg per day
Essential Fatty Acids	1000 mg per day
Garlic Extract	2 capsules 3 times per day
Taurine	1000 mg twice per day
Hawthorne Berry	250 – 500 mg per day
Vitamin B1	100-200 mg extra per day
Liquid Bio-electrical Trace Minerals	1 –2 ounces extra per day

Cardiomyopathy

A condition of the heart, which produces enlargement and ineffective cardiac performance. Cardiomyopathy may be caused by a variety of adjunct factors. Nutritionally, this condition has been linked back to a Selenium deficiency.

In fact, in China, Cardiomyopathy is treated very effectively with high doses of Selenium. If you have Cardiomyopathy, which is accompanied by Congestive Heart Failure, please see our further recommendations listed elsewhere under that heading.

Full Spectrum Nutrition Plus:

Selenium Chelate	1 – 10 mg per day
Vitamin E	400-800 IU extra per day

Hawthorn Berry	300-500 mg per day
Vitamin B1	100-200 mg per day
Magnesium	600-1000 mg per day

Cardiovascular Disease – See specific condition

Carpal Tunnel Syndrome

This debilitating condition is related to the process of Arthritis and is likely caused by prolonged nutrient deficiencies and specific joint stress.

Full Spectrum Nutrition Plus:

Vitamin B6	100 mg per day
Pantothenic Acid	500 mg per day
Calcium	1000 mg per day
Magnesium	500 mg per day
Zinc	25 mg per day
Glucosamine Sulfate	500 mg per day
Chondroitin Sulfate	500 mg per day
Essential Fatty Acids	1000 mg per day
B-Complex Stress Formula	As indicated on product label (take for three months)

DIET: Consume large amounts of pineapple, which contains bromelain, which reduces inflammation and swelling. Temporarily reduce sodium as it can retain fluids, aggravating this condition.

Cataracts

A cataract is the clouding of the lens in the eye that affects vision. Most cataracts are related to the aging process. By age 80, more than half of the American population either have a cataract or have had cataract surgery. Most age-related cataracts are the effect of clumping of the proteins in the lens. Other factors associated with cataract development are diabetes, smoking, alcohol use, and prolonged exposure to ultraviolet sunlight. A full-spectrum daily multiple that includes a minimum of 500 mg of vitamin C is recommended to lower the risk of cataract development. Specific nutrients also associated with delaying protein clumping in the lens:

Full Spectrum Nutrition Plus:

Zeaxanthin	3-4 mg
Lutein	7-12 mg

Product Recommendation – **Oculair** by Biosyntrx (see Appendix)

Celiac Disease

This rare disorder is thought to be an Autoimmune response to Gluten in foods and can be very debilitating. Grains containing Gluten such as wheat, barley, rye, and oats must be completely avoided. Symptoms of the condition such as abdominal swelling, irregular bowel movements, anemia, skin rash, and joint pain, become worse when these foods are eaten.

Over time the intestinal lining can become damaged and nutrient absorption is compromised. Liquid nutritional products, therefore, are of utmost importance in this situation.

Full Spectrum Liquid Nutrition Plus:

Protein Powder Supplement	
From rice or soy	25 – 35 grams per day
Extra B-Complex	50 mg per day
Vitamin K	As directed on product label
Zinc	25 mg per day
Essential Fatty Acids	2-4 grams per day
Vitamin C	1 –2 grams extra per day

DIET: Avoid all foods that contain gluten, which include barley, oats, rye or wheat. This condition causes mal-absorption, so be sure and consume a diet rich in whole fresh foods.

Cerebrovascular Disease – See Atherosclerosis and Hypertension

Cervical Dysplasia

The term Dysplasia indicates an abnormal cell development and in this case involves the lining of the uterus. This condition is considered to be one of pre-cancer and aggressive treatment is necessary to ensure that the condition does not progress.

Full Spectrum Nutrition Plus:

Folic Acid	15 – 30 mg per day
Beta Carotene	50,000 IU per day
Vitamin A	25,000 – 100,000 IU per day
Vitamin C	1 – 3 grams
Selenium	200 – 400 mcg per day
Vitamin B12	1 –5 mg per day
Gotu Kola (standardized)	1-3 capsules per day
Grape Seed Extract	200-300 mg per day

Chemical Allergies – See Allergies

Chemical Poisoning – See Heavy Metal Poisoning

Chicken Pox

This disease, like many infectious conditions may be improved and recovery time reduced by stimulating the immune system. In addition to Full Spectrum Nutrition, follow the protocol outlined under Immunodepression

Chlamydia – See Immunodepression

Cholecystitis – See Gallbladder Disease

Choleithiasis – See Gallbladder Disease

Cholesterol Elevation

While elevated Cholesterol is constantly implicated in Heart Disease, the fact remains that Cholesterol, at any level, has never caused one case of Heart Disease. This is not to say that elevated Cholesterol does not complicate the situation once Heart Disease has advanced.

Elevated Cholesterol is a sign of poor liver function and when the liver is cleansed and properly nourished, Cholesterol usually normalizes in a few months. (See the Appendix for our detoxifying and cleansing program.)

Full Spectrum Nutrition Plus:

Extra Liquid Trace Minerals	1 – 2 ounces per day
Vitamin C	3 grams per day
Lecithin Granules (not liquid)	1 Tbl 3 times per day
Essential Fatty Acids	1000 mg per day
Lipotropics	
Choline	
Inositol	
Methionine	1000 mg once or twice per day

DIET: Avoid all vegetable oils except olive oil. Foods that naturally lower cholesterol include apples, bananas, carrots grapefruit and cold-water fish.

EXERCISE: Get regular exercise three to four times per week.

Chronic Fatigue Syndrome/ Epstein Barr

These recently identified conditions, are thought to be related to a low- grade Chronic Viral Infection. This being the case, we should approach these conditions in much the same manner as with any invading pathogen and utilize immune stimulation while providing adjunct nutrients.

Full Spectrum Nutrition Plus:

Liquid Oxygen Flush	(see appendix)
Multi-Acidophilus	10 capsules per day on empty
	Stomach, after the oxy flush

After the flush add:

Take a combination of the following 3 to 4 times per day

Colostrum Concentrate	100mg
Beta- 1,3 Glucan	25 mg
Mushroom Mycelial Biomass	200 mg
Echinacea Purpurea leaf	25 mg
Astragalus Extract	50 mg
Pau D'Arco Extract	50 mg
Antioxidant combination of Coenzyme Q10, N-Acetyl Cysteine, Quercetin, and Grape Seed Extract	400-800 mg per day

DIET: Increase fiber to ensure adequate elimination of toxins.

Cirrhosis of the Liver

The liver has an unbelievable ability to heal and regenerate itself, but through constant and prolonged abuse deterioration can become chronic and a diagnosis of Cirrhosis is appropriate.

This degenerative, inflammatory disease results in the hardening of liver cells, producing scar tissue, which eventually takes over the entire organ causing liver failure.

Full Spectrum Nutrition Plus:

Lipotropics (non-stimulating)	
Choline, Inositol & Methionine	1000 mg combination 3 times/ day

High Potency	
B-Complex Stress Formula	As indicated on product label

Garlic	2 –4 capsules with each meal
L Cysteine	500 mg per day
Lecithin Granules	1 Tbl twice per day

Heavy Hitting Antioxidants

CoQ10, N-Acetyl Cysteine,	
Quercetin, Milk Thistle	400 mg 3 times per day

DIET: Consume a diet of at least 80 percent raw foods. Goat's milk is also very helpful. Juicing is particularly good for this condition as well. Do not consume vegetable oils except for olive oil. Consider a detoxification program. (see appendix)

Cold – See Common Cold

Cold Sores – See Herpes

Colitis

This condition is an acute inflammation and irritation of the Colon, which may become chronic if left unchecked. Colitis can strike at almost any age. There are many types of Colitis, some cases mild and others quite debilitating.

Causes of this condition range from allergies to foods, bad eating habits, excess stress, and intestinal bacteria imbalance. Once all food allergies have been eliminated consider the following:

Full Spectrum Nutrition Plus:

Increase Fiber	8 – 10 grams per day
Multi-Acidophilus	10 capsules daily
Liquid Oxygen	1 oz twice per day
Liquid Aloe Vera Concentrate	2 oz 3 times per day
Multi-Enzymes with Hcl	2 –4 with each meal

DIET: consume high fiber foods such as grains, unless flare-up is acute then be sure that fiber foods are very soft before consuming. If necessary, consume bland foods even baby foods during an acute phase.

EXERCISE: Light exercise often helps with colon action and will help to lower stress levels. Stress has been linked with this condition and stress management may also be indicated.

Common Cold

In spite of miraculous advances in conquering bacterial infections, the virus that causes the Common Cold has managed to escape the vast wisdom of medical science.

An occasional cold is not only normal, but is actually beneficial to the immune system. However, colds should be very infrequent and should never last more than 72 hours. If you get more than one cold per year and it lasts and lasts, it's a sign that your immune system is weakened and unable to respond quickly with antibody production.

Full Spectrum Nutrition Plus:

Take a combination of the following nutrients
Every two hours for two days...

Colostrum Concentrate	100 mg
Beta-1,3-D Glucan	25 mg
Mushroom Mycelial Biomass	200 mg
Echinacea Purpurea leaf	25 mg
Astragalus Extract	50 mg
Pau D'Arco Extract	50 mg
Vitamin C	1,000 mg every two hours
Vitamin A (natural only)	25,000 IU per day
Zinc Lozenges	1 every 4 hours

EXERCISE: Exercise should be reduced during a cold but on the other hand, you should not stay totally inactive either. Moving around and light exercise will actually help you to feel better and will likely shorten the length of the cold. Activity helps the immune system by circulating the lymphatic system.

DIET: consume lots of juices and fresh foods. Soups and other hot liquids help relieve nasal and sinus congestion.

Congestive Heart Failure

A symptom, more than a condition of its own, Congestive Heart Failure occurs most often after prolonged periods of high blood pressure, which results in heart damage. As the heart struggles to meet bodily demands, it often becomes enlarged and cannot function fully. This results in a buildup of water in the lungs and the lower extremities of the body. The treatment of this condition should begin with finding the cause and correcting it. The following nutrients will help strengthen the heartbeat.

Full Spectrum Nutrition Plus:

L-Carnitine	1000 mg 2 –3 times per day
CoEnzyme Q10	100 mg 2-3 times per day
Taurine	1000 mg per day
Hawthorn Berry	300-500 mg per day
Magnesium	600 – 1000 mg per day
Vitamin B1	150- 300 mg per day

Constipation

Constipation is a condition of sluggish bowels brought about by waste material exiting too slowly. As a result of constipation, the sufferer can develop Gas, Insomnia, Bad Breath, Varicose Veins, Indigestion, Diverticulitis, Bowel Cancer, and Hemorrhoids.

The most common cause of constipation is a lack of adequate fiber and fluids in the diet. Some medications can also cause constipation. It is important that the bowels move at least once per day to avoid reabsorbing potentially toxic substances from the feces.

Full Spectrum Nutrition Plus:

Aloe Vera Juice	6 ounces twice per day

Take a combination of the following herbs twice a day:

Cascara Extract	2 mg
Rhubarb Root	10 mg
Bukthorn Berry	10 mg
Elderberry	10 mg
Licorice Root Extract	50 mg
Garlic	50 mg
Quassia Bark	50 mg
Red Sage Root	50 mg
Increase Fiber	10 grams per day
Increase Water	8 – 10 glasses per day
Multi Acidophilus	5 capsules per day
Multi Enzymes	2 – 4 with each meal

DIET: Drink plenty of water! Eat high fiber foods such as fresh veggies, whole-grains and sweet potatoes. Avoid excessive fats until the condition has corrected itself.

EXERCISE: Regular exercise stimulates colon activity and often speeds up transit time of wastes in the intestines.

Copper Toxicity – See Heavy Metal Poisoning

Crohn's Disease

An Autoimmune condition, Crohn's Disease can be very dangerous if not properly controlled. Attention to diet and dietary restrictions are a must. Eliminate all possibility of allergies by testing and avoiding all offending foods. Crohn's Disease often strikes at a fairly young age, usually in the 20's. Since this disease causes malnutrition and absorption difficulties, liquid nutritional supplements are essential.

Full Spectrum Nutrition Plus:

Fiber	10 grams per day
Multi-Acidophilus	8-10 capsules per day
Aloe Vera Juice	6 ounces 3 times per day
Folic Acid	2 – 5 mg per day
Vitamin B12 (sublingual)	500 mcg 4 times per day
Calcium	1000 mg extra
Magnesium	500 mg extra
Zinc Gluconate	50 mg per day
Multi-Digestive Enzyme	2-3 with meals

DIET: consume alkaline veggies such as cabbage, carrots, celery, garlic, and spinach. Be sure to drink plenty of fluids such as juices and herb teas. Consider consuming papaya for better digestion. Avoid refined carbohydrates as these have been linked to Crohn's disease.

Cystic Fibrosis

This hereditary disease involves both the Endocrine and Exocrine glandular systems and is characterized by repeated lung infections and poor nutrient absorption. Again, for this condition, liquid nutritional formulas are an absolute must.

Full Spectrum Nutrition Plus:

Multi-Enzyme Formula	2- 4 capsules with each meal
Whole Food Enzymes	2 – 4 capsules with each meal
B-Complex Stress Formula	As indicated on label
Vitamin C	3-6 grams per day
Vitamin K	6 tablets per day
Zinc Gluconate	50 mg per day
Protein Powder Drink from rice or soy	25 grams per day

DIET: Ensure that you are ingesting enough protein. Remember that those with this condition need much higher levels of nutrients from diet and supplements.

Cystitis

A severe, often chronic infection of the bladder, Cystitis must be handled aggressively.

Full Spectrum Nutrition Plus:

Vitamin C	To bowel tolerance
Cranberry Juice	8 ox 3-6 times per day
Liquid Oxygen	1 ounce 3 times per day
Multi-Acidophilus	4 capsules twice per day
Bromelain	200 mg 3 times per day

Follow Immune Protocol under Immunodepression heading.

Dandruff

Dandruff, those embarrassing white flakes of skin that appear in the hair and on your clothes, is a product of dysfunctional Sebaceous Glands in the scalp, which have probably been damaged through free radical activity.

Full Spectrum Nutrition Plus:

Kelp Tablets	5 – 10 per day
Essential Fatty Acids	2 grams per day
Vitamin E	400 IU extra
Zinc Gluconate	25 mg per day
Vitamin A (natural only)	25,000 IU per day

DDT Poisoning – See Heavy Metal Poisoning

Dementia (Senility)

Age often brings with it many symptoms due to the deterioration of bodily function. As the brain ages, deterioration can take place as well. One of the best-proven remedies for Dementia is 'exercising' your brain in a challenging manner. The following nutrients have been shown to increase cognition and improve short-term memory.(see chapter 4, for a complete discussion of the memory)

Full Spectrum Nutrition Plus:

Folic Acid	5 – 10 mg daily for 1 week
Niacin	100 mg 3 times/ day for 1 week
Vitamin B12 (sublingual)	1000 mcg per day for 1 week

Follow-up after 1 week with:

Folic Acid	1 mg per day
Thiamin	100 mg 3 times per day
Vitamin B12	500 mcg per day
Zinc	50 mg per day
Phosphatidyl Choline	500 - 1000 mg per day
Phosphatidyl Serine	500 mg per day
5–Hydroxy-tryptophan (5-HTP)	25 mg per day

Depression

Symptoms of Depression include fatigue, insomnia, or frequent sleeping, moodiness, dark negative thoughts, loss of appetite, headaches, colon disorders, and feelings of worthlessness and despair.

Depression, especially if serious, should NEVER be self-treated. You need to be under the supervision of a qualified Orthomolecular Psychiatrist. Depression can be caused by many things and can range from minor to devastating. Nutrients involved in the stress response as well as those affecting brain chemistry are listed below.

Full Spectrum Nutrition Plus:

Stress B-Complex	double the label dosage
Vitamin B12 (sublingual)	500 mcg 3 –4 times per day
Magnesium	600 mg per day extra
Vitamin B1	100 – 200 mg per day
Vitamin B6	50 – 100 mg per day
Iron	50 mg per day for 1 week
Betaine Hydrochloride	300 mg with each meal
5-Hydroxy-Tryptophan (5-HTP)	200-400 mg per day
St. John's Wort	100 – 200 mg per day
Acetyl L-Carnitine	500 – 1000 mg per day
Phosphatidylserine	300 – 600 mg per day
Phenylalanine*	1000 mg at bed time

*Note: *do not take if you suffer from uncontrolled high blood pressure.*

DIET: Avoid refined carbohydrates, which can cause low blood sugar. Consume complex carbohydrates, which can help to relax the system. Do not consume artificial sweeteners, especially aspartame. Avoid alcohol, caffeine, and chocolate.

EXERCISE: Regular exercise increases the "feel good" hormones in the brain such as serotonin and the endorphins.

Dermatitis

An allergic reaction of the skin, which manifests as scaling, flaking, and itching. Dermatitis is caused by the skin's exposure to an offending substance such as poison ivy and other plants, certain creams, ointments, rubber, metals, and cosmetics. Avoidance of the offending substance is essential or the condition will worsen and spread.

Full Spectrum Nutrition Plus:

High Potency B-Complex	As indicated on product label
Kelp	5 – 10 tablets per day

Essential Fatty Acids	1000 mg per day
Zinc Gluconate	100 mg per day for 1 week

DIET: Avoid eggs, nuts, soy and dairy to excess. Some people do very well on a gluten-free diet. You may wish to try this for 4 to 6 weeks. Increase fiber in the diet by consuming high fiber foods. Check for food allergies. Consider doing a detoxification program every 3 to 6 months. (see appendix)

Diabetes Mellitus (Type-II diabetes)

The fastest growing epidemic in industrialized nations, Adult-Onset Diabetes accounts for 90% of all diabetes worldwide and is the product of over-consumption of refined carbohydrates and sugars. (See Chapter 4 for a complete discussion of this disease.)

Full Spectrum Nutrition Plus:

Chromium	200 mcg per meal
Vanadium	300 mcg per meal
Bitter Melon	50-100 mg per meal
Alpha Lipoic Acid	30 mg per meal
Gymnema Sylvestre	50 mg per meal
Syzqium Culmini	10 mg per meal
Hydroxycitric Acid	1200 mg per meal

Consider also taking a high potency antioxidant formula to prevent damage from free radicals generated by this disease.

EXERCISE: Regular exercise helps to increase insulin receptor site function and lower the need for insulin. Be sure and maintain the same level of exercise so your body can better regulate insulin requirements.

DIET: Controlling and restricting carbohydrate intake is essential for type II diabetes. If you have been consuming high amounts of carbohydrates, you will have to reduce them slowly to avoid a low blood sugar episode. (see chapter 4)

Diabetic Retinopathy

Type2 diabetes is an epidemic in this country. It now affects over 20% of the population over the age of 60 and almost 10% of the population over the age of 40. Both type1 and type2 diabetic patients are at high risk of developing diabetic cataracts and more serious retinopathies that can lead to complete loss of vision if not properly treated. A potent full-spectrum multiple is a <u>must</u> protocol for all diabetic patients. Additional diabetic/ocular disease specific nutrients include:

Zeaxanthin	3 - 12 mg
Lutein	7 - 12 mg
Chromium	150 mcg
Vanadium	150 mcg
Alpha Lipoic Acid	40 - 150 mg
Mixed flavanoid antioxidants	300 mg
N-acetyl-cysteine	100 mg
Good -quality Fish Oil	1000 mg

The formulas above are available from Biosyntrx: **Oculair** and **ZoOmega3** and **Zeaxanthin 4** (see Appendix)

Diarrhea

This condition can have many causes ranging from nothing more than the rapid elimination of a toxic substance to the result of a chronic chemical imbalance in the digestive system.

Loss of fluids can lead to dehydration so extra care must be given to adequate fluid replacement. If the condition persists, even after following the steps below, or if there is blood in the stool, see a qualified medical doctor immediately.

Full Spectrum Nutrition Plus:

Fasting	Eat nothing for 24 – 48 hours
Fluids	8-10 glasses of water daily

Multi-Acidophilus	10 capsules daily
Folic Acid	1 mg per day
Essential Fatty Acids	1000 mg per day
Multi-Enzymes with	
Hydrochloric acid	2 –6 per meal

Herbs such as Carob Pod Powder and Citrus Seed Extract are also helpful.

Diverticulitis – See Colitis

Drug Addiction (Substance Abuse)

This is a growing problem worldwide. While the single greatest factor is abusive behavior is society, it is believed to be, in part, a gross deficiency of the B–Complex nutrients. The following nutrient program can help reduce the cravings and speed along recovery.

Full Spectrum Nutrition Plus:

High potency B-Complex	2 –3 times the label dosage
B12 Injections	1cc per day
Calcium	1500 mg per day
Magnesium	750 mg per day
Antioxidant Compound with	
Coenzyme Q10, Milk Thistle,	
Quercetin, N-Acetyl Cysteine,	
Bilberry Extract and Grape Seed	400 mg 2 –3 times per day

If diet is poor...

High protein Liquid Meals	50 grams protein per day

GABA

(gamma-amino butyric acid)	As directed on product label
L-Phenylalanine*	1000 mg in the morning

*Note: *do not use this if you have uncontrolled high blood pressure.*

DIET: Increase protein intake by using a high quality protein, preferably from Whey protein. Whey is a natural anti-depressant and also increases immune function. Consider a detoxification program to help remove drug residue from the body. (see appendix)

EXERCISE: Endurance exercise helps to rid the body of toxins as well as improve mood by increasing the endorphins in the brain.

Dry Eyes

Dry Eye Syndrome, sometimes referred to as Tear Film Disorder by the eye care professional community, affects approximately 20% of the adult population over the age of 40. It is the most frequent patient complaint to eye doctors. This disease is commonly associated with a systemic inflammatory process, and like most degenerative eye disease, it is often related to health condition in the rest of the body, including dryness of other mucous membranes such as mouth, vagina, and joints. It's important to note that untreated dry eyes dramatically affect quality of vision. The following daily protocol controls dry eyes in about 80% of the dry eye population.

Full Spectrum Nutrition Plus:

Vitamin A	2000 IUs
Vitamin C	200 mg
Vitamin D	100 mg
Vitamin E	64 IUs
Vitamin B6	16 mg
Magnesium	40 mg
4:1 ratio of Black Currant Oil and Cod Liver Oil equaling 1600 mg per day	
Mucopolysaccharides	500 mg
Tumeric	200 mg
Lactoferrin	20 mg

This formula is available from Biosyntrx and is called **BioTears Oral GelCaps** (see Appendix)

Dumping Syndrome – See Irritable Bowel Syndrome

Dysmenorrehea

An all too common condition, Dysmenorrehea is the cause of more sick days among menstrual-age women than any other single factor. It is signified by excessive pain during menstruation. While the exact cause in unknown, increased Prostaglandins are thought to be part of the principle mechanism.

Full Spectrum Nutrition Plus:

Bilberry Extract	200 mg per day
Dong Quai	100 mg 3 times per day
Papain	2 –3 capsules with each meal
Bromelain	1-2 capsules with each meal
Feverfew	As indicated on product label

Dyspepsia – See Indigestion

Ear Infection/Ache

The most common cause for a doctor visit, ear infections send more children to the doctor than any other cause. Most ear infections will pass in a few days providing that the child's immune system is functioning properly. If not, then attention to the immune system must be primary.

Full Spectrum Nutrition Plus:

Liquid Oxygen	1 ounce twice daily – depending upon age
Vitamin C	To bowel tolerance
Vitamin A	5,000 to 25,000 IU – depending upon age

Consider the protocol under Immunodepression if there are repeated infections.

Ecchymoses – See Vasculitis

Eczema (Atopic Dermatitis)

This skin condition may be closely related to a fatty acid deficiency and/or specific food and airborne allergies. If control is difficult, it is essential to rule out all allergies.

Full Spectrum Nutrition Plus:

Vitamin C	3-5 grams
Zinc	100 mg for two weeks
Copper	2 mg for two weeks
Essential Fatty Acids	2 –3 grams
Vitamin A (from fish liver oil)	25,000 – 100,000 IU

If food allergies are present add:

Betaine Hydrochloride	100-400 mg per meal

Edema

This is a general term used for the accumulation of fluid in the body. Also called dropsy, edema may be caused by many underlying conditions. The best treatment for this problem is to address the causes behind it. The fluid is most often retained in the feet and ankles. Ongoing edema may be a sign of kidney, bladder, heart, or liver problems. Another major reason for edema is hypersensitivity to certain foods, especially intolerance to carbohydrates. If all other reasons are eliminated without finding the cause consider an allergy test and/or reduce the amount of carbohydrates in the body. A high protein diet, together with fresh fruits and vegetables, is very helpful. Exercise is also an important part of overall management.

Full Spectrum Nutrition Plus:

Protein	80-100 grams
Vitamin B6	50 mg 3 times per day
L- Carnitine	500 mg 2 times per day
L- Taurine	500 mg 2 times per day

Calcium/ Magnesium/ Potassium
(Lost during diuresis)   As needed

EXERCISE: Exercise regularly to keep fluids circulating in the body.

Emesis - See Nausea and Vomiting

Emphysema

An overall deterioration of the lungs and their ability to intake oxygen and exhale carbon dioxide, Emphysema is primarily caused by cigarette smoking. Other causes can include related lung disorders, repeated lung infections, and even long-term protein deficiency.

Full Spectrum Nutrition Plus:

Multi-purpose Enzyme	2-4 with each meal
Coenzyme Q10	50 mg twice per day
Germanium	200 mg per day
L-Cysteine/ L Methionine	500 –1000 mg twice per day
Protein	80 –100 grams per day
Vitamin A (from fish liver oil)	25,000-50,000 IU per day
Vitamin C	5-10 grams per day
Liquid Oxygen	1 ounce 3 times per day on an empty stomach

DIET: Consume mostly raw foods and use chicken, turkey and fish as the main sources of protein. Increase consumption of garlic.

EXERCISE. Regular exercise is very important. Try to exercise every day, either by walking or other activities you enjoy.

Endometriosis

This is a disorder results in the growth of cells normally lining the uterus to also grow elsewhere. This condition produces many symptoms and complications including severe pain in the uterus, lower back, and pelvic region.

Excessive bleeding together with large clots and shreds of tissue are also common symptoms. Nausea, vomiting, and constipation are common during the menses, and these individuals are frequently infertile. There are many theories, but few facts, as to the actual cause of this condition. Research, being conducted at several centers around the world, is 'shedding new light' on the cause of this condition.

Full Spectrum Nutrition Plus:

Vitamin E	800 –1200 IU per day
Chelated Iron	12-24 mg per day
Essential Fatty Acids	2-4 grams per day
Anti-Stress Nutrient Formula	As directed
Calcium (citrate/malate)	1500 mg
Magnesium	1000 mg
Potassium	100 – 400 mg per day
Lipotropics:	
Choline/Inostitol/Methionine	1000 mg twice per day
Vitamin B6	100 – 200 mg per day for 6 weeks

EXERCISE: A combination of endurance and aerobic exercise is best.

DIET: Avoid alcohol, caffeine, excessive animal fats and fried foods. Consider fasting once a month just before your anticipated menstrual period.

Environmental Toxicity

There are tens of thousands of foreign chemicals present in our immediate environment. They are in the water, food, air, and virtually everything found in our home and work environments. Detoxification of these chemical residues from the body is essential. (See Appendix for our cleanse and detoxification program)

Antioxidants are essential to prevent the massive free radical formation, which occurs when these toxins enter the internal environment of the body.

Full Spectrum Nutrition Plus:

Coenzyme Q10	30 –50 mg
Milk Thistle	100-200 mg
N-Acetyl Cysteine	200-400 mg
Garlic	2-4 capsules per meal
Vitamin A (from fish liver oil)	50,000-100,000 IU
Vitamin E	400-800 IU
Liquid Oxygen	1 ounce two or three times per day on empty stomach

Epilepsy

Caused by mild to massive electrical disturbances in the nerve impulses of the brain, epilepsy can result in seizures ranging from petit mal (mild) to grand mal (severe and extremely debilitating). While epilepsy is thought to be hereditary, it can also be suddenly induced by an infection, meningitis, malnutrition, hypoglycemia, head injuries, fever, or severe allergies. For this reason a diagnosis as to the type of epilepsy and probable cause is essential in building a specific support program

Full Spectrum Nutrition Plus:

Low Carbohydrate (Ketogenic) Diet	
Niacin	1-3 grams per day (work up slowly)
Vitamin B 6	100 mg per day
Copper chelate	2 mg per day
Magnesium	1000 mg on empty stomach

Note: if magnesium causes diarrhea, take either apple cider vinegar or Betaine Hydrochloride with it.

Vitamin B 12	200 mcg sublingual 3 times per day
L-Taurine	500 mg 3 times per day
L- Tyrosine	500 mg 3 times per day
High Potency B-Complex	50 mg combination, 3 times per day

DIET: A ketogenic diet (low carbohydrate) is often helpful in reducing the frequency and severity of seizures.

Epstein Barr Virus – See Chronic Fatigue Syndrome

Esophagitis – See Heartburn & Digestive Disorders

Flatulence

Lower intestinal gas is formed when fermented carbohydrates enter the small and large intestines, forming methane gases. This condition can also occur when there is a lack of natural bacterial in the Colon.

Full Spectrum Nutrition Plus:

Multi-purpose Enzyme	2-4 capsules per meal
Betaine Hyrochloride	100-200 mg per meal
Acidophilus	5-10 capsules per day on empty stomach

Fatigue (See also Chronic Fatigue Syndrome)

The biggest cause of fatigue is either a lack of adequate sleep or a diet high in fat and carbohydrates and low in protein. Drug abuse, including alcohol, caffeine, and tobacco, can steal precious energy and cause us to sleep less soundly at night. If the fatigue is severe, a medical examination is in order to expose the underlying cause, which may be another disease or the presence of a virus or bacterial infection. General lack of energy may be remedied with the following program.

Full Spectrum Nutrition Plus:

Extra Liquid Organic Source Minerals	1-2 ounces per day
High potency B-Complex	50 mg twice per day
Protein	80 – 100 grams per day

Iron	as needed
Zinc	50 mg per day
Folic Acid	400 mcg per day
Ginseng	per label indication
Vitamin B12 injections	per your physician

Fatty Liver

Like most problems with the liver, the Lipotropic Nutrients work the best in restoring function and fixing the problem.

Full Spectrum Nutrition Plus:

Lipotropics	
Choline	
Inositol	
Methionine	1000 mg 2 times per day
Lecithin Granules	1-2 tablespoons per day
Multi Antioxidants	400-800 mg per day

Fever

Fever is always caused by the presence of some pathogen, usually viral or bacterial. Fever, to a point, is beneficial and should be allowed to run its course providing it doesn't go too high. Fever is one of the body's best weapons against infection. Support by boosting the immune response is very helpful.

Full Spectrum Nutrition Plus: (as soon as the crisis period is over.)

Colostrum extract	200-500mg 4 to 6 times per day
Mushroom extract mix	100-200 mg 4 to 6 times per day
Astragallis	50 – 100 mg per day
Echinacea	100-300 mg per day
1-beta D Glucan	50 –200 mg per day

Fibrocystic Disease of the Breast – See protocol for Fatty Liver

Fibroid Tumor – See protocol for Fatty Liver

Fibromyalgia

This condition is relatively new, yet is appearing in epidemic numbers. There are many theories behind the cause of this, including a virus, although that has never been proven. My work with persons suffering from this condition has shown me that they are all very toxic. When their systems have been properly detoxified their symptoms all but disappear. My personal feeling is that this is a condition of hyper-toxicity and it manifests in persons who are unable to physically cope with the overload of toxins in the system.

Full Spectrum Nutrition Plus:

Toxi Cleanse	per label instructions
Liquid Oxygen	1 ounce 3 times per day
FibroEze	400 mg per day
Vitamin B-6	25 mg per day
Vitamin C	Bowel Tolerance
5-hydroxy Tryptophan (5-HTP)	50 mg 3 times per day

NOTE: FibroEze is available from Phoenix Nutritionals – www.phoenixnutritionals.com

DIET: It is important to eliminate any possible food allergies. Take an extensive allergy test and abstain from any offending foods.

Fibrositis – See Rheumatism

Flu – See Influenza

Food and Chemical Sensitivities – See Allergies

Fractures

A fracture is a break in the bone and may be simple or compound. Once the acute situation has been handled by medical personnel, the following protocol will help accelerate healing.

Full Spectrum Nutrition Plus:

Liquid Organic-Source Trace Minerals	2-4 oz per day
Liquid Oxygen	1 ounce 2 times per day
On an empty stomach	
Calcium	1000 –2000 mg per day
Magnesium	1000 mg per day
Boron	2-4 mg per day
Horsetail	per label instructions

Fungus

Fungus can take many forms both externally, such as under nails, or internally, such as Yeast Infections or Candidiasis.

Common sites for yeast infections are the mouth, skin, vagina, nails, or between the toes. While there are many causes of yeast and fungus infections, a depressed immune system, usually through stress, is the main cause. While using topical preparations, the following will help to kill the parasite off from the inside, while boosting the immune system.

Full Spectrum Nutrition Plus:

Liquid Oxygen	1 oz 3 times per day for 1 week 2 oz 3 times per day for 4 – 6 weeks
Multi-Acidophilus	10 capsules per day for 10 days on an empty stomach
Colostrum	200 –400 mg 3 times per day
Mushroom Extract	100-400 mg 3 times per day
Echinacea Extract	per label
Antiseptic Hydrogen Peroxide	topically to infected area

Gallbladder Disease/Disorder

Located directly under the liver, the Gallbladder serves as a storage site for bile, needed in the digestion of fat. A congested Gallbladder can inflame and even infect. This can be a serious condition and should be addressed medically as soon as possible.

Another condition of the gallbladder occurs when stones of calcium form in the organ and block the flow of bile. (See Gallstones protocol.) The following nutrients have been shown to assist the gallbladder in both maintenance and function.

Full Spectrum Nutrition Plus:

Vitamin C	2-4 grams per day
Vitamin E	400 IU
Choline	500 mg
Essential Fatty Acids	2-3 grams per day
Multi Digestive Enzyme	2-4 with each meal
Ox Bile	50-100 mg per meal
Curcumin	per label
Milk Thistle	100 mg per day

DIET: Avoid sugar and refined carbohydrates. Consider consuming as much apple juice as possible for a week during an incidence.

Gallstones

Stones, made up of calcium and other minerals, can form in various sites around the body such as the kidneys, bladder, and the Gallbladder. This usually occurs when the overall pH of the body is alkaline too much of the time.

Emphasis must therefore be placed upon increasing minerals while adjusting the pH of the body towards greater acidity at the same time.

Full Spectrum Nutrition Plus:

Calcium	1000-1500 mg per day
Magnesium	750-1000 mg per day

Boron	2 mg per day
Liquid Organic Trace Minerals	1 oz 2 times per day
Betaine Hydrochloride	100-400 mg per meal
Apple Cider Vinegar	2 tabl 2 or 3 times per day mixed with water
Lecithin Granules	2 tabl per day
Dietary Fiber	10-15 grams per day
Taurine	500 mg 2 times per day

Gingivitis

An advanced disease condition of the gums, Gingivitis involves bone loss through infection caused by the buildup of oral plaque. While nothing replaces regular cleaning and maintenance by your dentist, the following will help control the problem.

Full Spectrum Nutrition Plus:

Calcium/ Magnesium	2000 mg
Vitamin C	to Bowel Tolerance
Vitamin A (from fish liver oil)	25,000 –50,000 IU per day
Mouthwash & Toothpaste containing hydrogen peroxide	
Licorice Root	per label
Bloodroot	per label

Glaucoma

Glaucoma is the leading cause of blindness, not just vision loss, for people over the age of 40. It affects almost 4 million Americans and that number is rising. The genome project has identified genes specifically associated with retina cell death associated with nitric oxide radicals that contribute to the eye's fluid drainage system, which is associated with inner ocular pressure. As in the case of macular degeneration, specific nutrients appropriately control the activity of these genes and glaucoma risks. A full-spectrum multiple is recommended for the glaucoma patient. Specific nutrients associated with optic nerve health and inner ocular pressure control:

Full Spectrum Nutrition Plus:

Taurine	500 mg
Vitamin C	250 – 500 mg
Vitamin E	100-400 mg
Vitamin B6	30-60 mg
Lipoic Acid	100-150 mg
Ginkgo Biloba	20 - 40 mg
Magnesium	100 mg
Acetyl-L-Carnitine	200 mg
N-acetyl-cysteine	100 mg
Grape Seed Extract	30 mg
Bilberry	30 mg
Bioflavonoid Complex	510 mg
(quercetin, rutin, hesperiden)	
Omega3 fatty acids from fish oil```	1000 mg

The above protocol may be obtained from Biosyntrx. For this condition they recommend **Macula Complete** and **ZoOmega3** (see Appendix)

————

Gout

This genetic condition occurs primarily in males and is the result of excess uric acid forming in the blood. The uric acid forms crystals and settles in the joints of the body, most often the feet, creating extremely intense pain and inflammation. Since uric acid is the by-product of certain foods these must be limited at all times and complete eliminated during an outbreak.

Further, increasing urine output is also helpful in excreting the excess uric acid.

Full Spectrum Nutrition Plus:

Vitamin C	To Bowel Tolerance
High Potency B-Complex	50 mg 2 times per day
Pantothenic Acid	1000 mg per day

Vitamin E	400 IU per day
Multi-Purpose Enzyme	2-4 per meal
Folic Acid	5-10 mg per day
L-Cysteine	1 –2 grams per day
Essential Fatty Acids	3-5 grams per day

Avoid taking more than 10,000 IU of vitamin A during an attack and increase the consumption of water as much as possible.

DIET: Avoid purine foods including anchovies, asparagus, herring, meat gravies, mushrooms, mussels, organ meats, sardines, cauliflower, lentils, peas, and spinach. Reduce your overall intake of alcohol and never consume alcohol with purine foods as this greatly increases the production of uric acid.

Gum Disease – See Periodontal Disease & Gingivitis

Hair Loss

There are almost as many reasons for hair loss as there are people experiencing the problem. Nutrient deficiencies, stress, and hormone imbalances lead the list. Factors that also affect hair loss include acute illness, surgery, radiation, skin diseases, crash diets, diabetes, thyroid disorders, and many pharmaceuticals.

In treating severe hair loss, it is important to uncover the exact underlying cause. The following program will help to meet nutritional needs and eliminate obvious hair loss related deficiencies.

Full Spectrum Nutrition Plus:

Liquid Organic –Source Trace Minerals	1oz 2 times per day
Biotin	per label
Essential Fatty Acids	2-4 grams per day
High B-Complex	50 mg 2 times per day
MSM (organic sulfur)	100 mg 2 –3 times per day
Horsetail	2 tablets 2 times per day

Hay Fever – See also Allergies

Hay Fever or Allergic Rhinitis, is an allergic response, usually to airborne offenders such as dust, pollen, grasses and flowering plants.

It affects the mucous membranes of the nose, eyes, and throat. While treating the underlying allergy is essential the following nutrients will prevent infection by protecting the mucosal lining of the sinuses and throat.

Full Spectrum Nutrition Plus:

Vitamin A (from fish liver oil)	25,000 – 100,000+ IU per day
Coenzyme Q10	30 mg 2 –3 times per day
Vitamin C	to Bowel Tolerance
Liquid Oxygen	1 oz 2 –3 times per day
Vitamin E	400 – 800 IU per day

Headache

Headaches may be caused by dozens of situations and conditions from benign to acutely serious. If you have repeated headaches, I would recommend that you find out the cause behind the condition as this would make management much easier.

If you suffer from the occasional headache, it is most often due to stress or allergies. Typical offending foods and food substances that produce headaches include wheat, chocolate, MSG (monosodium glutamate), sulfites, sugar, processed meats, cold cuts, cheeses, sour cream, yogurt, alcohol, vinegar, or other marinated foods.

Many airborne allergies can contribute to headache by inflaming the sinuses and related tissues. If you have poor vertebral alignment, headaches can be a regular occurrence and you need to see a Chiropractor. Stress still remains the number one cause of headaches and efforts to manage and channel stress effectively are essential.

Full Spectrum Nutrition Plus:

Calcium	1500 mg per day
Magnesium	1000 mg per day
Acidophilus bacteria	1 tsp. daily

Stress B-Complex	2 –4 capsules 2 times per day
Vitamin C	1-3 grams
Essential Fatty Acids	1-2 grams
Gingko biloba extract	250-400 mg per day
Cayanne Pepper	as per label
Ginger	as per label
Lithium (organic)	20 mcg
Feverfew	as per label
Lavender	as per label

Hearing Impairment

While there are many causes for a loss of hearing, the following nutrients have proven to be very helpful in both restoring hearing and preventing further loss.

Full Spectrum Nutrition Plus:

Ginger	per label
Gingko Biloba	100-300 mg
Vitamin A (fish liver oil)	10,000 – 25,000 IU
Calcium	1000 mg
Fluoride	10-50 mg
Zinc sulfate	100-300 mg
Coenzyme Q10	30 mg 3 times per day
Essential Fatty Acids	1-2 grams per day

Rule out aluminum, lead and food poisoning.

Heartburn

This is one of the most misunderstood conditions of modern times. We are repeatedly told that heartburn is the result of excess stomach acid, when in fact, the exact opposite is most often the case.

The stomach is a naturally acidic organ. Hydrochloric Acid is produced in the stomach in the presence of protein foods. In truth, it is alkalinity that burns the stomach, not acidity. Heartburn is most often the result of too little stomach acid, causing food to ferment and form gases, resulting in further alkaline conditions.

Full Spectrum Nutrition Plus:

Multi-purpose enzymes	2-4 with each meal
Betaine Hydrochloride	100-400 mg with each meal
Licorice Root	1-2 capsules per meal

DIET: Try not to consume concentrated carbohydrates and concentrated proteins at the same meal. By eating them apart, many digestive disturbances can be eliminated.

EXERCISE: Regular exercise, especially light exercise like walking, after a meal will help stimulate stomach acids.

Heart Disease

The majority of all heart disease is caused by a condition known as Atherosclerosis (see Chapter 4). The following nutrients will help strengthen the heart muscle while assisting to regulate the heartbeat. Additionally, there are nutrients that assist the body in removing the fat and calcium buildup within the arteries.

Heartwise Oral Chelation Formula as per label (available from Phoenix Nutritionals – www.phoenixnutritionals.com

Folic Acid	2-5 mg
Niacin	1000 mg 2-3 times per day
work up slowly	
Essential Fatty Acids	2-3 grams per day
Vitamin B-6	25-50 mg per day
Pantethine	300 mg 2-4 times per day
Vitamin E	400-800 IU per day
L-Carnitine	1000 mg 2-3 times per day
Coenzyme Q10	30 mg 2-3 times per day

DIET: Eliminate all vegetable oils except olive oil. Limit overall fat intake, but do not follow a low fat diet. Ensure that adequate protein in ingested. (80-100 grams per day) Increase fiber in the diet by consuming high fiber foods.

EXERCISE: Exercise is vital to the health of your heart muscle. After clearing with your Doctor, begin an exercise program of low impact resistance and cardio at least 3 to 4 times per week.

Heavy Metal Poisoning

When base elements of potentially toxic nature enter the body they can build up within the soft tissues because our chemistry does not recognize them as readily as if they were present in naturally occurring organic compounds.

In fact, many of the so–called 'toxic minerals' are actually of benefit to the body, but they must be ingested in the form of organic compounds and not simply base heavy metals.

Regardless of the offending element, be it Lead, Cadmium, Mercury, Arsenic, or Aluminum, when you ingest organic trace mineral compounds they effectively *chelate*, or remove these heavy metal counterparts, from your body. This process can take anywhere from three to six months.

Full Spectrum Nutrition Plus:

Liquid Organic-Source Trace Minerals   2-4 oz per day
(Continue to take until diarrhea develops, then back off slowly)

Liquid Oxygen   1 oz 2 times per day

Heel or Bone Spurs

A bone spur occurs in the same manner an organ stone, such as a kidney or gallstone, does. When Calcium and Magnesium are deficient in the body, these minerals are leached from the bone. This Bone Calcium is very alkaline and easily forms heel or bone spurs when the chemistry of the body is also over alkaline.

This alkalinity can occur from eating a diet of dead, lifeless foods for years or it may be rapidly induced through gross calcium deficiency or conditions that produce Alkalosis. It is very common for people with Arthritis to have these conditions as well, since the cause of both disorders is essentially the same.

Full Spectrum Nutrition Plus:

Liquid Organic-Source Minerals	1-2 oz extra
Calcium	1500 mg
Magnesium	750 mg
Multi purpose enzymes	2-4 with each meal
Betaine Hydrochloride	100-300 mg per meal

DIET: Increase consumption of acid-forming foods such as proteins, and vinegar.

Hemophilia

Hemophilia is an obscure blood disorder found only in males. The disease prevents blood from clotting, and the individual is in constant threat of bleeding to death, even from a small cut. Internal bleeding is the biggest threat. There is no known cure for Hemophilia. The following nutrient program will assist in managing this difficult condition.

Full Spectrum Nutrition Plus:

Calcium	1500 mg
Magnesium	1000 mg
Raw Liver Nucleoprotein	5-10 tablets per day
Extra B-Complex	50 mg per day
Vitamin C	3 grams per day
Vitamin K	300 mcg per day

Hemorrhoids

Characterized by swollen tissues around the anus, which may protrude out of the rectum, Hemorrhoids can be both annoying and uncomfortable.

Full Spectrum Nutrition Plus:

Calcium Malate/Citrate	1000 mg
Magnesium	750 mg
Vitamin C	3 grams per day
Bioflavonoids	2 grams per day
Vitamin E	400 IU
Coenzyme Q10	100 mg per day
Increase natural fiber	4-8 grams per day
Colon Cleanse Product	as per label
Vitamin A (fish liver oil)	25,000 IU per day

Soaking in a bath of warm water and Witch Hazel may be helpful.

DIET: Increase fiber by taking a daily fiber formula and consuming high fiber foods.

EXERCISE: Regular exercise can strengthen the muscles of the sphincter

Hepatitis

There are several types of hepatitis. The most common form is Type A, which is spread through person to person contact. Type B is transmitted via serum or blood through contaminated syringes, needles, insects, and blood transfusions. Another strain, Hepatitis C, is often the most dangerous as it frequently becomes chronic and destroys the quality of life for the sufferer.

Full Spectrum Nutrition Plus:

High potency Stress B-Complex	as per label
Milk Thistle (Silymarin)	100-500 mg
N-Acetyl Cysteine	100-500 mg
Licorice Root	as per label
Folic Acid	2 mg per day
Coenzyme Q10	30 mg 3 times per day

Lipotropics

    Choline

    Inositol

    Methionine — 1000 mg 3 times per day

Multi-enzyme formula — 2-4 with each meal

Betaine Hydrochloride — 100-300 mg per meal

Vitamin C — 3-5 grams per day

High Protein Diet — 80 –100 grams per day

Herpes

There are two basic strains of the Herpes virus. Type I (Herpes Simplex) and is most often acquired during birth from the mother. Type II is Genital Herpes and is most often transmitted sexually from one person to another.

Like most viruses, once Herpes enters the body, it never leaves. It can become dormant but will usually surface again during periods of stress or immune suppression.

Full Spectrum Nutrition Plus:

L-Lysine — 1000-3000 mg per day during an outbreak

Vitamin A (fish liver oil) — 25,000 IU per day

Vitamin C — to bowel tolerance

Zinc Gluconate — 50-100 mg daily during an outbreak

Essential Fatty Acids — 1-3 grams extra

Multi Acidophilus — 5-8 capsules per day

Vitamin E oil topically

Herpes Zoster

Also known as shingles, this often painful disorder is caused by the same virus that causes chicken pox and it affects the endings of the nerve lines in the skin. Like most viruses, risk of an outbreak of shingles is greatest when you are under severe stress or have an immune compromise.

Full Spectrum Nutrition Plus:

L-Lysine	2-4 grams per day
Bilberry extract	200-400 mg per day
Vitamin C	2-4 grams extra per day
Adensoine Monophsphate	as per label
Vitamin B12	100 mg 3 times per day
Cayenne Pepper	as per label

High Blood Pressure

A very common occurrence, High Blood pressure or Hypertension is a result of modern stressful living and electrolyte nutrient imbalance. Efforts to control Hypertension must revolve around stress management and electrolyte nutrient intake.

Full Spectrum Nutrition Plus:

Calcium	1500 –3000 mg per day
Magnesium	1000 mg per day
Potassium	100-300 mg per day
L-Carnitine	500 mg 2-3 times per day
Essential Fatty Acids	2-3 grams
Garlic Concentrate	as per label
Selenium	200 mcg per day
Coenzyme Q10	30 mg 2 times per day
Taurine	1-3 grams per day

Eliminate heavy metal toxicity and possible allergies.

EXERCISE: Excess body weight is one of the single greatest causes of high blood pressure. Exercise can increase the flexibility of the vascular system while helping to normalize bodyweight.

High Cholesterol

While cholesterol has never actually caused a single case of Heart Disease in medical history, elevated Cholesterol and other fats in the blood are not necessarily healthy. Dietary intake of Cholesterol affects the overall Cholesterol levels in the blood only marginally in most people.

This is because the body produces far more Cholesterol than we can possibly consume from our diet. The problems with Cholesterol level regulation begin in the liver and must be managed by cleansing and nourishing this organ. (see chapter 4, for a complete discussion of cholesterol management)

Full Spectrum Nutrition Plus:

Lipotropics	
Choline	
Inositol	
Methionine	1-2 grams per day
Lecithin Granules	1-3 tablespoons per day
Multi Antioxidants	400mg per day
Increase Fiber	4-8 grams per day
Garlic Capsules	2 capsules 3 times per day
Pantethine	500-1000 mg per day
Essential Fatty Acids	1-3 grams per day extra
Guggulipids	100-300 mg
Gamma-oryzanol	250-500 mg
Red Yeast Extract	as per label

DIET: Avoid vegetable oils except for olive oil. Do not consume margarines or other synthetic, chemically altered fats.

HIV – See AIDS

Hot Flashes – See Menopause (Also Chapter 4)

Hyperactivity (See also ADD)

Hyperactivity usually occurs in children and teenagers, although, if left untreated, can carry on into adulthood. It is characterized by excessive nervousness and irritable behavior. Since the central nervous system is involved, our focus will be on nutrients governing this area.

Full Spectrum Nutrition Plus:

Niacin	500 mg to 2000 mg depending upon weight
High potency Stress B-Complex	2-8 capsules per day
Organic Liquid Trace Minerals	to bowel tolerance
Calcium	100-2000 mg per day
Magnesium	10-750 mg per day (depending upon weight)

Rule out food allergies
Rule out heavy metal poisoning

Hypertension – See High Blood Pressure

Hyperthyroid

An over-active thyroid gland produces excessive amounts of hormone, causing an overactive metabolic environment within the body. Often the body's digestion can speed up, causing mal-absorption. Symptoms of this disorder include nervousness, irritability, increased perspiration, fatigue, weakness, hair and weight loss, insomnia, brittle nails, low tolerance to heat, rapid heartbeat, and hand trembling.

Full Spectrum Nutrition Plus:

High potency Stress B-Complex	2-4 capsules 2-3 times per day
Vitamin C	to bowel tolerance

Hypoglycemia

One of the three phases of Carbohydrate Intolerance, technically known as Hyperinsulinemia, Hypoglycemia is characterized by low blood sugar levels, caused by an overproduction of insulin, from the pancreas. Hypoglycemics can be either overweight or underweight, depending upon a variety of factors. Like all disorders involving Insulin, Hypoglycemia also involves the adrenal glands, which frequently over-secrete adrenaline as a result of low blood sugar levels.

Symptoms of Hypoglycemia include fatigue, dizziness, headache, irritability, indigestion, obesity, and impaired memory. While proper diet is the key to managing this chronic condition, the following protocol will assist the body in normalizing blood sugar levels and improving insulin regulation. (see also chapter 4)

Full Spectrum Nutrition Plus:

High Protein Diet	100 grams per day
Low Carbohydrate Diet	60 grams per day or less
Vitamin C	2 – 4 grams
Pantothenic Acid	2000 – 3000 mg per day
Adrenal Glandulars	6-10 tablets per day
Vitamin E	400 IU extra
Chromium	500 mcg per day
Vanadium	200 –400 mcg per day
Bitter Melon	50-100 mg per day
Gymnema Sylvestre	25-50 mg per day
Hydroxycitric Acid	600-1200 mg per day

Our specialized formula is available from Phoenix Nutritionals, www.phoenixnutritionals.com

DIET: A controlled carbohydrate diet is essential. If overweight this is particularly important. If normal weight, choose carbohydrates of a complex nature.

EXERCISE: Regular exercise is important in stabilizing blood sugar levels. Try to maintain the same level of exercise regularly to help the body balance blood sugar and insulin.

Hypothyroid

When the thyroid gland under-produces hormone, a variety of symptoms can arise. These include fatigue, loss of appetite, obesity, painful menstrual periods, weakness, dry/scaly skin, yellow bumps on the eyelids, frequent infections, depression, hair loss, and intolerance to the cold.

You can easily test your thyroid with a regular fever thermometer. Before you go to bed at night, shake down a thermometer and place it by your bed. When you first wake up in the morning, before moving about at all, place the thermometer under your arm for 10 minutes. You must remain still and quiet. If the temperature is consistently at 97.6 F or lower, it is a good indication that your thyroid is not producing enough hormone.

If it is low on a regular basis you may need Armour Thyroid Extract, which is available only by prescription from your doctor. The following protocol will help support thyroid function and may even adjust thyroid production if it is not too low.

Be sure to avoid anything with Chlorine or Fluoride, since these substances are not only carcinogenic, but block the action of Iodine, necessary for proper thyroid function.

Full Spectrum Nutrition Plus:

Kelp (seaweed)	10-15 Tablets daily
L-Tyrosine	500-1000 mg daily
Raw Thyroid Glandular	4-8 tablet per day
High Potency Stress B-Complex	30 –100 mg per day

The Institute has recently developed a unique formulation for those with under-active thyroid. Contact them for further information. (see Appendix)

Hysterectomy - See Chapter 4

Immunodepression

Our immune system is really the army of the body, providing protection against invading pathogens, which can cause harm to our health and well-being.

For years, medical science simply took for granted that the immune system did its job. Through the prominence of such conditions as AIDS and Cancer, we can see just how devastating it can be when the immune system fails or is prevented from functioning.

Through the tens of thousands of toxins in our environment, our immune system is constantly on overload, having to build antibodies to the many thousands of byproducts produced when these poisons are broken down internally.

Full Spectrum Nutrition Plus:

Colostrum Concentrate

Mycelium Mushroom Extracts   Beta – 1 D Glucan

Take this combination together according to your health care professional

Echinacea	as per label
Astragallus Membranaceus Extract	as per label
Panax Ginseng	as per label
Garlic Extract	4-8 capsules
Multi Antioxidants	400-800 mg per day
Dimethylglycine	100-400 mg per day
Selenium	200 mcg extra
L-Ornithine	500 mg 2 times per day
Zinc	50-100 mg per day
Beta Carotene	10,000 – 25,000 IU per day
Olive Leaf Extract	500 –1000 mg per day
Glycerol monolaurate	1000 mg per day
Goldenseal	1-4 capsule per day
Pantethine	500-1000 mg per day

To help prevent infections

Vitamin A	25,000 – 100,000 IU
Coenzyme Q10	30 mg

Be sure and rule out Heavy Metal Toxicity. If Heavy Metal Toxicity exists, it will be necessary to *chelate* or remove these offending substances. (See section on Heavy Metal Poisoning.)

Impotence

Difficulty in obtaining or maintaining an erection is becoming an increasing problem, even among younger men. There are some organic, physical reasons for this problem such as peripheral vascular disease and low sperm count, but for the vast majority of men it is a nutrient deficiency. I suggest the following protocol, but if it doesn't produce results within 30 days, see your physician and explore other possible causes.

Full Spectrum Nutrition Plus:

Yohimbine	100-400 mg
Note: Do not use if you have uncontrolled High Blood Pressure	
Gingko biloba	50- 100 mg
L-Arginine	500 mg 3 times per day
Zinc	50 mg extra
Octacosanol	per label
Raw Orchic Glandular	4-8 tablets per day
Ginseng	per label
Tribulus Terrestris	750 mg 1 or 2 times per day

NOTE: The Institute has developed a special combination of these nutrients. Contact them for further information on this formula. (see Appendix)

Indigestion (Dyspepsia)

Most symptoms of indigestion, which include feelings of fullness after a meal, bloating, belching, gas, and heartburn are caused by a lack of natural Hydrochloric Acid in the stomach. This lack of acids prevents the proper breakdown of protein foods leading to protein and mineral deficiencies.

Further, the lack of Hydrochloric Acid prevents the production of specific enzymes, involved in further digestion of foods. Taking antacids, while often producing relief, does nothing to improve digestion or assimilation of food.

The following program will not only bring relief, but also solve the problem as well by increasing the absorption of both foods and nutrients.

Full Spectrum Nutrition Plus:

Betaine Hydrochloride	100-300 mg per meal
Multi-Purpose Enzyme Precursor Containing	
Pancreatin	
Papain	
Bromelain	
Ox Bile	100-300 mg per meal

In severe cases of Over Alkalinity, Apple Cider Vinegar (2 Tbl) and water, taken two or three times per day is often helpful.

DIET: Avoid concentrated carbohydrates and concentrated proteins at the same meal.

Infections (See also Immunodepression)

Infections are a normal part of living. In fact an occasional bout with an invading bug actually stimulates the Immune System into greater function. However, when infections are prolonged and/or occur often, it is a sign of immune weakness and the Immune System needs to be both stimulated and nourished. Follow the protocol under Immunodepression. For topical infections follow the treatment suggestions below.

Full Spectrum Nutrition Plus:

Liquid Oxygen	1 ounce two or three times per day On an empty stomach

Use 3% on skin infections but not on open wounds.

Infertility (Men) – See Impotence in Chapter 4

Infertility (Women)

The inability to become pregnant after a long period of regular sexual activity usually signals hormonal problems. Some of the more frequent causes in women include pelvic disease, Chlamydia infection (untreated), and allergic reactions to their partner's sperm.

Since there are so many possible causes, it is wise to seek the advice of a qualified physician. If all the physical causes have been eliminated, the following program will support the woman's body nutritionally and put her in the best possible hormonal position to conceive.

Full Spectrum Nutrition Plus:

Folic Acid	400 mcg extra
Vitamin B6	50 mg extra
Zinc	50 –100 mg per day
Vitamin E	400 – 800 IU extra
Ovarian Glandular Extract	4-8 tablets per day
L-Arginine	4 grams per day
Iron	10-20 mg per day
Vitamin B12	100-300 mcg per day

Since stress is often involved in hormone imbalance, a high potency Stress B–complex formula, taken two or three times per day is often helpful.

Inflammation

When the body reacts to trauma or infection, swelling and pain is often the result. Inflammation may be either internal or external and involve almost any organ or other tissue.

Full Spectrum Nutrition Plus:

Vitamin C	To Bowel Tolerance
Bioflavonoids	3 –6 grams per day
Antioxidant Combination	400-800 mg per day during inflammation period
Bromelain	200-500 mg 3 times per day on empty stomach
Organic Source Trace Minerals	1 –3 ounces extra during inflammation
Horsetail Extract	per label
Curcumin	as per label
MSM	as per label

Inflammatory Bowel Disease (Irritable Bowel Syndrome)

This condition, which is directly tied into unmanageable stress, is becoming more and more common. Twice as many women suffer from this problem as men. IBD involves the muscular contraction of intestines and when these contractions are not smooth, it affects the movement of waste material to the bowel.

Symptoms include constipation alternating with rapid onset diarrhea, abdominal pain and cramping, and an excess production of mucus in the stool. Food allergies are also often at the heart of this problem so it is important to eliminate all offending foods.

Stress, the cardinal player in this condition, interferes with the acid/alkaline balance often causing spontaneous dumping of the contents of the Colon by flooding it with water.

Full Spectrum Nutrition Plus:

Essential Fatty Acids	3-6 grams extra
Fiber	3-6 grams
Peppermint Extract	2 capsules per day
Ginger Root Extract	3 capsules with each meal
Multi-Purpose Enzymes	2 –6 or more with each meal
High Potency Stress B-Complex	2-4 capsules 2 or 3 times per day
L-Glutamine	3-5 grams per day
Cascara sagrada	per label
Chamomile	per label

Eliminate all food allergens.

It is also important to learn to manage and reduce the stress your life.

Influenza – See Immunodepression

Insect Bite

Localized insect bites can be soothed and healed by applying 3% Hydrogen Peroxide to the affected area several times per day. A paste made from baking soda and applied to the skin is often helpful as well.

Insomnia

Sleeplessness is occasionally experienced by everyone and is little cause for concern. If, however, this condition occurs night after night, the underlying cause should be sought. Since there are many causes for this condition, you should seek the advice of a qualified health care practitioner. Poor nutritional habits and excess stress can also contribute to this condition.

Full Spectrum Nutrition Plus:

Calcium Lactate	1000 mg before bed
Magnesium	1000 mg before bed
Valerian Root Capsules	2-6 capsules 1 hour before bed

If stress is the underlying cause:

Kava Kava Extract	2-4 capsules 2 times per day
High Potency B-Complex	3 capsules 2 or 3 times per day

Melatonin	per label
Passion Flower Extract	per label

EXERCISE: Regular exercise can often greatly improve sleep patterns.

Intermittent Claudication

This condition, often associated with Atherosclerosis and other heart and circulatory disorders, is characterized by a weakness in the legs. This weakness occurs most often during exercise and may be accompanied by cramps or spasms in the calves. Intermittent Claudication occurs only at certain times, usually after an extended period of walking. (See also protocol for Atherosclerosis.)

Full Spectrum Nutrition Plus:

Bilberry Extract	4-8 capsules per day
Bromelain	300-500 mg per day

Gingko biloba	100 mg per day
Vitamin E	400 –800 IU extra
Inositol	500 – 1000 mg
Essential Fatty Acids	3-5 grams per day
Centella asiatica	per label
Hawthorn Berry	per label
Horsechestnut	per label
Ruscus aculeatus	per label

Irritable Bowel Syndrome – See Inflammatory Bowel Disease

Jaundice

Jaundice is caused by an obstruction of the flow of bile from the liver. This can be a sign of serious Liver Disease and should be addressed by a qualified physician. Nutrients to support the liver are as follows.

Full Spectrum Nutrition Plus:

Milk Thistle	100 – 400 mg per day
N-acetyl Cysteine	200-600 mg per day
Lipotropics	
Choline	
Inositol	
Methionine	1000 mg of combination 3 times per day

Kidney & Bladder Problems

Since the kidneys and bladder are responsible for elimination of waste fluids from the body, they must be kept in good health to avoid infections. There are several types of infections of the kidneys, many of them serious and require immediate medical attention. To avoid most of these situations, it is important to keep the bladder healthy and free from pathogens since many kidney problems result from previous bladder infections.

The following nutrients will help strengthen both the kidneys and bladder and assist with proper function.

Full Spectrum Nutrition Plus:

Water	6-8 ounce glass every hour during the day
Acidophilus capsules	5 capsules daily
Vitamin B6	50 mg 3 times per day during infection
Vitamin C	to bowel tolerance
Dandelion Root	per label
Calcium	1000 mg extra
L-Arginine	500 mg 3 times per day
Vitamin A (natural only)	25,000 – 50,000 IU per day
Zinc	50 mg per day
Choline & Inositol	1000 mg per day

FOR men: Saw Palmetto & Pygeum Africanum

FOR women: Black Cohosh & Mexican Yam

Kidney Stones

Stones in the kidneys and bladder as well as other deposits, such as heel spurs, are caused by minerals (especially calcium) dropping out of solution and forming crystals.

There are two main causes for this problem. Firstly, an over alkaline digestive system, which cannot properly acidify these minerals. Secondly, the over-consumption of sugar foods. When Insulin is present in the blood stream in large amounts, it accelerates the excretion of Calcium.

Full Spectrum Nutrition Plus:

To Acidify:

Betaine Hydrochloride	200-400 mg per meal
Apple Cider Vinegar	1Tbl 3 times per day in water

Nutritional Support:

Calcium Citrate/Malate only	1000 mg total per day
Magnesium Chelate	300 mg 3 times per day
Vitamin B6	50 mg 2 times per day during problems
Vitamin A	25,000 IU per day
Vitamin C	to bowel tolerance
Potassium	100 mg per day
L-Lysine	300 mg 2 times per day
Ginkgo Biloba Extract	per label
Goldenrod	per label
Rose hips	per label
Cranberry Juice or Capsules	8 oz 4 times per day or Label dose 4 times per day

---

Lead Poisoning – See Heavy Metal Poisoning

Learning Disabilities – See Attention Deficit Disorders

Leg Ulcers

Wounds that do not heal, primarily due to poor circulation, develop an erosion and ulceration is often the result. Diabetes and other diseases, which destroy circulation, are often at the cause of ulcers that will not heal.

Full Spectrum Nutrition Plus:

Liquid Oxygen	1 oz 3 –4 times per day on empty stomach
Hyperbaric Oxygen Treatments	as needed
Coenzyme Q 10	30 mg 2- 3 times per day
DMG (Dimethylglycine)	100 mg 3 times per day
Vitamin C	to bowel tolerance

Vitamin E	400 – 800 IU extra
Garlic Extract	4 capsules 3 times per day

Leukemia – See Cancer

Leukorrhea

This is a vaginal discharge resulting from, either, an infection, likely Chlamydia, or a yeast infection, such as Candida Albicans. Other causes can include nutrient deficiencies, especially the B-complex group.

Full Spectrum Nutrition Plus:

High Potency B-Complex	per label
Garlic Extract	2 capsules 3 or 4 times per day
Essential Fatty Acids	4-5 grams per day
Acidophilus	3 capsules 3 –4 times per day
Vitamin C	to bowel tolerance
Vitamin A (natural only)	25,000 – 50,000 IU per day
Liquid Oxygen Flush	See Chapter 4, under Candida

Lupus

This disease belongs to a group of illnesses called Autoimmune Disorders. This means that the immune system of the patient is actually attacking itself. Since the Immune System is already over-active, it is essential that these individuals DO NOT take any supplements that heavily stimulate the Immune System, as this can make the condition much worse.

There are two types of Lupus, Systemic Lupus Erythematosus, which affects organs and joints, and Discord Lupus Erythematosus, which is a skin disease. Various theories exist as to the cause of this autoimmune problem.

Full Spectrum Nutrition Plus:

Vitamin C	to bowel tolerance
Essential Fatty Acids	4-6 grams per day

Selenium	500 mcg
Multi-enzymes	2-4 with each meal
Alfalfa Capsules	per label
Niacin	25 mg 2 times per day
Pantothenic Acid	500 mg 2 times per day
Vitamin A (Fish liver oil)	25,000 IU per day
L-Cysteine	500 mg 3 times per day
Zinc	50 – 100 mg per day
Organic Sulfur	per label
DHEA	25 mg per day

Lyme Disease – See Immunodepression

Macular Degeneration

Age-related macular degeneration is a degenerative condition of the macula (the central retina). It is the most common cause of vision loss in Americans aged 50 or older, particularly in blue-eyed, post-menopausal females. Macular Degeneration is associated with arterial damage, which decreases blood flow into the capillaries that nourish the retina. The genome project has identified a number of genes associated with an increased risk of developing age-related macular degeneration. Clinical studies suggest that disease risk associated with these genes can be lowered by lifestyle choices that include moderate exercise, smoking cessation, UV protection and the daily intake of a potent full-spectrum multiple, including these additional nutrients, which are specifically associated with macula health:

Lutein	3 – 12 mg
Zeaxanthin	4 mg

These two plant based nutrients make up the macula pigment (the eyes' natural sunglasses).

Acetyl-L-carnitine	200 mg
Lipoic Acid	150 mg
CoQ10	20 mg

N-acetyl-cysteine	100 mg
Omega 3 fatty acids from fish oil	1000 mg

Supplements for the eyes are available from Biosyntrx. For this condition they recommend **Macula Complete** and **ZoOmega3** and **Zeaxanthin 4** (for resources see the Appendix)

Manic-Depressive Disorder

This disorder of brain chemistry is characterized by extreme mood swings, from excitement and elation to the depths of depression.

It is important to understand that no disorder involving brain chemistry imbalances should be self-treated. The chemistry of the brain is very tricky and ignorant experimentation can lead to a much worse condition.

We have done considerable work in this area of psycho nutrition, but I have decided not to publish our protocols due to the risk of attempts at self-management. If you suffer from this or any brain chemistry disorder, it is essential that you be under the care of a health care practitioner that understands both the disorder and the alternative methods of management involved.

If you have a health care practitioner, I am happy to share my experiences and the results of my work directly with them.

Melanoma – See Cancer

Memory Improvement (see also Chapter 4)

We all experience a temporary loss of memory from time to time. The most common cause of short term and brief memory loss is fatigue and excess stress. When memory recall becomes a more regular occurrence this is often a sign of underlying nutritional deficiencies, which are leading to an altered biochemistry. The following protocol represents the latest research into substances that have been shown to improve the memory response.

Full Spectrum Nutrition Plus:

L-Carnitine	100-300 mg
DMAE	150-300 mg
Gotu Kola	50 mg
Pantothenic Acid	150 mg
Phosphatidyl Serine	200-400 mg
Phosphatidyl Choline	200-400 mg
Vitamin B6	10-20 mg
Vitamin B12	100-300 mcg
Choline Bitartrite	200-400 mg
1-Pyroglutamic Acid	150-300 mg

Meniere's Syndrome

This condition of the inner ear can have many causes such as allergies, clogged arteries, poor circulation, and spasms. Symptoms of Meniere's included ringing in the ears, loss of hearing, nausea, and loss of balance. The following program represents a combination of the latest nutritional research on managing this annoying condition.

Full Spectrum Nutrition Plus:

Manganese	5 mg per day
Coenzyme Q10	100 mg per day
Vitamin A (natural)	25,000 IU per day
Vitamin D	200 IU extra
Calcium	1000 mg
Essential Fatty Acids	2-4 grams per day
Fluoride	per label
Zinc	100 mg per day
Valerian Root	per label
Kava Kava	per label

Meningitis – See Immunodepression

Menopause – See Chapter 4

Menstrual Cramps

The following program is especially helpful for the cramping often experienced during menstruation.

Full Spectrum Nutrition Plus:

Niacin	100 mg total per day
	100 mg every 3 hours during cramping
Vitamin E	400 IU extra
Iron	18 mg
Magnesium	100 mg 4 times per day
Bilberry Extract	100 mg 3 times per day

Menorrhagia

Characterized by long and excessive menstrual periods, this condition can be very debilitating, causing excessive iron deficiency and other nutrient loss. This condition often is a complication of Uterine Fibromyomata and other Uterine Disorders.

Full Spectrum Nutrition Plus:

Vitamin A (from fish liver oil)	25,000 IU 2 times per day
Iron	100 mg daily for 15 days
Manganese	5 mg per day
Bioflavonoids	1000 mg 3 times per day
Vitamin C	to bowel tolerance

Mercury Toxicity – See Heavy Metal Poisoning

Migraine Headaches

A headache of extreme severity, migraines are usually caused by either a chemical imbalance in brain chemistry or stress, which constricts the arteries of the brain putting pressure on nerves.

Allergies are also a common cause of migraine and other headaches and therefore should be either ruled out or managed accordingly. The majority of migraine headache sufferers are women (75%).

Migraine headaches may be distinguished from other types of headache by vomiting, blurred vision, tingling and numbness in the limbs, seeing stars, sparks, or flashes, and sometimes speech disorders.

Full Spectrum Nutrition Plus:

Liquid Oxygen	1 ounce 2-3 times per day
	2 ounces at the onset of headache
DMG (Dimethylglycine)	per label
Magnesium	200 – 400 mg per day
Essential Fatty Acids	2 grams per day
Feverfew	25-75 mg per day
Niacin	take enough to flush just as headache begins

DIET: Reduce or eliminate refined carbohydrates from the diet. Consume complex carbohydrates and a relatively high protein diet. (100 grams or more per day)

EXERCISE: Regular exercise has been shown to reduce the both frequency and intensity of migraines.

Mitral Valve Prolapse

This is one of the most common heart valve problems, often involving lesions on the surface of the valves themselves. The following program is helpful in supporting the heart muscle with many types of valve disturbances.

Full Spectrum Nutrition Plus:

Magnesium	600 –1000 mg per day extra
L-Carnitine	2-4 grams per day
Selenium	200-400 mcg
Coenzyme Q10	100-200 mg
Potassium	300 –800 mg per day
Hawthorn berry	250-500 mg
Taurine	2-3 grams per day
Vitamin C	1-2 grams per day

Mononucleosis – See Immunodepression

Motion Sickness

Motion sickness can occur while in a car, airplane, or boat. Severe sufferers can experience motion sickness while riding in an elevator or watching a turning object. Symptoms of motion sickness include cold sweats, nausea, vomiting, and dizziness.

Full Spectrum Nutrition Plus:

Charcoal Tablets	5 tablets 1 hour before travel
Ginger Root Capsules	2-4 capsules every 2 hours during travel
Magnesium	500 mg before travel
Vitamin B6	50 mg before travel
Liquid Oxygen	2 ounces before travel and as needed Take on an empty stomach

Mouth and Gum Disorders – See Periodontal Disease

Multiple Sclerosis

This disease affects the central nervous system and is a progressive autoimmune condition. There are many causes for this disease such as allergies, environmental exposure, and many others that have not yet been identified.

Since it is an autoimmune condition, sufferers should avoid immune stimulants of all kinds. Currently there is no cure for MS. The late Dr. Hans Neiper of Germany discovered the best treatment methods for control of this condition. His work continues through his Foundation.

Full Spectrum Nutrition Plus:

Liquid Organic Source Trace Minerals	2-4 ounces per day
Essential Fatty Acids	4-10 grams per day
Multi-Antioxidants	400-1200 mg per day
Multi Enzymes with Hydrochloric Acid	3-6 capsules per meal
AEP Salts:	
Calcium	
Magnesium	
Potassium	3-6 capsules per day
Octacosanol	25-50 mg
Vitamin B12 (as methylcobalamin)	10-30 mg per day
Gingko Biloba	100 mg per day
High Potency B-Complex Stress	per label
Liquid Oxygen	1 oz 3 times per day
on an empty stomach	
Kelp	10-15 tablets per day

DIET: Eliminate all possible food allergies as these can actually cause similar symptoms as MS. Avoid all foods that are processed or that contain food additives. Consume at least 64 ounces of water daily. Increase fiber by consuming high fiber foods.

Muscle Cramps

The most common cause of muscle cramping is an imbalance or deficiency of the electrolyte minerals, calcium, magnesium, and, to some extent, potassium. Another cause of this phenomenon is a vitamin E deficiency. Most muscle cramps occur at night and this variety is almost exclusively caused by a calcium/magnesium deficit.

Full Spectrum Nutrition Plus:

Calcium	1500 mg per day
	500 mg a bedtime
Magnesium	1000 mg per day
Potassium	100 mg 2 or 3 times per day
High Potency Stress B-Complex	per label
Vitamin E	200-400 IU extra

Check if Sodium levels are low. If so, salt tablets may be helpful, especially during warm weather.

Muscular Dystrophy (see also Myopathy)

This genetic condition involves the destruction and atrophy of skeletal muscles. Symptoms include loss of strength and deformity. While the exact cause is still unknown, errors in metabolism are involved.

Full Spectrum Nutrition Plus:

Selenium	200 – 1000 mcg per day
Vitamin E	200-400 IU extra
Free Form Amino Acids	per label
Choline	3,000 – 10,000 mg per day
Liquid Organic Trace Minerals	2-4 oz per day

Myasthenia Gravis – See Myopathy

Myocardial Infarction – See Chapter 4

Myopathy

This is a wasting away of skeletal muscle associated with many diseases such as Muscular Dystrophy.

Full Spectrum Nutrition Plus:

Riboflavin (B2)	100-200 mg per day
Vitamin A (natural)	25,000 IU per day
Vitamin E	400-800 IU per day
Magnesium	200 mg 3 times per day
Selenium	500 mcg
Phosphatidyl Choline	1000 mg per day
Vitamin B6	50 mg 2 times per day
Coenzyme Q10	50 mg 3 times per day
Vitamin C	2-4 grams per day

Nail Problems

The fingernails have often been called a mirror to the inside of the body. Many problems with fingernails often stem from a lack of quality protein in the diet.

Deficiencies of Vitamin A or Calcium can cause the nail to become dry and brittle. Ridges in the nail can either be caused from damage to the nail bed or a lack of B-Complex nutrients. White marks on the nails are a sign of Zinc deficiency. Low protein consumption and/or Vitamin C deficiencies can lead to hangnails. Insufficient amounts of natural stomach acid can cause fingernails to split or peel.

Full Spectrum Nutrition Plus:

Protein	80 grams per day
Vitamin A	25,000 IU
Gelatin/ Chondroitin sulfate	400 mg per day
Zinc	25- 50 mg per day
B-Complex	25 mg per day
Horsetail	per label
Vitamin C	2-3 grams per day

Nausea (During Pregnancy) – See Motion Sickness

Nausea (w/ Vomiting) – See Motion Sickness

Neuritis

This painful condition is the result of an inflammation of the nerves in a particular grouping. Prolonged Neuritis can lead to nerve deterioration. Symptoms include pain, tingling, loss of sensation, swelling, and redness of the affected area(s).

There are many causes for this condition, which include nutritional deficiencies, but may also be a side effect from a bone fracture, nerve infection, or diseases such as diabetes or gout. Toxic metals, such as Mercury, Lead, or Cadmium, in the body can also cause this condition and should be eliminated through Chelation.

Full Spectrum Nutrition Plus:

Lecithin Granules	1 Tablespoon 2 or 3 times per day
Vitamin B1	100 mg 2 times per day during flair up
High potency Stress B-Complex	per label
Calcium	2000 mg daily
Magnesium	500 mg daily
Increase fluid intake and avoid caffeine	

Neuromuscular Degeneration

When the impulses from the nerves have difficulty signaling muscle response, a variety of neuromuscular conditions are suspected. The following program will support nerve impulse and strengthen function.

Full Spectrum Nutrition Plus:

Folic Acid	800-1200 mcg
Vitamin B6	50 mg 3 times per day
Vitamin B12	500 mcg 3 or 4 times per day
Calcium	2000 mg
Magnesium	750 mg

Free Form Amino Acids	per label
L-Carnitine	500 mg 3 times per day
Coenzyme Q10	50 mg 2 times per day

Be sure and rule out allergies such as Gluten as well as heavy metal poisoning.

Nickel Toxicity – See Heavy Metal Poisoning

Night Blindness

If your vision is normally stable, with or without glasses, during the daylight hours but you have difficulty seeing well at night, due to the reflection and glare of bright lights, this condition is referred to as 'night blindness'. This condition can be a signal of more serious eye trouble but generally it is a symptom of Vitamin A deficiency.

Full Spectrum Nutrition Plus:

Vitamin A (from fish liver oil)	25,000 – 100,000+ per day
Leutin	per label

Obesity

It is important to determine the cause of your weight gain and then to plan a proper eating program based on the way your body handles food. (I have written a book covering this subject – contact The Institute for availability.) Once you understand the right type of diet for your body chemistry, the following nutrients are often helpful.

Full Spectrum Nutrition Plus:

Essential Fatty Acids	1-2 grams per day
L-Carnitine	1000-2000 mg per day
Phenylalanine*	500-1000 mg at bedtime

*Note: Do not take if you have uncontrolled high blood pressure.

Choline	1000 mg

Inositol	1500 mg
Methionine	400-800 mg
Conjugated Linoleic Acid	2-4 grams per day

EXERCISE: Regular exercise in the form of both resistance and aerobic activities is essential for increasing metabolism and losing unwanted weight.

DIET: It is almost impossible to lose weight without some form of dietary program. The biggest problem most dieters make is to follow a weight loss program that is not right for their metabolism. The Institute offers weight management evaluation programs to help you determine the right type of diet program for your body. (see appendix)

Osteoarthritis – See Arthritis

Osteoporosis

Osteoporosis is a condition, which results in the thinning of bone tissue and a loss of bone density. The leaching or depletion of Calcium and other minerals from the bone tissue results in Osteoporosis.

Although Osteoporosis primarily affects women, men do suffer from this condition as well. We previously thought that estrogen depletion was the chief causes of this condition. While hormone imbalance during and after menopause certainly does play a part, we now know that micro trace mineral deficiencies are at the root of the problem.

Full Spectrum Nutrition Plus:

Multi-Enzymes with Hydrochloric Acid	4-6 capsules with each meal
Calcium (citrate/malate)	1000-1500 mg per day
Magnesium	750 mg per day
Manganese	per label
Copper	2 mg
Zinc	10 mg
Boron	2-4 mg
Vitamin D	400-600 mg

Strontium	per label
Horsetail	per label

Otosclerosis – See Inner Ear Dysfunction

Overweight – See Obesity

Pain

Pain is nature's way of telling us that there is something wrong with the body. All too frequently we take drugs designed to alleviate the pain, but we do not look to find the cause of the discomfort.

Neglect and continued abuse can lead to the problem worsening. Once the cause of the pain has been determined and properly addressed, the following nutrients may help you naturally manage the pain until the underlying cause has an opportunity to correct itself.

Full Spectrum Nutrition Plus:

dl- Phenylalanine*	500 mg 3 times per day

*Note: do not take if you have uncontrolled high blood pressure

Curcumin	per label

Topical Pain Relief

Capsaicin Cream	as needed

Pancreatitis

An inflammation or infection of the Pancreas, which is often caused by Pancreatic Stones, scarring, or even cancer. This condition can either be acute or become chronic.

Full Spectrum Nutrition Plus:

Chromium	300-400 mcg
Pancreas Glandular Extract	4-10 tablets
Stress B-Complex	per label

If infection is present, use protocol under Immunodepression.

Parasites/Amebas

The biggest reason parasites and other similar organisms take up residence within the human body is due to a deficiency of Hydrochloric Acid in the stomach as well as a lack of available Oxygen within the body.

This Oxygen Deficiency is caused by lack of exercise, lung disorders, advanced age, or other disease. Fortunately, regardless of the invading parasitic organism, most all of them are anaerobic in nature and are effectively destroyed with a Liquid Oxygen Flush.

Full Spectrum Nutrition Plus:

| Liquid Oxygen* | 1 ounce 3 times per day |
| | Then 2 ounces 3 times per day after 1 week |

Stay at a total of 6 ounces per day for a period of 4 to 6 weeks.
> *Note: Liquid oxygen must be taken on an empty stomach, 30 minutes before, or three hours after a meal.

| Acidophilus | 10 capsules per day on empty stomach for ten days after the liquid oxygen flush. |

Consider also using a short duration of immune boosting nutrients as discussed under Immunodepression.

Parkinson's Disease

This degenerative disease affects the nervous system. While the exact cause is still not fully understood, we do know that there is an imbalance between two chemicals, Dopamine and Acetylcholine.

Symptoms of this condition include shaking, drooling, loss of appetite, shuffling gait, tremors, and impaired speech. The most common pharmaceutical for the management of this disease is Levodopa.

If you are taking this drug be sure NOT take Vitamin B6 as they interact, causing an elevation of Dopamine in the brain. Levodopa must be carefully administered, since it can produce serious side effects. Evidence has shown that taking Vitamin B6 alone, in mega doses, is often as effective as Levodopa and much safer.

Full Spectrum Nutrition Plus: (with low B6 if taking levodopa)

Calcium	1500 mg
Magnesium	1000 mg
Lecithin Granules	1 tbsp. 3 times per day
Folic Acid	400 –800 mcg
Vitamin B6	300-1000 mg per day

Note: Do not take B6 if you are taking the medication Levodopa.

Vitamin C	2-4 grams
Vitamin E	up to 3,000 IU
Essential Fatty Acids	4-8 grams
Stress B-Complex	100 mg 3 times per day

Rule out the possibility of Heavy Metal Poisoning by taking a Hair Mineral Analysis Test. (Contact The Institute of Nutritional Science)

Pellagra

This is a vitamin disease caused by prolonged and severe deficiency of the B-Complex nutrients. Full Spectrum Nutrition and B-Complex Vitamins will completely cure the disorder.

Full Spectrum Nutrition Plus:

B-complex

Peptic Ulcers

The stomach lining ulcerates primarily when the natural stomach pH is disturbed for long periods of time. We often think that ulcers are caused by stomach acid, but this is not true. Stomach acid can irritate an open ulcer, once it has developed, but it is actually a lack of stomach acids combined with an infection that produces this disorder.

Emphasis must be placed upon healing the open ulceration then re-establishing the proper pH of the stomach with enzymes and Betaine Hydrochloride.

Full Spectrum Nutrition Plus:

Multi – Enzymes	3-4 with each meal
Bilberry Extract	200-500 mg
Licorice Root Extract	per label
Rhubarb	per label
Fatty Acids	2-4 grams
Vitamin A (natural only)	50,000 – 100,000 IU
Vitamin C	2-4 grams
Organic Aluminum (from plant sources)	1-3 ounces per day
Bismuth	150 mg 4 times per day
Zinc	25-50 mg 2 or 3 times per day

EXERCISE: Since stress is often linked to this condition, regular exercise can help to lower stress levels and increase the brain chemicals that make us feel better.

DIET: if your ulcer is severe, consider a diet of very bland foods, even baby foods until the situation improves.

Periodontal Disease

This is a general term for infections and other disease pathology of the gums and supporting tissues around the teeth. When addressing these conditions, we must place emphasis upon both the infection, usually present, as well as the rebuilding of bone, which holds teeth in place.

The Standard American Diet (SAD Diet) provides so many soft foods that plaque, which builds up on the teeth, never gets cleaned off. This leads to infection and inflammation, which can result in one of two major gum problems, Gingivitis and eventually, Pyorrhea (periodontitis).

Full Spectrum Nutrition Plus:

Coenzyme Q10	50 mg 2 or 3 times per day
Vitamin C	4 – 10 grams

Calcium	1000 – 1500 mg
Magnesium	800 mg
Phosphorus	as per label
Folic Acid	1 mg per day
Vitamin A (natural only)	10,000 – 20,000 IU
Zinc	50 mg
Centella Asiatica	2-4 capsule per day
Licorice Root	per label
Bloodroot	per label
Chlorella	1 tsp. per day

Ensure you have adequate Hydrochloric Acid production in the stomach

Rule out leaking dental fillings, which can lead to Mercury poisoning, by taking a Hair Mineral Analysis Test.

Peripheral Vascular Disease

This deterioration of the vascular system can lead to inflammation and infection of the vascular system. When this condition exists, you may also have Atherosclerosis and Varicose Veins.

Full Spectrum Nutrition Plus:

Bilberry Extract	100 mg 4 times per day
Hawthorn Berry	250-500 mg
Gingko Biloba	50 mg 3 times per day
Horsechestnut	50 mg 3 times per day
Bromelain	250 – 500 mg 3 times per day on empty stomach
Zinc	50 mg
Magnesium	200 mg extra 2-3 times per day
Essential Fatty Acids	2-4 Grams
Inositol	500 mg 2 times per day
Vitamin E	400-1400 IU extra
Vitamin A (natural only)	25,000 IU

Phlebitis

This condition is caused by an inflammation of the veins, often causing blood clots. It occurs mostly, as a result of a trauma to the blood vessel wall, an infection, prolonged sitting, standing or inactivity.

Full Spectrum Nutrition Plus:

Vitamin E	800 – 1200 IU
High Potency B-Complex	50 mg 2 times per day
Vitamin C w/bioflavonoids	to bowel tolerance
Essential Fatty Acids	3-6 grams per day
Increase Fiber	10-20 grams
Water	64 oz per day

Pneumonia

This condition of the lungs may be caused by a variety of viruses, bacteria or even fungi. When the body is compromised with other infections, or during the presence of chronic diseases or prolonged inactivity, pneumonia is more likely to occur. Age is also a factor. Since there is most often an infection of some sort at the root of pneumonia, immune-boosting supplements should be considered. (See protocol for Immunodepression.)

Full Spectrum Nutrition Plus:

Immune building protocol	
Vitamin A	25,000- 100,000 IU
Vitamin C	3-10 grams
Acidophilus ..if taking antibiotics	10 capsules per day on empty stomach
Raw Thymus Extract	500 mg 3 times per day
Zinc	50 mg
Antioxidant Mix	400 mg 2-3 times per day

Polyps

Polyps are non-cancerous growths, which may grow on any mucous lining such as bladder, cervix, large intestine, and the sinuses. Since those with Polyps are much more likely to develop Cancer, attention to the management and surgical removal, if necessary, is of paramount importance. (See protocol for Immunodepression.)

Full Spectrum Nutrition Plus:

Beta Carotene	25,000 IU
Vitamin A (natural only)	25,000 IU
Vitamin C	5-10 grams
Vitamin E	400 IU extra
Multi-Antioxidant Mix	400 mg 2 or 3 times per day

Pregnancy

The period of pregnancy lasts about 280 days, and for most women, this is a happy time with very little complication. The most common problems during pregnancy are morning sickness, indigestion, hemorrhoids, and hemorrhage. These are addressed in the following protocol.

Full Spectrum Nutrition Plus:

Ginger Root (morning sickness)	3-5 capsules 3 or 4 times per day
Increase Fiber	10 grams per day
Exercise (walking)	1 mile per day
Essential Fatty Acids	2 grams extra
Vitamin K	100 mg per day
Folic Acid	400 mcg extra per day
Potassium	100 mg 2 times per day
Iron	10-14 mg extra
Protein	100 grams per day minimum

Note: a lack of protein is the main cause of toxemia of pregnancy, especially during the last trimester.

EXERCISE: Regular exercise is important during pregnancy and will allow for a much easier delivery

Pregnancy Toxemia (See also Pregnancy)

Usually occurring during the last trimester, this is almost often caused by a lack of protein in the diet. The typical symptom is edema of the hands and feet.

Full Spectrum Nutrition Plus:

Protein	100-150 grams per day
Liquid Amino Acids	per label
Vitamin B6	25 –50 mg per day (stop after birth)
Water	64 or more oz per day

Premenstrual Syndrome

PMS is another disorder of the hormone balance of the body and, oddly enough, is related to and shares many of the same causes as symptoms of the Menopause.

Typical effects of PMS include headaches, bloating, backache, breast swelling, fatigue, irritability, and emotional outbursts, which can be severe enough to produce anger, violence, and even thoughts of suicide.

In the past, doctors thought that women with these symptoms were psychotic and recommended either psychopharmacology or that they be institutionalized. Thankfully, today we realize that these symptoms are not only very real but they have a biochemical origin as well. This means that they can be effectively treated with diet and nutritional supplements.

Full Spectrum Nutrition Plus:

Progesterone Cream	per label
Calcium	1500 mg
Magnesium	1000 mg
Vitamin B 6	50 mg 3 times per day

Essential Fatty Acids	4-6 grams per day
High potency Stress B-Complex	4 capsules 2 times per day
Corn silk	2 capsules 3 times per day
Gingko biloba	150 mg per day
Vitamin A (natural only)	100,000 to 200,000 IU per day
Tyrosine	3-6 grams per day in the morning
Choline	200 mg
Inositol	1000 – 1500 mg
GABA	500 – 2000 mg per day
Black cohosh	25 mg 2 times per day
DHEA	20 mg per day

Prostatitis – See Chapter 4

Prostate Enlargement – See Chapter 4

Psoriasis

This condition, often hereditary, is the result of an over replication of the cells in the outer layer of the skin. Most often it is a lack of fats and fatty acids in the diet. For example, a prolonged very low fat diet can induce this condition.

Full Spectrum Nutrition Plus:

Essential Fatty Acids	2-6 grams per day
Multi-Enzymes	as needed per meal
Vitamin A (from fish liver oil)	50,000 –100,000 IU
Vitamin B12	500 –1000 mcg
Selenium	200 mcg extra
Hypoallergenic cream with Selenium	apply topically 2or 3 times per day
Capsaicin	per label
Sarsaparilla	per label
Milk Thistle	200 mg
Lecithin Capsules	2 capsules with each meal

Rule out the possibility of food allergies by taking a RAST blood test. Also, test for a lack of Hydrochloric Acid in the stomach by taking a pH test. (see Appendix to contact The Institute about Diagnostic Testing)

Puppura – See Peripheral Vascular Disease

Raynaud's Disease – See Peripheral Vascular Disease

Restless Leg Syndrome

This is a symptom of nervousness or inner stress that is not managed. See recommendations under stress management as well.

Full Spectrum Nutrition Plus:

Folic Acid	50 mcg 3 times per day
Calcium	1500 mg
Magnesium	800 mg
Vitamin E	400 IU extra
Iron	10 mg
L-Tryptophan (if you can find it) or 5-Hydroxy Tryptophan (5-HTP)	per label
High Potency Stress B-Complex	4 capsules 2 or 3 times per day

Retinopathy – See Macular Degeneration

Rheumatic Fever – See Immunodepression

Rheumatism – See also Arthritis

An inflammatory disorder of joints and connective tissue, rheumatism can be very painful and debilitating.

Full Spectrum Nutrition Plus:

Vitamin B1	200 mg per day
Vitamin B6	50 mg 3 times per day
Vitamin E	400-800 IU
Copper	2-3 mg per day
5-Hydroxy Tryptophan	per label
Selenium	200 mcg extra
Magnesium	800 mg

Be sure to rule out the possibility of food allergies by taking a RAST blood test.

Rheumatoid Arthritis – See Also Arthritis

This is an autoimmune disease, which results in the destruction of cartilage and connective tissues due to over–activity of the immune system. As with all autoimmune conditions, do not use any immune stimulants of any kind.

Full Spectrum Nutrition Plus:

Chicken Cartilage	Double the label suggestion
Bromelain	1000 mg for 60 days then 500 mg thereafter
Liquid Oxygen	2-3 oz per day
	Take on an empty stomach
MSM (organic sulfur)	per label

Follow arthritis protocol listed under Arthritis

Capsaicin	per label
Devils Claw	per label
Feverfew	per label
Ginger Root Extract	per label
Pantothenic Acid	500 mg 4 times per day
Vitamin A	25,000 IU
Vitamin C	to bowel tolerance

Copper Salicylate	1-3 tablets per day
	For 10 days only
Colloidal Gold	per label
L-Histidine	1000 mg 2 or 3 times per day
Essential Fatty Acids	2-6 grams
Quercitin	200 mg per day
Bromelain	2 capsules 3 or 4 times per day

Rule out the possibility of food allergies by taking a RAST allergy test. Also, ensure adequate Hydrochloric Acid in stomach. To check your acid/alkaline levels take a pH test.

Scleroderma

This is a rare autoimmune disease affecting the blood vessels and connective tissue of the body. The disease produces fibrous degeneration of the connective tissue of the skin, lungs, and internal organs. Most of the cases of Scleroderma occur in middle-aged females.

Full Spectrum Nutrition Plus:

Bromelain	150 –500 mg 3 times per day
Gotu Kola	twice label suggestion
Vitamin E	800 IU with each meal
	Decrease to a total of 1600 IU after a week
	Then down to 800 IU after two weeks
Essential Fatty Acids	4-6 grams per day
Para-amino Benzoic Acid	4 grams 2 or 3 times per day
Bovine Cartilage	6-12 capsules per day

Seborrhea – See Seborrheic Dermatitis

Seborrheic Dermatitis

This condition is caused by a malfunction of the Sebaceous Glands, which secrete oil. The most likely spots for flare-ups to occur are on the scalp, face, or chest, but can occur anywhere on the skin. This condition is frequently caused by a combination of Vitamin A and Essential Fatty Acid Deficiencies.

Full Spectrum Nutrition Plus:

Essential Fatty Acids	4-8 grams per day
Vitamin A (from fish liver oil)	50,000 IU
Vitamin E	400-800 IU extra
Folic Acid	2 mg per day
Vitamin B12	500 mcg 3 times per day under tongue
Selenium	200 mcg extra
Lithium	per physicians instruction

Be sure and rule out the possibility of a Hydrochloric Acid deficiency in the stomach. Take a pH test to determine your acid/alkaline levels. (Contact The Institute for Testing)

Senility (Senile Dementia)

Senility is really a very rare disorder, most often affecting the elderly. Many times this condition is misdiagnosed and really turns out to be something else such as nutrient deficiencies due to mal-absorption, drug overdose, depression, thyroid deficiency, and liver or kidney disorders.

Full Spectrum Nutrition Plus:

Multi Enzymes with HCl	2-4 with each meal
Protein	at least 60 grams per day
High Potency B-Complex	100 mg 3 times per day
Vitamin B12	2,000 mcg daily
Choline	1000 mg 2 or 3 times per day
Niacin	25-50 mg 3 times per day
Antioxidant Multi Formula	400 –1200 mg per day

Shingles – See Herpes Zoster

Sinusitis

An inflammation and infection of the Sinuses, Sinusitis is most often the result of either a respiratory infection or repeated irritation from airborne allergies. Symptoms of this condition include loss of the sense of smell, pain and tenderness in the face, fever, headache, earache, and toothache. If the cause is another infection, treatment of both is essential. (Use the Immunodepression program.)

Full Spectrum Nutrition Plus:

Vitamin A (from fish liver oil)	25,000 –100,000 + IU per day
Vitamin C	2-4 grams

Skin Cancer (See also Cancer)

Over- exposure to radiation, primarily from the sun, is the biggest single cause of most skin cancers. The lighter your skin, the more likely you will develop skin cancer due to over-exposure to sunlight. It is essential to use a sunscreen and limit your exposure to the sun if you are fair skinned, since you have minimal protective pigmentation.

Full Spectrum Nutrition Plus:

Multi Anti-oxidants	400 –1600 mg per day
DMG	per label
Liquid Oxygen	1 oz 3 or 4 times per day on empty stomach
Essential Fatty Acids	2 grams with each meal
Germanium	200 mg per day
Coenzyme Q10	100 mg per day
Selenium	200 mcg extra
Vitamin A (from fish liver oil)	50,000 –100,000 IU per day
Vitamin E	800 –1000 IU

Sore Throat – See Immunodepression

Spasmodic Colon – See Colitis

Sports Injuries

Most sports related injuries involve soft tissues, bones and connective tissue, or both. Healing of these types of injuries may be accelerated by aggressive nutrition with an emphasis upon liquid organic mineral compounds.

Full Spectrum Nutrition Plus:

Liquid Organic Source Trace Minerals	3-5 oz per day
Vitamin C	3-6 grams
Bioflavonoids	2-4 grams
Coenzyme Q10	100 mg per day
Glucosamine Sulfate	400 mg 2 times per day
Bromelain	200-400 mg 3 times per day
	On an empty stomach

Stress and Anxiety

Excess stress is almost a given in today's society. Each of us is trying to cram 90 minutes into every hour, resulting in stress related illnesses including anxiety, mood swings, aggressive behavior, and depression.

Nutrition can play an important role in managing stress from the physical angle but stress management from the mental or emotional side is also essential.

Full Spectrum Nutrition Plus:

Vitamin C	to bowel tolerance
Vitamin B12	500 mcg 3 times per day
Pantothenic Acid	1000-2000 mg per day
Adrenal Glandular Extract	2-4 tablets 3 times per day
Calcium	1500-2000 mg per day
Magnesium	800-1000 mg per day

EXERCISE: Regular exercise can be one of the greatest de-stressors. When combined with the Stress nutrients above, the results are often fairly rapid.

Stroke

A Stroke, or Cerebral Hemorrhage, is caused by the rupturing of a blood vessel in the brain and is a common source of debilitation and death. The most common cause of this condition is elevated blood pressure. The best treatment for stroke is prevention by keeping blood pressure down and managing stress effectively. If you have had a Stroke, it is essential that you get the right treatment as soon as possible. Hyperbaric Oxygen treatments are one of the best methods of helping restore brain function.

Full Spectrum Nutrition Plus:

Vitamin E	400-1200 IU
Essential Fatty Acids	3-6 grams
Multi-Antioxidant Mix	800 –1200 mg per day
Liquid Oxygen	1 oz 3 or 4 times per day on empty stomach

Sunburn

Overexposure to the sun can lead to painful burning of the upper layers of the skin. If you are fair skinned, it is important to limit your exposure to the sun and stay completely out of the sun during peek radiation periods, which are from 10 AM until 2 PM.

Full Spectrum Nutrition Plus:

Liquid Organic Source Trace Minerals	1 oz 2 or 3 times per day
Apply liquid trace minerals topically to burned area	2 or 3 times per day
Vitamin C	3-4 grams
Vitamin A	25,000 IU
Vitamin E	400 IU extra
Apply vitamin E directly on skin	once or twice per day
Aloe Vera Gel	apply as needed to skin

Temperomandibular Joint Syndrome (TMJ)

This common condition affects over 20 million people worldwide. The causes of TMJ are poor bite, grinding of teeth, and stress. If you are under more stress than you can manage, you must consider dealing with this issue independently of the following protocol.

Full Spectrum Nutrition Plus:

Calcium	2000 mg
Magnesium	1500 mg in divided doses
Stress B-Complex	2-4 capsules 2or 3 times per day
Co Enzyme Q10	30 mg 3 times per day
L-Tyrosine	500-1000 mg on empty stomach 1 hour before bed
Vitamin C	1000 mg extra
Vitamin B6	25 mg taken with the Tyrosine

Tendon Problems – See Sports Injuries

Tendinitis – See Inflammation

Thrombophlebitis – See Peripheral Vascular Disease

Thrush – See Candidiasis and Yeast Infection in Chapter 4

Thyroid – See either Hyperthyroid (overactive) or Hypothyroid (underactive)

Tinnitus

This condition of the middle ear causes a ringing in the ears, which may be anything from barely noticeable to almost deafening. This can be caused by repeated or prolonged acoustic trauma, Meniere's disease, Otosclerosis, or a physiological blockage to the ear passages.

Full Spectrum Nutrition Plus:

Essential Fatty Acids	2-4 grams per day
Vitamin A (natural only)	25,000 IU
Zinc	50 mg
Calcium	1500 mg
Magnesium	700 mg
Potassium	100 mg

DIET: It is important to reduce refined carbohydrates and sugars from the diet. Also, rule out the possibility of any allergies by taking a RAST blood test.

Tonsillitis – See Immunodepression

Toxicity – See Heavy Metal Poisoning

Triglycerides Elevated

Excess triglycerides, unlike cholesterol, are caused by a combination of the over-consumption of sugar and refined carbohydrates and a lack of activity or exercise. Reduce sugar and sugar forming foods in the diet and exercise at least three times per week for 30 minutes each time.

Full Spectrum Nutrition Plus:

Essential Fatty Acids	2-4 grams per day
Chromium	200-400 mcg
Vanadium	500+ mcg per day
Aspartic Acid	300 mg per day
Selenium	500 mcg
Vitamin C	to bowel tolerance

EXERCISE: Excess triglycerides in the blood are caused by an over-consumption of refined carbohydrates and a lack of exercise. Get at least 30 minutes of exercise 3 to 4 times per week.

DIET: Reduce or eliminate refined sugars and starches in the diet.

Tuberculosis – See Immunodepression

Ulcers, Stomach & Duodenal (See also indigestion)

Ulcers of the Stomach and Duodenum are caused by an imbalance in the pH of the organ. When the pH of the stomach becomes alkaline, it compromises the integrity of the stomach lining. When bacteria are present in an alkaline stomach environment, the tissues of that organ are highly susceptible to infection since the bacteria cannot be effectively killed off. Once an ulcer has formed, even the smallest amount of naturally occurring stomach acid will irritate the open sore.

Full Spectrum Nutrition Plus:

Vitamin A (from fish liver oil)	100,000 – 200,000 IU
Bioflavonoids	2 –3 grams per day
Multi-enzyme without HCl	2- 4 with each meal
Vitamin B6	100 mg per day during healing
Zinc	50 mg per day
Vitamin B12	500 mcg per day during healing
Gamma oryzanol	500-1000 mg per day
Glutamine	1000-3000 mg
Pantethine	500-1000 mg
Licorice Root	1-2 caps with each meal
Cat's claw extract	1-2 caps with each meal

Rule out the possibility of food allergies by taking a RAST blood test.

Urinary Tract Infections – See Kidney and Bladder Infections

Urticaria (See also allergies)

Also known as Hives, this is a serious skin rash caused by an allergic reaction to a variety of substances, but most often foods are responsible. The best treatment is identifying and avoiding the offending substances. The use of antihistamines is frequently required.

Full Spectrum Nutrition Plus:

Beta Carotene	20,000 IU
Niacin	25 mg 2 or 3 times per day
Vitamin B12	200 mcg sublingual 3 times per day
Magnesium	500 mg extra

Rule out the possibility of food allergies by taking a RAST blood test.

Vaginitis

This condition is most often caused by a bacteria or yeast infection. Other causes may be excessive douching or a nutrient deficiency. Symptoms include burning and itching along with a vaginal discharge. Antibiotic abuse can also lead to this condition.

Full Spectrum Nutrition Plus:

Multi-Acidophilus	10 capsules per day for 10 days on empty stomach
Liquid Oxygen	1 ounce 3 times per day on empty stomach
Garlic Capsules	2 capsules with each meal
Essential Fatty Acids	2-4 grams per day
High Potency B-Complex	50 mg 2 times per day

Varicose Veins – See Peripheral Vascular Disease

Vasculitis – See Peripheral Vascular Disease

Venous Insufficiency – See Peripheral Vascular Disease

Vericose Veins – See Peripheral Vascular Disease

Vertigo – See Inner Ear Dysfunction

Extreme dizziness, Vertigo is usually the result of an inner ear dysfunction.

Viral Infections – See Immunodepression

Vitiligo

This is a skin condition, identified by white patches, which is caused by a loss of melanin or skin pigment in the area. Sometimes thyroid problems can be at the heart of this problem and should be considered.

Full Spectrum Nutrition Plus:

Para-amino Benzoic Acid (PABA)	100-200 mg 3 times per day
Pantothenic Acid	200 mg 2 times per day
Essential Fatty Acids	2-4 grams
Copper	2 mg per day
L-Phenylalanine*	500 mg 2 times per day

*Note: Do not use if you have uncontrolled high blood pressure.

Vitamin C	2-4 grams per day
High Potency Stress B-Complex	2 capsules 2 times per day

Weakened Immune System – See Immunodepression

Worms

These are a variety of parasites that live in the gastrointestinal tract. They are most common in children.

Full Spectrum Nutrition Plus:

Garlic Capsules	2 capsules 3 times per day with meals
Liquid Oxygen	½ to 1 oz 3 or 4 times per day on an empty stomach
Pumpkin Extract	per label

Wound Healing

Slow wound healing can be the result of a deficient immune system or the side effect of chronic diseases such as Diabetes. If the immune system is depressed, follow the protocol under Immunodepression as well as the following.

Full Spectrum Nutrition Plus:

Aloe Vera	apply topically
Bromelain	100 mg 3 times per day
Gotu kola	per label
Vitamin A	10,000 – 25, 000 IU per day
Vitamin C	2-3 grams
Zinc	50 mg
Essential Fatty Acids	2-4 grams

Yeast Infection – See Candidiasis in Chapter 4

ABOUT THE AUTHOR

K. STEVEN WHITING, PHD, is an Orthomolecular Nutritionist. His degrees include a Masters in Psychology as well as a Doctorate in Biochemistry. Over three decades of research, and practical experience with thousands of clients in the field of human nutrition have earned him an international reputation in protecting and preserving human health and well being.

His commitment and dedication within the nutrition field has led him into extensive research into such chronic conditions as Heart Disease, Arthritis, Diabetes, Osteoporosis, Prostate problems, Memory loss, Fibromyalgia, and Thyroid issues, to name but a few. The result of this research has been pivotal in the development of nutritional protocols for the prevention, management and reversal of these conditions.

In 1991, Dr. Whiting founded The Institute of Nutritional Science, an international organization, with offices in Den Haag, The Netherlands, Spain, London England, and San Diego, California, USA. The purpose of The Institute is to gather information and conduct research on how natural supplements can prevent, manage or reverse disease conditions.

Author, Lecturer, Teacher, and Consultant, Dr. Whiting is dedicated to helping others in helping themselves toward a more healthful existence, through better understanding of the nutritional needs of the body. He has formulated unique products for such companies as Curves Fitness Centers.

He is committed to empowering individuals with the very latest nutritional information, safe in the knowledge that this will serve to enhance both the quality and quantity of life for everyone in the years ahead.

Author Photo by: Jennifer Thomas

APPENDIX
& RESOURCES

M any of the protocols and recommendations in this book are based on the use of specific formulas, which I have found to be the most effective. While I am not employed, in any capacity, by these companies, I have been instrumental in helping to develop the formulas they currently offer. These are the same products we use with our clients and patients, at our clinics and Centers around the world. You can obtain these formulas for yourself, by contacting these companies directly.

Full Spectrum Nutrition & Targeted Formulas for Specific Needs:

Phoenix Nutritionals
Telephone: 1-800-440-2390
Website: www.phoenixnutritionals.com
Address: 9528 Miramar Road #215, San Diego, CA 92126
Email Address: questions@phoenixnutritionals.com

Targeted Formulas For The Eyes:

To order Targeted Nutrition Supplements for the Eyes:
Biosyntrx, Inc
151-A Riverchase Way
Lexington, SC 29072
www.biosyntrx.com
Customer Service - 1800-688-6815

For Questions regarding Supplements for the Eyes:

Ellen Troyer, MT MA
Biosyntrx Chief Research Officer

719-227-7888 – phone
etroyer@biosyntrx.com

Custom Supplement Programs, Weight Management Programs, Nutrient Evaluation Testing, Educational Booklets and to reach Dr. Whiting:

The Institute of Nutritional Science
Telephone: 1-888-454-8464
Websites: www.healthyinformation.com (main)
www.chronicdiseasealternatives.com (Free Special Reports)
Free Newsletter: www.healthyinformation.com
Email Address: askthedoc@healthyinformation.com

Institute of Nutritional Science Foundation Europe
Telephone +31 575 552 661
Address: Larenseweg 2, 7251 JL Vorden, The Netherlands

TEN-DAY FASTING
PROGRAM FOR
DEEPER DETOXIFICIATION

Throughout this book, a great deal of emphasis has been placed upon the benefits of detoxification of the body when dealing with specific health challenges. The following program has been used by me and with my clients, for many years, with great results. If you have any questions about fasting, consult your Health Care Provider before you begin.

Cleansing the Body of Unwanted Toxins

While excess toxic buildup occurs in every chronic disease process, I can think of no other condition wherein this problem plays a more direct role in the actual disease than in the case of all types of arthritis. In fact, it has been said by many that arthritis is a disease of toxicity. Because of the direct role that toxic waste plays in this particular disease process, it is essential that the body be cleansed of these unwanted poisons, if we are to expect to see any real improvement in the condition. The best way to rapidly, yet safely, remove these toxins from the soft tissues of the body is through a modified fast which causes the liver, kidney, colon and bowel to dump their stored toxins into the blood stream for eventual elimination via the urine and feces. The following fast should be undertaken as soon as possible:

Needed:

1. Between 12 and 15 fresh lemons daily for 3 days
2. About 3 quarts of distilled water per day for 3 days
3. A multi-herbal formula consisting of fiber, Celery, Cascara sagrada, Irish most, Peppermint, Senna, Bromelain, Anise, Ginger, Turkey rhubarb and Chlorophyll.

(A combination fiber and herbal powder formula is available from Phoenix Nutritonals, 1-800-440-2390)

4. Additional fiber tablets

5. Honey to taste

Day One

Make up one and one half cups of freshly squeezed lemon juice. Add this to two or three quarts of distilled water and mix in a little honey for taste. This will be your total intake of fluid and food of any kind for the entire day. Sip this mixture slowly throughout the day. If you become excessively thirsty or develop a headache this first day, make up another quart of the lemon and honey water and continue sipping it as needed. In addition, take 1 teaspoon of the fiber/herbal mixture in at least 6 to 8 ounces of the lemon water twice per day.

Day Two

Continue as on day one, making up another fresh batch of the lemon-honey distilled water mixture. Take one teaspoon of the fiber/herbal mixture twice per day as in day one.

Day Three

Repeat the lemon and honey water. Take the fiber/herbal powder as in days one and two.

Days Four and Five

*Day four marks the end of the concentrated cleansing program, but continue to follow the outline given for days four and five in order to reap the full benefits of the program and to avoid shocking your body. Stop using the lemon water mix. Today, through day 10, use just one teaspoon of the fiber/herbal powder in 6 to 8 ounces of juice per day. Drink any amount of tomato juice or carrot juice. You may also use white grape juice if diluted with 50% water. DO NOT CONSUME ANY CITRUS JUICES OF ANY KIND. Fresh non-distilled spring water may be taken in any quantity.

Days Six and Seven

Continue as with days four and five but you may now add fruits and vegetables. Use the fiber/herbal powder once per day as above.

Days Eight and Nine

Add yogurt and/or cottage cheese to your diet. Use the fiber/ herbal powder once a day as above.

Days Ten and Forward

Add whole protein foods such as chicken or fish slowly, for instance, at one meal per day. Gradually return to your normal protein intake over the next few days. Stop taking the fiber/herbal powder today.

This fast is not only safe and easy but very effective in removing the buildup of toxins that can contribute to all chronic degenerative diseases, especially arthritis. It is important to remember that you MUST consume the stated amount of the lemon and honey water during the first three days of the program. If you have a medical condition such as diabetes, hypoglycemia or other challenge, which would prevent you from fasting, you can use the ToxiCleanse herbal formula without the fast. Simply take one teaspoon in 8 oz of fluid once per day for 14 days.

INSTRUCTIONS
FOR COMPLETING THE
OXY FLUSH

The Oxy Flush Program is designed to detoxify the body from unwanted poisons as well as eliminate such organisums as candida/yeast, parasites and low grade bacteria/virus. This program is recommended in chapter 4 in our discussion of candida/yeast.

Following you will find the exact instructions for completing my Oxy Flush, as described in the section on Candida & systemic yeast.

Be sure to follow the instructions exactly and do not run out of liquid oxygen before you have completed the full cycle. To do so may greatly inhibit your results.

1. **Begin by taking one ounce (one capful) of liquid oxygen three times per day.** (Note that the liquid oxygen MUST be taken on an empty stomach, 30 minutes before eating. Ideal times are upon awakening, 30 minutes before lunch, and, either 30 minutes before the evening meal, or before bed.)

2. **After 2 weeks, increase the oxygen to two ounces three times a day**, also on an empty stomach. Continue this for the next four weeks.

3. After four weeks at a total of six ounces per day, stop the oxygen altogether and **take 10 capsules of acidophilus, together, on an empty stomach, for ten days.**

This completes one cycle. This will arrest yeast and candida, as well a low-grade virus and bacterial activity about 70 percent of the time. For about 20 percent of sufferers, a second cycle will be necessary in order to complete kill off the yeast, especially if it is systemic and you have had it for some time. If a second cycle is necessary, wait 30 days and repeat the above program again.

Should you have any questions, feel free to contact us at The Institute (see Appendix)

NOTE: The products that Dr. Whiting refers to in this protocol are:

LiquiDaily Oxy Aloe

MegaDoph Acidophilus

Both these products are available from Phoenix Nutritionals (see Appendix)

THE NUTRIENT
EVALUATION TEST

This test, designed by The Institute of Nutritional Science, has been developed to identify hidden nutrient deficiencies in the living system of the human body.

The test consists of yes or no questions, in several categories. These are based on the symptomology of the body, in that specific symptoms are the result of specific nutrient deficiencies.

Once completed, this test is scanned through our computer system, which correlates each symptom against known nutrient deficiencies. We then can use this information to help design a custom program of Full Spectrum and Targeted nutritional supplements to fit the specific needs of each individual.

If you are interested in taking this test, you can order a copy at The Institute's Website: www.healthyinformation.com

The Coupon, on the next page, offers you the opportunity to take our Nutrient Profile tests at a substantial discount. The results of these test will allow our Staff to design a Custom Supplement Program just for your body.

HOW TO GET MORE
THAN 50% OFF A CUSTOM NUTRITION PROGRAM

As a purchaser of this book, you are entitled to an important health benefit that can help you take full advantage of what you have learned about improving (and prolonging) your life through the correct use of nutrients.

The Institute of Nutritional Science in San Diego, California, would like to make it as easy as possible for you to get a professional nutrient evaluation and a recommended personal nutrient program.

This evaluation will answer questions you have probably had on your mind for a while, including:

- What are the best supplements for me?
- How do I know what my body needs?
- How can I get everything I need?
- What about addressing my individual health challenges?
- What about a customized weight loss program?

You have the choice of two different evaluations. The purpose of these evaluations is to help you enjoy better health and longevity by following programs custom tailored to your body's individual needs.

Here are the two programs you can get at a special reduced fee:

1. Nutrient Evaluation Testing and Custom Supplement Program (normally $40.00)
2. Weight Management Testing and Custom Weight Loss Programs (normally $20.00)

311

As a purchaser of this book, you are entitled to a 60% reduction of the regular cost of either custom evaluation.

It's easy to get your evaluation. Just call The Institute at **1–888–454–8464** and mention Code HL9439 or go to the following webpage to order:

www.healthyinformation.com

Start taking advantage of the Science of Diet and Nutrition right away.

Remember, you don't have to settle for a generic health program. A customized diet and supplement program for you and your family is available today!

REFERENCES

Chapter 1

1. Burr, ML et al, Dietary fiber, blood pressure and plasma cholestero. Nutrtional Research, 1985; 5:465-472

2. Garrison, R.H. Jr. Somer, E., The Nutrition Desk Reference, 1985. Keats Publishing: New Canaan, Ct.

3. Erasmus, Udo, Fats and Oils, Alive Books

4. Heber D, Bowerman, S., Applying science to changing dietary patterns. J. Nutr. 2001: 131: 3121S-6S

5. Yeager, Selene and the Editors of Prevention Magazine: The New Foods For Health. New York: Banam Books, 1999

6. Carper, Jean, Food, Your Miracle Medicine. New York: HarperCollins, 1993.

7. Simopoulos AP. The Mediterranean diets: what is so special about the diet of Greece? The Scientific evidence. J Nutr 2001: 131: 3065S-73S.

8. Robbins, John. The Food Revolution: How Your Diet Can Help Save Your Life and the World. Berkeley, Ca.: Conari Press, 2001

9. Schlosser, Eric. Fast Food Nation: The Dark Side of the All American Meal. Boston: Houghton Mifflin, 2001.

10. Rissler, Jane, and Mellon, Margaret. The Ecological Risks of Engineered Crops Cambridge Mass.: MIT Press 1996.

11. Steinman, D. Diet for a Poisoned Planet. New York: Ballantine Books, 1990.

12. Trevisan, M. et al. Consumption of olive oil, butter and vegetable oils and coronary heart disease risk factors. JAMA, 263 No. 5; Feb, 1990: 688-692.

13. Friedman, M. Ed. Nutritional and Toxicological Consequences of Food Processing. New York: Plenum Press, 1991.

14. Winter, RA Consumer's Dictionary of Food Additives. New York: Crown Publishing 1989.

Chapter 3

1. Hill, R. et al. The discovery of vitamins, in The Chemistry of Life. Cambridge: Cambridge University Press, 1970.

2. Mertz, W. A balanced approach to nutrition for health: the need for biologically essential minerals and vitamins, Journal of the American Dietetic Association 94: 1259-1262, 1994.

3. McCarthy, MA., & Matthews, RH., Conserving Nutrients in Foods. Administrative report No 384. Hyattsville, MD: Nutrition Monitoring Division, Human Nutrition Information Service, U.S. Dept. of Agriculture. 1988.
4. National Research Council, Recommended Dietary Allowances, 10th Ed. Washington DC, National Academy Press. 1989.
5. Goodhart RS & Shils, ME., Modern Nutrition in Health and Disease, Philadelphia: Lea & Febiger, 1980.
6. Orten, JM., & Neuhaus, OW., Human Biochemistry. St. Louis: The CV Mosby Co. 1994.
7. Cooper, K. Advanced Nutritional Therapies. Nashville Tenn: Thomas Nelson Publishers, 1998.
8. Brin, M. Drugs and Environmental Chemicals in Relation fo Vitamin Needs. In Nutrition and Drug Interrelations, ed. J Hathcock. New York: Academic Press 1978.
9. Tucker, DM, et al. Nutritonal Status and Brain Function in Aging. Am J. Clin.Nutr. 52 (1990): 93-102.
10. Packer L. Protective role of vitamin E in biological systems. Am J Clin Nutr. 53 no. 4 1991: 1050S-1055S

Chapter 4

Heart Disease

1. Benditt, EP, University of Washington, School of Medicine. American Journal of Pathology 1974.
2. McGill, HC, The Geographic Pathology of Atherosclerosis. Laboratory Investigation. Vol 18, 5, May 1968
3. The Pathogenesis of Atherosclerosis. Edited by RW Wissler and JC Geer. The Williams & Wilkins Company, 1972.
4. Benditt, EP and Benditt, JM, Evidence For A MonoClonal Origin of Human Atherosclerotic Plaques. Proceedings of the National Academy of Sciences of the United States of America. Vol 70: (6) 1753-1756; June 1993.
5. Benditt, EP, Implications of the MonoClonal Character of Human Atherosclerotic Plaques. Beitrage zur Pathologie, Vol 158: (4) 405-416; 1976.
6. Yudkin, J Dietary Fat and Dietary Sugar in Relation to Ischemic Heart Disease and Diabetes. Lancet, 4-5; 1964.
7. Yudkin, J, Levels of Dietary Sucrose in Patients with Occlusive Atherosclerotic Disease. Lancet 6-8; 1964.
8. Yudkin, J, Diet and Coronary Thrombosis. Lancet 155-62, 1957.
9. Blankenhorn, DH, et al. The Influence of Diet on the appearance of New Lesions in Human Coronary Arteries. JAMA, 1990; 263: 1646-1652.
10. Witztum, JL, The Oxidation Hypothesis of Atherosclerosis. Lancet, 344: 793-5; 1994.
11. Scharts, CJ, et al. The Pathogenesis of Atherosclerosis: An Overview. Clin Cardiol 14(1): 1-16; 1991.
12. Ross, R. The Pathogenesis of Atherosclerosis - An Update. NEJM 314(8): 488-500; 1986.
13. Steinberg, D, et al. Beyond Cholesterol. NEJM, 320(14); 915-24; 1989.
14. Goodnight, SH, et al. Polyunsaturated Fatty Acids, Hyperlipidemia and Thrombosis. Arteriosclerosis. 2: 87-113; 1982.

15. Newbold, HL, Reducing the Serum Cholesterol Level With a Diet High in Animal Fat. Southern Med J. 81(1); 61-63; 1988.

16. Gorringe, JAL, Why Blame Butter?: A Discussion Paper. J Royal Soc Med, 79: 661-663; 1986.

17. Klurfeld, DM and Kritchevsky, D, The Western Diet: An Examination of its Relationship with Chronic Disease. J Am Coll Nutr, 5: 477-485; 1986.

18. Eaton, SB, et al. Stone Agers in the Fast Lane: Chronic Degenerative Diseases in Evolutionary Perspective. Am J Med, 84: 739-49; 1988.

19. Mensink, RP and Katan, MB, Effect of Monounsaturated Fatty Acids verses Complex Carbohydrates on High-Density Lipoprotein in Healthy Men and Women. Lancet, 122-5; 1987.

20. Ginsberg, H, et al. Induction of Hypertriglyceridemia by a Low-Fat Diet. J Clin Endocrinol Metab, 42: 729-35; 1976.

21. Leaf, DA, Omega-3 Fatty Acids and Coronary Artery Disease. Postgrad Med, 85(8); 237-42; 1989.

22. Mann, GV, et al. Journal of Atherosclerosis Research, 1964.

23. Ball, KP, et al. Lancet 1965.

24. Rose, GA. British Journal of Medicine 1965.

25. Malhorta, SL. American Journal of Atherosclerosis Research, 1964.

26. Hunter, JD. Atiu and Mitiaro Natives of Polynesia. Federation Proceedings, 21:36; 1962.

27. Cohen, AM. Jews Living in Yemen. American Heart Journal, 1963.

Diabetes & Hypoglycemia

1. Lowenstein & Preger. *Diabetes - New Look At An Old Problem.* Harper & Row

2. West & Kalbfleisch. Influence of Nutritional factors on Prevalence of Diabetes. *Diabetes.* 1971;20: 99-108

3. Yudkin, J. Dietary Fat and dietary sugar in relation to ischemic heart-disease and diabetes. Lancet. 1964; 4-5

4. Durrington, PN. Is insulin atherogenic? *Diabetic Medicine.* 1992; 9: 597-600

5. Yudkin, J. Medical problems from modern diet. *J Royal Coll of Physicians of London.* 1975; 9(2): 161-164

6. Allred, JB. Too Much of A Good Thing? *J Amer Dietetic Assoc.* 1995; 95(4): 417-418

7. Cohen, MP, et al. High Prevalence of Diabetes in Young Adult Ethiopian Immigrants to Israel. *Diabetes.* 1988; 37: 824-828

8. Paolisso, G. et al. Pharmacologic Doses of Vitamin E Improve Insulin Action in Healthy Subjects and Non-insulin-dependent Diabetic Patients. *Am J Clin Nutr.* 1993; 57: 650-656

9. Urberg, M. And Zemel, MB. Evidence for Synergism Between Chromium and Nicotinic Acid in the Control of Glucose Tolerance in Elderly Humans. *Metabolism.*1987; 36(9): 896-899

10. Moan, A, et al. Mental Stress Increases Glucose Uptake During Hyperinsulinemia: Associations with Sympathetic and Cardiovascular Responsiveness. *Metabolism.* 1995; 44(10): 1303-1307

11. Nicholson, AL, and Yudkin, J. The Nutritional Value of the Low-Carbohydrate Diet Used in the Treatment of Obesity. *Proc Nutr Soc.* 1968; 28(1):13 A

12. Klurfeld, DM and Kritchevsky, D. The Western Diet: An Examination of its Relationship With Chronic Disease. *J Am Coll Nutr.* 1986; 5: 477-485

13. Mouratoff, GJ and Scott, EM. Diabetes Mellitus in Eskimos After a Decade. *JAMA.* 1973; 226(11): 1345-1346

14. O'Dea, K. Westernisation, Insulin Resistance and Diabetes in Australian Aborigines. *Med J Aust.* 1991; 155: 258-264

15. Yudkin, J. Evolutionary and Historical Changes in Dietary Carbohydrates. *Am J Clin Nutr.* 1967; 20(2): 108-115

16. Garg, A, et al. Effects of Varying Carbohydrate Content of Diet in Patients with Non-insulin-dependent Diabetes Mellitus. *JAMA.* 1994; 271(18): 1421-1428

17. Cahill, GF and Boston, MD. Physiology of Insulin in Man. *Diabetes.* 1971; 20(12): 785-799

18. Hollenbeck, CB and Coulston, AM. Effects of Dietary Carbohydrate and Fat Intake on Glucose and Lipoprotein Metabolism in Individuals with Diabetes Mellitus. *Diabetes Care.* 1991; 14: 744-785

19. Chen, YD, et al. Why do Low-fat High-carbohydrate Diets Accentuate Postprandial Lipemia in Patients with NIDDM? *Diabetes Care.* 1995; 18(1): 10-16

20. Farquhar, JW, et al. Glucose Insulin and Triglyceride Responses to High and Low Carbohydrate Diets in Man. *J Clin Invest.* 1966; 45(10): 1648-1656

21. Zimmet, PZ. Hyperinsulinemia - How Innocent a Bystander. *Diabetes Care.* 1993; 16(3): 56-70

Arthritis

1. Sperling, RI et al. Arthritis and Rheumatism 25: 133 (1983)

2. Lee, TH, et al. New Eng. J Med 312 (19) 1217-24, May 1985.

3. Kremer, J et al, Clin Res. 33: A778, 1985.

4. McCormick, JN et al, Lancet 2:508, 1977

5. Aaseth, J, et al, Selenium In Biology and Medicine May 1980.

6. McKenzie, LS, et al, Osteoarthrosis: Uncertain Rationale for Anti-inflammatory Drug Therapy. Lancet 1:908-909, 1976.

7. Vidal y Plana, RR, et al, Articular Cartilage Pharmacology: In Vitro Studies on Glucosamine and Non-steroidal Anti-inflammatory Drugs. Pharmacological Research Communications. 10(6): 557-569, 1978.

8. Arthritis Information: Osteoarthritis. Atlanta, GA. The Arthritis Foundation, Brochure No. 4040, May 1995.

9. Liang MH and Fortin, P, Management of Osteoarthritis of the Hip and Knee. JAMA 325(2): 125-127, 1991.

10. Mueller-Fabbender, H, et al. Glucosamine Sulfate Compared to Ibuprofen in Osteoarthritis of the Knee. Osteoarthritis and Cartilage 2:61 - 69, 1994.

11. Crolle, G and D'Este, E. Glucosamine Sulphate for the Management of arthosis: A Controlled Clinical Investigation. Current Medical Research and Opinion 7(2): 104-109, 1980.

12. Tapadinhas, MJ, et al, Oral Glucosamine Sulphate in the Management of Arthosis: Report on a Multi-centre Open Investigation in Portugal. Pharmatherapeutica. 3(3): 157-168, 1982.

13. Piptone, VR, Chondroprotection with Chondroitin Sulfate. Drugs in Experimental and Clinical Research 17(1): 3-7, 1991.

14. Mazieres, B, et al. Le Chondroitin Sulfate Dayns le Traitement de la Gonarthrose et de la Coxarthrose. Rev. Rheum Mal Osteoartic 59(7-8): 466-472, 1992.

15. Kerzberg, EM, et al. Combination of Glycosaminoglycans and Acetylsalicylic Acid in Knee Osteoarthrosis. Scandinavian Journal of Rheumatology.

16. Gay, G. Another Side Effect of NSAIDs. JAMA 264(20): 2677-2678, Nov. 1990.

17. Sandler, DP. Analgesic Use and Chronic Renal Disease. New Eng. J. Med. 320: 1238-1243, 1989.

18. Fredericks, Carlton; Arthritis: Don't Learn to Live With It, Grosset & Dunlap, New York. 1981.
19. Charnot, A, et al, Ann. Endocrinol. 32:397, 1971.

Menopause

1.   Adlercreutz, H., et al. Soybean phytoestrogen intake and cancer risk. J. Nutrition 125:757-770.
2.   Adlercreutz H., Mazur W. Phytoestrogens and western diseases. Annuals Med 29: 95-120 1997.
3.   Blatt MHG., et al. Vitamin E and climacteric syndrome: Failure of effective control as measured by menopausal index. Arch Intern Med 91:792-9, 1953.
4.   Finkler, RS. The effect of vitamin E in the menopause. J Clin Endocrinol Metab 9: 89-94, 1949.
5.   Clemetson, CAB, et al. Capillary strength and the menstrual cycle. Ann NY Acad Sci 93: 277-300, 1962.
6.   Smith, CJ. Non-hormonal control of vaso-motor flushing in menopausal patients. Chic Med 67(5): 193-5, 1964.
7.   Miksicek RJ. Interaction of naturally occurring nonsteroidal estrogens with expressed recombinant human estrogen receptor. Journal of Steroid Biochemistry and Molecular Biology. 49: 153-160, 1994.
8.   Joannou, GE., et al. A urinary profile study of dietary phytoestrogens. The identification and mode of metabolism of new isoflavonoids. J Steroid Bio and Molecular Biology, 54: 167-184, 1995.
9.   Ingram D., et al. Case control study of phyto-oestrogens an breast cancer. Lancet, 350: 990-994, 1997.
10. Cassidy, A., et al. Biological effects of a diet of soy protein rich in isoflavones on the menstrual cycle of premenopausal women. Am J Clin Nutr. 60: 333-340, 1994.
11. Horoschak, A., Nocturnal leg cramps, easy bruisability and epistaxis in menopausal patients: Treated with hesperidin and ascorbic acid. Del State Med J. January 1959, pp. 19-22.
12. Wilcox G., et al. Oestrogenic effects of plant foods in postmenopausal women. Br Med J 301:905-6, 1990.
13. Thompson J. et al. Relationship between nocturnal plasma oestrogen concentration and free plasma tryptophan in perimenopausal women. J Endocrinol 72(3): 395-6, 1977.
14. Duker EM, et al. Effects of extracts from Cimicifuga racemosa on gonadotropin release in menopause women and ovariectomized rats. Plant Med 57(5): 420-4, 1991.
15. Zhy DPQ. Dong quai. Am J Chin Med 15(3-4): 117-25, 1987.
16. Costello CH, Lynn, EV. Estrogenic substances from plants: I. Glycyrrhiza. J Am Pharm Soc 39: 177-80, 1950.
17. Kumagai, A. et al. Effect of glycyrrhizin on estrogen action. Endocrinol Japan 14: 34-8, 1967.
18. Kaldas Rs, Hughes, CL. Reproductive and general metabolic effects of phytoestrogens in mammals. Reprod Toxicol 3: 81-9, 1989.
19. Rose, DP. Dietary fiber, phytoestrogens, and breast cancer. Nutrition 8: 47-51, 1992.
20. Messina, M., Barnes, S. The roles of soy products in reducing risk of cancer. J Natl Cancer Inst. 83: 541-6, 1991.

Prostate & Impotence

1. Braeckman, J, The extract of Serenoa Repens in the Treatment of Benign Prostatic Hyperplasia: a Multi center Open Study. Current Therapeutic Research, July 1994; 55: 776-85.

2. Carroll, KK and Khor, HT, Dietary Fat in Relation to Tumorigeneses. Prog. Biochem Pharmacol., 1975; 10: 308-53.

3. Carrilla E, et al, Binding of Permixon, a new treatment for prostatic benign hyperplasia, to the cytosolic androgen receptor in the rat prostate. J Steroid Biochem 1984; 20: 521-23.

4. Champault, G, et al, A Double-Blind Trial of an Extract of the Plant Serenoa Repens in benign Prostatic Hyperplasia. British Journal of Clinical Pharmacology, 1984; 18: 461-62.

5. Wynder EL, et al. Nutrition and prostate cancer: a proposal for dietary intervention. Natr Cancer. 1994; 22: 1-10.

6. Pusateri, DJ et al. Dietary and Hormonal Evaluation of Men at Different Risks for Prostate Cancer, Plasma and Fecal Hormone - Nutrient Interrelationships. Am J Clin Nutr. 1990; 51: 371-77.

7. Vitramo J, and Huttunen, J. Vitamin A and Prostatic Cancer. Ann Med. 1992; 24: 143-44.

8. Marchand L, et al. Vegetable and Fruit Consumption in Relation to Prostate Cancer Risk in Hawaii: a Reevaluation of the Effect of Dietary Beta-Carotene. Am J Epidemiol. 1991; 133: 215-19.

9. Oshi K, et al. A Case-Control Study of Prostatic Cancer with Reference to Dietary Habits. Prostate 12: 179-90. 1988.

10. Carter JP, et al. Hypothesis: Dietary Management May Improve Survival from Nutritional Linked Cancers Based on Analysis of Representative Cases. J Am Coll Nutr. 3: 209-29. 1993.

11. Dumrau, F., Benign Prostatic Hyperplasia: Amino Acid Therapy for Symptomatic Relief. American Journal of Geriatrics, 1962; 10: 426-30.

12. Lu-Yao, GL, et al. An Assessment of Radical Prostatectomy. JAMA, 1993; 269 (20) 2633 - 36.

13. Tripoli, V. Et al. Treatment of Prostatic Hypertrophy with Serenoa Repens Extract. Med Praxis, 1983; 4: 41-46.

14. Rhodes, L et al. Comparison of Finasteride (Proscar), a 5–alpha–reductase Inhibitor and Various Commercial Plant Extracts in Vitro and in Vivo 5-Alpha-reductase Inhibition. The Prostate 1993; 22: 43-51.

15. Johansson, JE, et al. Natural History of Localized Prostatic Cancer. Lancet, 1989; 799-803.

16. Flemming , C, et al. A Decision Analysis of Alternative Treatment Strategies for Clinically Localized Prostate Cancer. JAMA 1993; 269 (20): 2650-58

17. Tasca A, et al. Treatment of Obstructive Symptomology Caused by Prostatic Adenoma with an Extract of Serenoa repens. Double-blind Clinical Study vs Placebo. Minerva Urol Nefrol 1985; 37: 87-97.

18. Mattei FM, et al. Serenoa repens extract in the Medical Treatment of Benign Prostatic Hypertrophy. Urologia 1988; 55: 547-52.

19. Hart JP, and Cooper, WL: Vitamin F in the Treatment of Prostatic Hyperplasia (No.1) Lee Foundation for Nutritional Research, Milwaukee, WI 1941.

20. Scott WW. The Lipids of the Prostatic Fluid, Seminal Plasma and Enlarged Prostate Gland of Man. J Urol. 1945; 53: 712-8.

21. Fahim M, et al. Zinc Treatment for the Reduction of Hyperplasia of the Prostate. Fed Proc 1976; 35: 361.

22. Judd AM, et al. Zinc Acutely, Selectively and Reversibly Inhibits Pituitary Prolactin Secretion. Brain Res 1984; 294: 190-2.

23. Vescovi PP, et al. Pyridoxine (vitamin B-6) Decreases Opioids-Induced Hyperprolactinemia. Horm Metab Res 1985; 17: 46-7.

24. Pansadoro V and Benincasa, A. Prostatic Hypertrophy: Results Obtained with Pygeum africanum extract. Minerva Med 1972; 11: 119-44.

25. Carani C, et al. Urological and Sexual Evaluation of Treatment of Benign Prostatic Disease Using Pygeum africanum at High Dose. Arch Ital Urol Nefrol Androl 1991; 63: 341-5.
26. Netter A, et al. Effect of Zinc Administration on Plasma Testosterone, Dihydrotestosterone and Sperm Count. Arch Androl 1981; 7: 69-73.
27. Prodromos PN, et al. Cranberry Juice in the Treatment of Urinary Tract Infections. Southwest Med 1968; 47: 17.
28. Kahn, DH, et al. Effect of Cranberry Juice on Urine. J Am Dietetic Assoc 1967; 51: 251.
29. Frohne V. Untersuchungen zur Frage der Harndesifizierenden Wirkungen von Barentraubenblatt-extracten. Planta Medical 1970- 18: 1-25.
30. Wynder, D, et al. Nutrition and Prostate Cancer: A Proposal for Dietary Intervention. Nutrition and Cancer 1994; 22: 4-1

Cholesterol

1. Maritz FJ. Efficacy and danger of statin therapy. Cardiovasc J S Afr. 2002 13 (4) 200-203,
2. Singh, RB, et al. Hypolipidemic and antioxidant effects of Commiphora mukul as an adjunct to dietary therapy in patients with hypercholesterolemia. Cardiovasc Drugs Ther 1994 8 (4) 659-664.
3. Ghorai M., et al. A comparative study on hypocholesterolaemic effect of allicin, whole germinated seeds of Bengal gram and guggulipid of gum guggul. Phytother Res 2000 14 (3) 200-202.
4. Binaghi, P. et al. Evaluation of the cholesterol-lowering effectiveness of pantethine in women in perimenopausal age. Minerva Med. 1990 81(6): 475-479.
5. Prisco, D., et al. Effect of oral treatment with pantethine on platelet and plasma phospholipids in IIa hyperlipoproteinemia. Angiology 1987 38 (3) 241-247.
6. Arsenio, L., et al. Clinical use of pantethine by parenteral route in the treatment of hyperlipidemia. Acta Biomed Ateneo Parmense. 1987 58 (5-6) 143-152.
7. Moghadasian, MH, and Frohlich, JJ. Effects of dietary phyosterols on cholesterol metabolism and atherosclerosis: clinical and experimental evidence. Am J Med. 1999 107 (6): 588-594.
8. Plat, J. and Mensink, RP. Effects of plant sterols on lipid metabolism and cardiovascular risk. Nutr. Metab Cardiovasc Dis. 2001 11(1): 31-40.
9. Whittaker, MH. Effects of dietary phytosterols on cholesterol metabolism and atherosclerosis: clinical and experimental evidence. Am J Med 2000 109(7) 600-601.
10. De Graaf, J. et al. Consumption of tall oil-derived phytosterols in a chocolate matrix significantly decreases plasma total and low-density lipoprotein-cholesterol levels. Br J Nutr. 2002 88(5): 479-488.
11. Szapary, PO et al. Guggulipid for the treatment of hypercholesterolemia: a randomized controlled trial. JAMA 2003 13, 290(6): 765-772.
12. Leontowicz, M. et al. Apple and Pear Peel and Pulp and their influence on plasma lipids and antioxidant potentials in rats fed cholesterol-containing diets. J Agric Food Chem. 2003 10;51(19):5780-5785.
13. Kerckhoffs, DA. et al. Cholesterol-lowering effect of beta-glucan from oat bran in mildly hypercholesterolemic subjects may decrease when beta-glucan is incorporated into bread and cookies. Am J Clin Nutr. 2003 78(2):221-227.
14. Comparison of the effects of inositol hexanicotinate and nicotinic acid on lipid levels. Functional Medicine Vol 21, Dec 2001.

Candida/Yeast

1. Jay B.E. et al. The Super saturation of Biologic fluids with Oxygen by the Decomposition of Hydrogen Peroxide. Texas Rpts. Biol and Med 1964; 22: 106–109.
2. Shenep JL., et al. Lack of Antibacterial Activity after Intravenous Hydrogen Peroxide Infusion in Experimental Escherichia Coli Sepses. Inefct. Immun 1985; 48: 607–610.
3. Snyder LM., et al. Effect of Hydrogen Peroxide Exposure on Normal Human Erthrocyte Deformability, Cross-linking. J. Clin Invest. 1985; 76: 1971–1977.
4. Lebedev, LV., Levine AO., et al. Regional Oxygenation in the Treatment of Severe Destructive forms of Obliterating Diseases of the Extremity Arteries. Vestn. Khir 1984; 132: 85–88.
5. Levine PH., et al. Release of Hydrogen Peroxide by Granulocytes as a Modulator of Platelate Reactions. J. Clin Invest. 1976; 57: 955–963.
6. Crook, William The Yeast Connection: A Medical Breakthrough. Random House, New York, 1992
7. Crook, William Yeast Connection Cookbook: A Guide to Good Nutrition. Professional Books, 1989.
8. Truss, Orian, Tissue Injury Induced by Candida Albicans, Mental and Neurologic Manifestations. J. Ortho Psy, 7: (1)
9. Truss, Orian, Restoration of Immunologic Competence to Candida Albicans. J. Ortho Psy. 9 (4).
10. Truss, Orian, The Role of Candida Albicans in Human Illness. J. Ortho Psy. 10: (4).
11. Schmidt, Michael A. Tired of Being Tired: Overcoming Chronic Fatigue and Low Energy. Frog Ltd., Berkley, CA. 1995.

Fibromyalgia

1. Abraham GE, Flechas JD. Hypothesis: Management of fibromyalgia: rational for the use of magnesium and malic acid. J Nutr Med 3:49-59, 1991
2. Caruso I, et al. Double-blind study of 5-hydroxytryptophan versus placebo in the treatment of primary fibromyalgia syndrome. J Int Med Res 18 (3): 201-209.
3. Eisinger J, et al. Donnees actuelles sur les fibromyalgies: traitment des fibromyalgies primitives par la cocarboxylase. Lyon Med Med 24: 11585-6, 1988 (in French)
4. Eisinger J, et al. Glycolysis abnormalities in fibromyalgia J Am Coll Nutr 13 (2): 144-148, 1994
5. Eisinger J., et al. Selenium and magnesium status in fibromyalgia. Magnes Res 7(3-4):285-288, 1994.
6. Moldofsky H, Warsh JJ. Plasma tryptophan and musculoskeletal pain in non–articular rheumatism. Pain 5(1):65-71, 1978.
7. Romano TJ, Stiller JW. Magnesium deficiency in fibromyalgia syndrome. J Nutr Med 4:165-167, 1994.
8. Yunus B, et al. Plasma tryptophan and other amino acids in primary fibromyalgia: acontrolled study. J Rheumatol 19(1):90-94, 1992.

Memory

1. Parkin, AJ Human Memory: Novelty, Association and the Brain. Current Biology 7 (12): 1997
2. Quillfeldt, JA, et al. Different Brian Areas are Involved in Memory Expression at Different Times form Training. Neurobiology of Learning and Memory 66 (2): 97-101, 1996.

3. Smanson, JC. The Biological Basis of Phosphatidylserine Pharmacology. Clinical Trials Journal 24 (1): 108 1987.
4. Christianson, SA & Loftus, EF. Memory for Traumatic Events. Applied Cognitive Psychology.
5. Small, GW. et al. Predictors of Cognitive Change in Middle-aged and Older Adults with Memory Loss. American Journal of Psychiatry. 152 (12): 1757-1764, 1995.
6. Petersen, RC., et al. Memory Function in Normal Aging. Neurology 42 (2) 396-401, 1992.
7. Kidd, PM. Phosphatidylserine (PS): Number-One Brain Booster. New Canaan, Conn: Keats Publishing 1998.
8. Toffano, GA, et al. Pharmacokinetics of Radiolabelled Brain Phosphatidylserine. Clinical Trials Journal 24 (1): 18024, 1987.
9. Folch, J. The Chemical Structure of Phosphatidylserine. Journal of Biological Chemistry 174: 439-450, 1948.
10. Caffarra, P & Santamaria, V. The Effects of Phosphatidylserine in Patients with Mild Cognitive Decline. Clinical Trials Journal 24 (1): 109-114, 1987.
11. Sinforiani, E., et al. Cognitive Decline in Ageing Brain. Therapeutic Approach with Phosphatidylserine. Clinical Trials Journal 24 (1): 115- 124. 1987.
12. Crook, TH. et al. Effects of Phosphatidylserine in Age-associated Memory Impairment. Neurology 41 (5): 644-649, 1991.
13. Crook, TH., et al. Effects of Phosphatidylserine in Alzheimer's Disease. Psychopharmacology Bulletin 28 (1): 61066, 1992.
14. Maylor, EA, & Rabbitt, PM. Effect of Alcohol on Rate of Forgetting. Psychopharmacology (Germany) 91 (2): 230-235, 1987.
15. Pritz-Hohmeier, S., et al. Effect of In Vivo Application of the Ginkgo biloba Extract on the Susceptibility of Mammalian Retinal Cells to Proteolytic Enzymes. Ophthalmic Research. 26 (2): 80-86, 1994.
16. Winter, JC. The Effects of an Extract of Ginkgo biloba on Cognitive Behavior and Longevity in the Rat. Physiology and Behavior. 63 (3): 425-433. 1998.
17. Le Bars, PL., et al. A Placebo-controlled, Double-blind Randomized Trial of an Extract of Ginkgo biloba for Dementia. Journal of the American Medical Association. 278 (16): 1327-1332, 1997.
18. Meck, WH., et al. Pre and Postnatal Choline Supplementation Produces Long-term Facilitation of Spatial Memory. Developmental Psychobiology 21 (4): 339-353. 1988.
19. Ladd, SL., et al. Effect of Phosphatidylcholine on Explicit Memory. Clinical Neuropharmacology. 16 (6): 540-549, 1993.
20. Vasterling, JJ., et al. Attention and Memory Dysfunction in Post-traumatic Stress Disorder. Neuropsychology 12 (1): 125-133, 1998.
21. Bremner, JD., et al. Functional Neuroanatomical Correlates of the Effects of Stress on Memory. Journal of Traumatic Stress 8 (4): 527-553, 1995.

Chapter 5

The following is only a partial list of the references used for this chapter. There were literally hundreds of studies that went into the protocols recommended.

1. Stillians, AW Pyridoxine in treatment of acne vulgaris. J Invest Dermatol 7:150-151, 1946.
2. Plewig G, et al. Action of isotretinoin in acne rosacea and gram-negative folliculitis. J Invest Dermatol 86:390-393, 1986.

3. Bogden JD, et al. Micronutrient status and human immunodeficiency virus (HIV) infection. Ann NY Acad Sci 587: 189-195, 1990.
4. Shambaugh, jGE Jr. Zinc and AIDS. J Appl Nutr 40(20): 138-139, 1989.
5. Baines, M. Detection and incidence of B and C vitamin deficiency in alcohol-related illness. Ann Clin Biochem 15:307-312, 1978.
6. Cleary, JP, Niacinamide and addictions. Letter. J Nutr Med 1: 83-84, 1990.
7. Simon, SW. Vitamin B12 therapy in allergy and chronic dematoses. J Allergy 2: 183-185, 1951.
8. Clemetson, CA Histamine and ascorbic acid in human blood. J Nutr 110(4):662-668, 1980.
9. Reed, JD et al. Nutrition and sickle cell disease. Am J Hematol 24(4): 441-55, 1987.
10. Wray D. A double blind trial of systemic zinc sulfate in recurrent aphthous stomatitis. Oral Surg 53(5): 559-561, 1977.
11. Meyer, EC et al. Vitamin E and benign breast disease. Surgery 107(%): 549-551, 1990.
12. Gately, CA, Mansel RE. Managemetn of the painful and nodular breast. Br Med Bull 47(2):284-294, 1991.
13. Schwartz J, Weiss ST. Dietary factors and their relation to respiratory symptoms. The Second National Health and Nutrition Examination Survey. Am J Epidemiol 132(1): 67-76, 1990.
14. Truss CO. Metabolic abnormalities in patients with chronic candidiasis: The acetaldehyde hypothesis. J Orthomol Psychiatry 13: 66-93, 1984.
15. Fujii T. The clinical effects of vitamin E on purpuras due to vascular defects. J Vitaminology 18: 125-130, 1972.
16. Cox BD, Butterfield WJ. Vitamin C supplements and diabetic cutaneious capillary fragility. Br Med J 3:205, 1975.
17. Roden DM. Magnesium treatment of ventricular arrhythmias. Am J Cardiol 63(14):43G-46G, 1989.
18. Fujioka T, et al. Antiarrhythmic action of coenzyme Q10 in diabetics. Tohoku J Exp Med. 141 (suppl): 453-463, 1983.
19. Driskell JA et al. Effectiveness of pyridoxine hydrochloride treatment on carpal tunnel patients. Nutr Rep Int 34: 1031-1040, 1986.
20. Devamanoharan, P, et al. Prevention of selenite cataract by vitamin C. Exp Eye Res 52: 563-568.
21. Bhat KS. Plasma calcium and trace minerals in human subject with mature cataract. Nutr Rep Int 37:157-163, 1988.
22. Butterworth CE. Et al. Improvement in cervical dysplasia associated with folic acid therapy in usuers of oral contraceptives. Am J Clin Nutr 35: 73-82, 1982.
23. Palan PR et al. Plasma levels of antioxidant beta-carotene and alpha-tocopherol in uterine cervix dysplasias and cancer. Nutr Cancer 15:13-20, 1991.
24. Altura, BM, Altura BT. Biochemistry and pathophysiology of congestive heart failure: Is there a role for magnesium? Magnesium 5(3): 134-143, 1986. Azuma J et al. Double-blind randomized crossover trial of taurine in congestive heart failure. Curr Ther Res 34(4): 543-557, 1983.
25. Gorbach SL. Bismuth therapy in gastrointestinal diseases. Gastroenterology 99(3):863-875, 1990.
26. Morse PF et al. Meta-analysis of placebo-controlled studies of the efficacy of Epogram in the treatment of atopic exzema: relationship between plasma essential fatty changes and treatment response. Br J Dermatol 121:75-90, 1989
27. Asregadoo ER. Blood levels of thiamine and ascorbic acid in chronic open-angle glaucoma. Ann Ophthalmol 11(7): 1095-1100, 1979.

28. Campbell RE, Pruitt FW. The effect of vitamin B12 and folic acid in the treatment of viral hepatitis. Am J Med Sci 229:8-15, 1955.

29. McCune MA et al. Treatment of recurrent herpes simplex infections with L-lysine monohydrochloride Cutis 34(4): 366-373, 1984.

30. Zureick M. Treatment of shingles and herpes with vitamin C intravenously. J de Praticiens 64:586-, 1950.

31. Digiese V, et al. Effect of coenzyme Q10 on essential arterial hypertension Curr Ther Res 47:841-845, 1990.

32. Shansky, A. Vitamin B3 in the alleviation of hypglycemia. Drug Cosmetic Industry 129(4):68, 1981.

33. Gugliano D, Torella R. Prostaglandin E1 inhibits glucose-induced insulin secretion in man. Prostaglandins Med 48:302, 1979.

34. Bernstein J et al. Depression of lymphocyte transformation following oral glucose ingestion. Am J Clin Nutr. 30:613, 1977.

35. Cohen B, et al. Revesal of postoperative immunosuppresion in man by vitamin A. Surg Gynecol Obstet 149: 658-662, 1979.

36. Anderson R. The immunostimulatory, anti-inflammatory and anti-allergic properties of ascorbate. Adv Nutr Res 6:19-45, 1984.

37. Chandra RK. Trace element regulation of immunity and infection. J Am Coll Nutr 4 (1): 5-16, 1985.

38. Reynolds JV, et al. Immunomodulary mechanisms of arginine. Surgery 104(2): 142-151, 1988.

39. Pinnock CB et al. Vitamin A status in children who are prone to respiratory tract infections. Aust Paediatr J 22(2): 95-99, 1986.

40. Carr AB et al. Vitamin C and the common cold: Using identical twins as controls. Med J Aust 2: 411-412, 1981.

41. Baer MT et al. Nitrogen utilization, enzyme activity, glucose intolerance and leukocyte chemataxis in human experimental zinc depletion. Am J Clin Nutr 41(6): 1220-1235, 1985.

42. Roberts P. et al. Vitamin C and inflammation. Med Biol 62:88, 1984.

43. Cichoke AJ, Marty L. The use of proteolytic enzymes with soft tissue athletic injuries. Am Chiropractor, October 1981, P 32.

44. Romeo G. The therapeutic effect of vitamins A and E in neurosensory hearing loss. Acta Vitaminol Enzymol 7 Suppl: 85-92, 1985

45. Moser M et al. A double-blind clinical trial of hydroxyethylrutosides in Meniere's disease. J Laryngol Otol 98(3): 265-272, 1984.

46. Mitwalli A et al. Control of hyperoxaluria with large doses of pyridoxine in patients with kidney stones. Int Urol Nephrol 20(4): 353-359, 1988.

47. Welsh AL Lupus erythematosus: Treatment by combined use of massive amounts of pantothenic acid and vitamin E. Arch Dermatol Syphilol 70:1810198, 1954.

48. Katz ML et al. Dietary vitamins A and E influence retinyl ester composition and content of the retinal pigment epithelium Biochim Biophys Acta 824(3):432-441, 1987.

49. Newsome DA et al. Oral zinc in macular degeneration. Arch Ophthalmol 106(2):192-198, 1988.

50. Wright JV et al. Improvement of vision in macular degeneration associated with intravenous zinc and selenium therapy: two cases J Nutr Med 1:133-138, 1990.

51. Sotonishi T et al. Treatment of climacteric complaints with gamma oryzanol plus tocopherol. Folha Med (Brazil) 77(2): 235, 1978.

52. Wilcox G et al. Oestrogenic effects of plant foods in postmenopausal women. Br Med J 301: 905-906, 1990

53. Reynolds, EH, Linnell JC.Vitamin B12 deficiency, demyelination and multiple sclerosis. Lancet 2-920, 1987

54. Mai J. et al. High dose antioxidant supplementation to MS patients. Biol Trace Element Res 24:109, 1990.

55. Wolfgram, F et al. Serum linoleic acid in multiple sclerosis. Neurology 25(8): 786-788, 1975.

56. Page EW, Page EP, Leg crams in pregnancy: Etiology and treatment. Obstet Gynecol 1(94):1953.

57. Milhorat AT Bartels WE.The defect in utilization of tocopherol in progressive muscular dystrophy. Science. 101:93-94, 1945

58. Tomasi LG. Reversibility of human myopathy caused by vitamin E deficiency. Neurology 29:1182, 1979.

59. Nurmikko T et al. Attentuation of tourniquet-induced pain in man by D-phenylalanine, a putative inhibitor of enkephalin degradation. Acupunct Electrother Res. 12 (3-4):185-191, 1987.

60. Reilly DK et al. On-off effects in Parkinson's disease: a controlled investigation of ascorbil acid therapy. Adv Neurol 37:51-60, 1983.

61. Snider SR. Octacosanol in parkinsonism. Letter Ann Neurol 16(6):723, 1984.

62. Rubinoff, AB et al.Vitamin C and oral health.J Can Dent Assoc 55(9):705-707, 1989.

63. Khmelevski IuV et al. Effect of vitamins A, E, and K on the indices of the glutathione antiperoxidase system in gingival tissues in periodontosis.Vopr Pitan (4): 54-56, 1985.

64. Piesse JW.Vitamin E and peripheral vascular disease. Int Clin Nutr Rev 4(4):178-182, 1984.

65. Brevetti G et al. Increases in walking distance in patients with peripheral vascular disease treated with L-carnitine: A double-blind, cross-over study. Circulation 77(4):767-773, 1988.

66. Chuong CJ, et al.Vitamin A levels in premenstrual syndrome. Fertil Steril 54(4):643-647, 1990.

67. Doll H et al. Pyridoxine and the premenstrual syndrome: A randomized crossover trial. JR Coll Gen Pract 39:364-368, 1989.

68. Morimoto S et al.Therapeutic effect of 1,25-dihydroxyvitamin D3 for psoriasis: Report of five cases. Calcif Tissue Inter 38: 119-122, 1986.

69. Dochao A et al.Therapeutic effects of vitamin D and vitamin A in psoriasis: A 20-year experiment. Actas Dermosifiliogr 66(3-4):121-130, 1975.

70. DiGiacomo RA et al. Fish-oil dietary supplementation in patients with Raynaud's phenomenon: da double-blind, controlled, prospective study. Am J Med 86:158-164, 1989.

71. Ellis JM Folkers K. Clinical aspects of treatment of carpal tunnnel syndrome with vitamin B6. Ann NY Acad Sci 585:302-320, 1990.

72. Barton-Wright EC, Elliott WA.The pantothenic acid metabolism of rheumatoid arthritis. Lancet 2: 862-863, 1963.

73. Honkanen V et al.Vitamins A and E, retinol binding protein and zinc in rheumatoid arthritis. Clin Exp Rheumatol 7:465-469, 1989.

74. Block MT.Vitamin E in the treatment of diseases of the skin. Clin Med Jan. 1953.

75. Gey GO, et al. Effect of ascorbic acid on endurance performance and athletic injury. JAMA 211(1):105, 1970.

76. Shimomura Y et al. Protective effect of coenzyme Q10 on exercise-induced muscular injury. Biochem Biophys Res Commun 176:349-355, 1991.

77. Salomon P et al.Treatment of ulcerative colitis with fish oil in n-3-omega fatty acid: an open trial. J Clin Gastroenterol 12(2):157-161, 1990.

78. Alvarez OM Gilbreath RL,Thiamin influence on collagen during the granulation of skin wounds. J Surg Res 32:24-31, 1982.

79. Werbach, MR, M.D. Nutritional Influences on Illness.Tarzana, CAL Third Line Press 1991.

80. Pizzorno, JE and Murray, MT. A Textbook of Natural Medicine. Seattle, WA: John Bastyr College Publications. 1989.
81. Taylor, R. Management of Constipation. High Fiber Diets Work. British Medical Journal 300. No. 6731 1990: 1063-1064.
82. Foushee DB, et al. Garlic as a natural agent for the treatment of hypertension. Cytobios 34 nos. 135-136 1982: 145-152.

CPSIA information can be obtained at www.ICGtesting.com
Printed in the USA
BVOW060113260313

316425BV00003B/7/A